WORKBOOK

EMERGENCY CARE

11th Edition

WORKBOOK

Bob Elling

EMERGENCY CARE

11th Edition

Daniel Limmer

Michael F. O'Keefe

Medical Editor

Edward T. Dickinson, MD, FACEP

Legacy Authors
Harvey D. Grant
Robert H. Murray, Jr.
J. David Bergeron

Upper Saddle River, New Jersey 07458

Dedicated to my two beautiful daughters: Laura and Caitlin. And to my lovely wife Kirsten. May you always maintain humility as your accomplishments meet the stars!

B.E.

Publisher: Julie Levin Alexander
Publisher's Assistant: Regina Bruno
Executive Editor: Marlene McHugh Pratt
Acquisitions Editor: Sladjana Repic
Senior Managing Editor for Development: Lois Berlowitz
Project Manager: Triple SSS Press Media Development, Inc.
Editorial Assistant: Sean Karpowicz
Director of Marketing: Karen Allman
Executive Marketing Manager: Katrin Beacom
Marketing Specialist: Michael Sirinides
Managing Editor for Production: Patrick Walsh
Production Liaison: Faye Gemmellaro
Production Editor: Erin Melloy, S4Carlisle Publishing Services
Manufacturing Manager: Ilene Sanford
Manufacturing Buyer: Pat Brown
Senior Design Coordinator: Christopher Weigand
Cover Design: Delgado and Company, Inc.
Front Cover Image: Shutterstock/Craig Hosterman
Back Cover Image: Getty Images/Mike Powell
Executive Marketing Manager: Katrin Beacom
Printer/Binder: Bind-Rite Graphics
Cover Printer: Phoenix Color
Composition: S4Carlisle Publishing Services

Pearson Education Ltd., London
Pearson Education Australia Pty. Limited
Pearson Education Singapore, Pte. Ltd.
Pearson Education North Asia Ltd., Hong Kong
Pearson Education Canada, Inc.
Pearson Educación de Mexico, S.A. de C.V.
Pearson Education—Japan
Pearson Education Malaysia, Pte. Ltd
Pearson Education, Upper Saddle River, New Jersey

NOTICE ON CARE PROCEDURES

This workbook reflects current EMS practices based on the 1994 U.S. Department of Transportation's EMT-Basic National Standard Curriculum. It is the intent of the authors and publisher that this workbook be used as part of a formal Emergency Medical Technician education program taught by qualified instructors and supervised by a licensed physician. The procedures described in this workbook are based upon consultation with EMS and medical authorities. The authors and publisher have taken care to make certain that these procedures reflect currently accepted clinical practice; however, they cannot be considered absolute recommendations.

The material in this workbook contains the most current information available at the time of publication. However, federal, state, and local guidelines concerning clinical practices, including, without limitation, those governing infection control and Standard Precautions, change rapidly. The reader should note, therefore, that new regulations may require changes in some procedures.

It is the responsibility of the reader to familiarize himself or herself with the policies and procedures set by federal, state, and local agencies as well as the institution or agency where the reader may be employed. The author and the publisher of this workbook disclaim any liability, loss, or risk resulting directly or indirectly from the suggested procedures and theory, from any undetected errors, or from the reader's misunderstanding of the text. It is the reader's responsibility to stay informed of any new changes or recommendations made by any federal, state, and local agency as well as by his or her employing institution or agency.

If when reading this workbook you find an error, have an idea for how to improve it, or simply want to share your comments with us, please send your letter to one of the following addresses below.

Managing Editor
Brady/Pearson Health Science
Pearson Education
One Lake Street
Upper Saddle River, New Jersey 07458

bobelling@usa.net

NOTICE ON BCLS PROCEDURES

The national standards for BCLS are reviewed and revised on a regular basis and may change slightly after this book is printed. It is important that you know the most current procedures for CPR, both for the classroom and your patients. The most current information may always be downloaded from www.bradybooks.com or obtained from your instructor.

10 9 8 7 6 5

ISBN 10:   0-13-500863-8
ISBN 13: 978-0-13-500863-8

Contents

Introduction vii

©2009 Pearson Education, Inc.
Emergency Care, 11th Ed.

Introduction

► **OVERVIEW**

This workbook is designed to accompany the textbook *Emergency Care,* 11th Edition. The workbook covers the course knowledge and U.S. Department of Transportation (DOT) skill objectives to which all standardized testing instruments are referenced. In all areas where the textbook goes beyond the DOT objectives to present current trends in medical care, this workbook also follows along very closely. It is neither meant to replace the text nor is it meant to be a substitute for a well-designed course in emergency care.

This is a self-instructional workbook. It has been designed to allow you to work at your own pace and evaluate your own progress. To benefit from this workbook, follow the procedures in this introduction. Thousands of EMT students before you have used prior editions of this workbook as part of their emergency medical training. The system works, having helped them to learn and excel on state and national certification and registration examinations. By doing your best on each chapter, you, as well as those patients to whom you deliver emergency care, will benefit.

This edition continues the emphasis of the 1994 U.S. DOT curriculum on patient assessment. In addition, there are a number of updated sections and new features in this workbook. Additional Case Studies have been added and the EMT-Basic Performance Checklists have been updated. Two new reference features have been added to the workbook: reference to http://www.prenhall.com/EMTAchieve, an online test preparation product by Brady, and reference to Brady's *Pocket Reference for BLS Providers.*

► **FEATURES**

Each chapter in this workbook contains these elements:

- **Match Terminology/Definitions**—In this section, you are asked to match chapter terminology with appropriate definitions, which are included in the chapter's running text, appear in the chapter glossary, or both. The terms have been placed in alphabetical order so that after reading the definitions you can quickly select the appropriate term.
- **Multiple-Choice Review**—This section provides on average 25 to 45 questions. Emphasis is placed on multiple-choice

questions, since this is the format of state and national exams used for certification or registration. Practice in answering multiple-choice questions can help improve your understanding of the material as well as your course grades. These multiple-choice questions generally appear in the sequential order that the topics appear in the textbook, enabling you to build on prior knowledge. When similar questions appear in the three Interim Exams, the order is scrambled, as is done on state and national exams.

- **Complete the Following**—This section focuses on your recalling and listing specific information on chapter objectives, such as the signs and symptoms of shock or the five stages of grief.
- **Label the Diagram/Photograph and Complete the Chart**—In some chapters, you are asked to study a visual and to identify its content or to complete a partially filled-in chart. These diagrams, photographs, and charts correspond to those in the textbook.
- **Street Scenes Discussion**—Each chapter of the textbook has a section called Street Scenes. These scenarios are designed to apply what you have learned in the chapter to a situation that could easily be found in your work as an EMT. In the workbook, you are asked to reread the Street Scenes and then use the knowledge you have obtained thus far in your course to answer a few more questions.
- **Web Simulations**—Using the Internet, a number of cases have been designed to complement the topics in the textbook and workbook. These are referred to in the workbook, and the Internet URL is listed.
- **Case Study**—After every few chapters, a case study requires you to synthesize information that you have learned up to that particular point in the course and to apply this knowledge to a real-life situation. As each step of the case is presented, you are asked a series of questions that build on the facts of the case.
- **Answer Key**—The Answer Key at the back of the workbook provides answers for all of the above-mentioned workbook elements. For the Street Scenes Discussion questions, rationales appear for each answer. For the Multiple-Choice Review questions, rationales are provided where appropriate along

with the textbook page reference where each topic is discussed.

- **EMT Skills Performance Checklists**—Most workbook chapters include a listing of the EMT skills that incorporate national standards or the DOT EMT curriculum description of a method of doing each skill. These checklists are from the *Pocket Reference for BLS Providers*. This handy pocket-sized reference contains checklists that detail the steps followed in the performance of EMT skills and also many of the medical terms, abbreviations, anatomical charts, and reference tools used in the field.

▶ STEPS FOR SUCCESS

To get the most out of this workbook, you should complete the following eight steps:

Step 1—Learn the Course Objectives

Each chapter of the textbook begins with objectives that were developed as a part of the U.S. Department of Transportation's EMT 1994 training curriculum. Most state and national certifying examinations are based on these course objectives. To score well on those exams, you must learn the objectives of the course. Use the objectives in the textbook in the following way:

1. Read them over.
2. Read the text.
3. Reread the objective in the form of a question.
4. Write down your answer to each question on a blank piece of paper.
5. Perform a self-assessment or ask your instructor to assess how well you understand the material in the chapter.

Step 2—Learn the Language of the EMT

Emergency Medical Services (EMS) is clearly a medical field, and as such it is necessary for the EMT to learn and understand the language of medicine. This will help you communicate with the other members of the health care team in a clear, concise, and accurate manner. In addition, learning the language of medicine will facilitate your understanding of medical and trade journal articles as you work to keep current in the constantly changing EMS field.

First, review the medical terminology in the text and then put aside the text. Next, test your understanding of the terminology by completing the Match Terminology/Definitions exercise in each workbook chapter. Complete the entire matching exercise before checking your answers against the Answer Key. For those terms you were unable to match, write down the word on one side of a 3″ × 5″ card and write the definition on the other side of the card. Carry these cards in your pocket and refer to them frequently to help you learn the terms.

Step 3—Learn the Structure of the Body

The language of medicine also includes learning the names and locations of the structures of the human body. Imagine being unable to control serious bleeding because you could not find the pressure point in the arm! To help you learn the structures of the body, in workbook chapters in which it is appropriate, anatomical drawings and diagrams are provided. For example, the drawing of the respiratory system in the workbook has blank numbered lines that point to each of the system's different structures. Label each structure as requested and check your answers in the back of the workbook. For those you miss, go to the textbook page suggested and study the body structure again.

Step 4—Answer the Multiple-Choice Questions

For each Multiple-Choice Review, complete the entire exercise at one sitting. Read each question and all the answer choices before you mark your answer. If you jump to a conclusion without fully reading the question, you could answer incorrectly. Also, watch out for questions with negative expressions or the word "except." You will notice that the author has minimized the use of "all of the above" as an answer to questions in this edition. This was done to ensure that exam items mirror those used in standardized tests. Once you have completed the exercise, refer to the Answer Key to check your performance. A textbook page reference has been provided for the theory or principle tested in each question. Many answers have an "author's comment" whenever it is appropriate to clarify the answer to a question.

You will need to practice reading, and not reading into, multiple-choice questions. If it has been many years since you took a standardized test, leave extra time to review this section of each workbook chapter. If you notice any trends in your performance on these questions, you may wish to consult your instructor for "test-taking assistance."

Step 5—Use the Street Scenes Discussion and Web Simulations on the Internet

Step 6—Review the EMT Skill Performance Checklists

Whenever a skill is introduced in the chapter, a checklist has been included in the workbook.

©2009 Pearson Education, Inc.
Emergency Care, 11th Ed.

Work in pairs and use these checklists to test each other.

Step 7—Take the Interim Exams

Once you have completed each individual workbook chapter, move on to the next chapter and repeat steps one to five. Interim Exams appear after Modules 2, 4, and 8 and are similar to the interim exams your instructor may give in the EMT course. Each exam covers material in the chapters that precede it. Therefore, when you have completed all of the material preceding an exam, it's time to take the Interim Exam.

Also be sure to review the extra materials in the Appendix sections that appear at the end of the workbook.

Step 8—Pay Close Attention to the Case Studies

The case studies integrated in the workbook help you synthesize your knowledge and apply it to real-life situations. They actually put you at a scene and require you to think quickly and accurately. Answers at the back of the workbook will help you sort out any problems you confront.

So that's it in eight simple steps. It will take your time and commitment to work through each of the steps. Since this is a self-instructional workbook, it will be up to you to reward yourself for doing well on chapters. At the same time, you need to be honest with yourself. If you are having difficulty with a chapter, let your instructor know immediately so he or she can offer additional assistance.

It is the hope of the *Emergency Care* authors and development team that using this workbook as an integral part of your EMT training package will help you improve your understanding of the material and enhance your performance in the field. After all, isn't quality patient care what EMS is all about? See you in the streets!

▶ **ACKNOWLEDGMENTS**

The authors of the *Emergency Care Workbook,* 11th Edition, would like to thank the publishing team led by Julie Alexander, Sladjana Repic, Marlene Pratt, and Lois Berlowitz for all their hard work and support on the Emergency Care series. Appreciation is extended to Dan Limmer and Mike O'Keefe for their friendship and confidence and the opportunity to partake in this important project. Gratitude is extended to Triple SSS Press Media Development for excellent developmental guidance. And last, but not least, a special thanks to our dear friend and mentor J. David Bergeron.

▶ **ABOUT THE AUTHOR**

Bob Elling, MPA, REMT-P, has been involved in EMS since 1975. He is an active paramedic with the Town of Colonie (NY), National Faculty for the AHA, and Regional Faculty for the NYS Bureau of EMS. Bob has served as a paramedic and lieutenant for NYC EMS, Program Director for the Hudson Valley Community College's Institute of Prehospital Emergency Medicine, Associate Director of the NYS EMS Program, the Education Coordinator for PULSE: Emergency Medical Update, and as the AHA Guidelines 2005 BLS Editor. He is an author/coauthor of these Brady books: *Pocket Reference for BLS Providers, MedReview for the EMT-B, Essentials of Emergency Care, Paramedic Care: Principles & Practice Workbook Volume 5, EMT Achieve: Basic Test Preparation,* and *EMT Achieve: Online First Responder Test Preparation.*

You can reach him at his e-mail address: bobelling@usa.net.

CHAPTER 1

Introduction to Emergency Medical Care

MATCH TERMINOLOGY/ DEFINITIONS

A. State laws that allow an EMS system to exist

B. A process of continuous self-review with the purpose of identifying and correcting aspects of the system that require improvement

C. The provision for physician input and direction of patient care, training, and quality assurance of an emergency medical service or system

D. A system designed to get trained personnel to the patient as quickly as possible and to provide emergency care on the scene, en route to the hospital, and in the hospital

E. Policy or protocol issued by a Medical Director that authorizes EMTs or others to perform particular skills in certain situations

F. Lists of steps, developed by the Medical Director of an EMS system, that are to be taken in different situations

G. A communications system that has the capability of automatically identifying the caller's phone number and location

H. A system for telephone access to report emergencies in which a dispatcher answers the call, takes the information, and alerts EMS or the fire or police departments as needed

I. An EMT or other person authorized by a Medical Director to give medications and provide emergency care

J. A physician who assumes the ultimate responsibility for the patient-care aspects of the EMS system

_____ **1.** Designated agent

_____ **2.** EMS system

_____ **3.** Enabling legislation

_____ **4.** Enhanced 911

_____ **5.** Medical direction

_____ **6.** Medical Director

_____ **7.** 911 system

_____ **8.** Protocols

_____ **9.** Quality improvement

_____ **10.** Standing order

MULTIPLE-CHOICE REVIEW

_____ 1. The earliest documented emergency medical service was in:
A. England in the 1890s.
B. France in the 1790s.
C. Seattle in the 1970s.
D. Miami in the 1960s.

_____ 2. In 1966, the _____ charged the United States _____ with developing EMS standards.
A. Uniform Traffic Act, Department of Transportation
B. President, Fire Academy
C. National Highway Safety Act, Department of Transportation
D. American Medical Association, Department of Health and Human Services

_____ 3. Of the following, which is not a major component in the National Highway Traffic Safety Administration's EMS system assessment standards?
A. Transportation
B. Computerization
C. Communications
D. Evaluation

_____ 4. An example of a specialty hospital in the EMS system is a(n):
A. emergency department.
B. correctional facility.
C. poison control center.
D. primary care center.

_____ 5. National levels of EMS training include all of the following except:
A. advanced first aid.
B. First Responder.
C. EMT-Intermediate.
D. EMT-Paramedic.

_____ 6. The major emphasis of the curriculum for the EMT deals with _____ of the ill or injured patient in the prehospital setting.
A. immediate life-threatening care
B. interpretation of electrocardiograms
C. assessment and care
D. techniques of advanced airway care

_____ 7. Patient care provided by the EMT should be:
A. delayed until transportation.
B. based on assessment findings.
C. guided by the service's attorney.
D. based upon the diagnosis of the patient.

_____ 8. An example of assuring continuity during the transfer of care of the patient would be:
A. providing pertinent patient information to the hospital staff.
B. performing more hospital procedures in the field.
C. only giving a report directly to a physician.
D. none of the above.

_____ 9. Patient advocacy is:
A. assessing your patient.
B. abandoning your patient.
C. executing your primary responsibility as an EMT.
D. speaking up for your patient.

_____ 10. Good personality traits are very important to the EMT. You should be:
A. cooperative and resourceful.
B. cunning and inventive.
C. respectful and condescending.
D. emotionally stable and shy.

_____ 11. If an EMT is not in control of personal habits, he or she might:
A. contaminate the patient's wounds.
B. make inappropriate decisions.
C. render improper care.
D. do all of the above.

©2009 Pearson Education, Inc.
Emergency Care, 11th Ed.

_____ 12. To prevent violating patient confidentiality, the EMT should:
   A. communicate with medical direction.
   B. perform an accurate interview.
   C. avoid inappropriate conversation.
   D. develop the ability to listen to others.

_____ 13. Way(s) in which an EMT may further his or her EMS education include:
   A. rereading the EMT textbook.
   C. attending EMS conferences.
   B. repeating the EMT course.
   D. all the above.

_____ 14. A process of continuous self-review of all aspects of an EMS system for the purpose of identifying and correcting aspects of the system that require improvement is called:
   A. off-line medical direction.
   C. quality improvement.
   B. patient advocacy.
   D. continuing education.

_____ 15. Obtaining feedback from patients and the hospital staff is a means of:
   A. obtaining on-line medical direction.
   B. providing quality improvement.
   C. determining what is wrong with patients.
   D. avoiding charges of negligence.

_____ 16. Participation in continuing education and keeping carefully written documentation are examples of the EMT's role in:
   A. patient advocacy.
   C. quality improvement.
   B. medical direction.
   D. transfer of care.

_____ 17. Every EMS system should have a:
   A. minimum of three EMTs on each vehicle.
   B. call review on a monthly basis.
   C. contract with the local hospital.
   D. Medical Director.

_____ 18. An EMT is operating as the Medical Director's:
   A. employee.
   C. designated agent.
   B. replacement.
   D. peer.

_____ 19. The difference between on-line (direct) and off-line (indirect) medical direction is that:
   A. off-line does not need protocols.
   B. off-line orders are given by the on-duty physician, usually over the radio or phone.
   C. on-line uses standing orders.
   D. on-line orders are given by the on-duty physician, usually over the radio or phone.

_____ 20. An example of a medication carried by EMTs that may require a physician consultation to administer is:
   A. lidocaine.
   C. oxygen.
   B. activated charcoal.
   D. aspirin.

_____ 21. An example of a community health initiative that EMTs may be involved in would be:
   A. flag day parade.
   B. participating in injury prevention.
   C. planning new training curriculums.
   D. lobbying for EMS grants.

_____ 22. It is the responsibility of the EMT to treat patients:
   A. as quickly as possible.
   B. in their community or district.
   C. in a nonjudgmental and fair manner.
   D. who are insured or injured at work.

_____ **23.** An example of clinical decision making that is within the practice of the EMT is:
- **A.** determining the patient's diagnosis.
- **B.** advising the patient which medications to take.
- **C.** deciding which hospital to transport to.
- **D.** none of the above.

_____ **24.** In the near future, the designation "First Responder" will change to:
- **A.** Paramedic.
- **B.** Advanced EMT.
- **C.** Emergency Medical Technician.
- **D.** Emergency Medical Responder.

COMPLETE THE FOLLOWING

1. List at least six of the categories and standards of an EMS system established by the National Highway Traffic Safety Administration.

A. _____   **D.** _____

B. _____   **E.** _____

C. _____   **F.** _____

2. List the six types of specialty hospitals.

A. _____   **D.** _____

B. _____   **E.** _____

C. _____   **F.** _____

3. List the four levels of EMS certification and new name changes.

A. _____   **C.** _____

B. _____   **D.** _____

STREET SCENES DISCUSSION

Review the Street Scene on p. 19 in the textbook. Then answer the question below.

What responsibilities of the EMT are illustrated in this scenario?

ON THE WEB

To help you review and practice basic skills, visit the *Emergency Care 11th Ed. Companion Website* at www.prenhall.com/limmer. For Online Test Preparation, visit www.prenhall.com/emtachieve.

The Well-Being of the EMT

MATCH TERMINOLOGY/ DEFINITIONS

A. A form of infection control based on the presumption that all body fluids are infectious

B. Mental health professionals and peer counselors who work as a team to provide emotional and psychological support to EMS personnel who are or have been involved in a highly stressful incident

C. The removal or cleansing of dangerous chemicals or other dangerous or infectious materials

D. Equipment that protects the EMS worker from infection and/or from hazardous materials and the dangers of rescue operations

E. The organisms that cause infection, such as viruses and bacteria

F. An emergency involving multiple patients

G. When a patient mentally tries to postpone death for a short time

H. The release of a harmful substance into the environment

I. A state of physical and/or psychological arousal to a stimulus

J. When a patient gets upset and questions, "Why me?"

K. Injections given to a rescuer that are designed to prevent him or her from getting a disease

L. When a patient puts off dealing with the inevitable end of the process of dying

M. A potentially infectious material

N. A high-efficiency particulate air respirator or mask designed to reduce the spread of tuberculosis (TB)

O. Test that determines if a person has been exposed to TB

_____ **1.** Anger

_____ **2.** Bargaining

_____ **3.** Biohazard

_____ **4.** Body substance isolation (BSI)/ Standard Precautions

_____ **5.** Critical incident stress management (CISM) teams

_____ **6.** Decontamination

_____ **7.** Denial

_____ **8.** Stress

_____ **9.** Hazardous-material incident

_____ **10.** HEPA

_____ **11.** Immunizations

_____ **12.** MCI

_____ **13.** Pathogens

_____ **14.** Personal protective equipment (PPE)

_____ **15.** PPD test

MULTIPLE-CHOICE REVIEW

_____ 1. The most critical job of the EMT is to:
   A. stay physically safe and emotionally well.
   B. immediately assess the patient and call the hospital.
   C. provide medical advice to friends and community members.
   D. check the unit at the end of each shift.

_____ 2. An organism that causes infection is referred to as a(n):
   A. airborne.   C. allergen.
   B. bloodborne.   D. pathogen.

_____ 3. Precautions the EMT should take when dealing with all patients are known as:
   A. universal precautions.   C. standard precautions.
   B. general isolation.   D. quarantine isolation.

_____ 4. To provide body substance isolation, the EMT may need to use:
   A. hand washing and SCBA.
   B. HEPA mask and shoe covers.
   C. disposable gloves and eye protection.
   D. paper gown and leather gloves.

_____ 5. An EMT should routinely wear a mask when treating a patient with:
   A. hepatitis B or C.   C. AIDS.
   B. potential for blood or fluid spatter.   D. all of the above.

_____ 6. When an EMT covers a patient's mouth and nose with a mask to prevent the spread of an airborne disease, he or she should:
   A. monitor the respirations and airway closely.
   B. write "TB alert" on the patient's prehospital care report.
   C. wear a surgical mask to reduce the spread of TB.
   D. notify his or her supervisor prior to transporting the patient.

_____ 7. All of the following are ways the EMT can plan safety precautions in advance of the call except:
   A. keeping his or her tetanus immunization current.
   B. maintaining a list of communicable patients.
   C. verifying immune status.
   D. obtaining the hepatitis B vaccine.

_____ 8. It is suggested that all EMTs be immunized with all of the following vaccines except:
   A. tetanus.   C. purified protein derivative.
   B. hepatitis B or C.   D. measles.

_____ 9. A federal organization responsible for issuing guidelines for employee safety around biohazards is called the:
   A. Food and Drug Administration.
   B. Federal Communications Commission.
   C. Occupational Safety and Health Administration.
   D. Public Health Service.

_____ 10. Every employer of EMTs must provide free of charge:
   A. a yearly physical examination.   C. a hepatitis B vaccination.
   B. a life insurance policy.   D. universal health insurance.

_____ 11. A federal act that establishes procedures by which emergency response workers can find out if they have been exposed to life-threatening infectious diseases is:
   A. OSHA 1910.1030.   C. NFPA 1207.
   B. Ryan White CARE Act.   D. OSHA 1910.1200.

©2009 Pearson Education, Inc.
Emergency Care, 11th Ed.

_____ 12. After contact with the blood or body fluids of a patient, an EMT may submit a request for a determination of exposure to his or her:
   A. employer.
   B. Medical Director.
   C. designated officer.
   D. local hospital.

_____ 13. Always assume that any person with:
   A. a cold has a bloodborne disease.
   B. a productive cough has TB.
   C. a fever has typhoid.
   D. dehydration and sores has AIDS.

_____ 14. Which of the following is true about treating a contaminated patient at a hazardous-material incident?
   A. Take the patient to the ambulance.
   B. Bring the patient to the hospital.
   C. Wear an SCBA when treating the patient.
   D. Delay treatment until the patient is decontaminated.

_____ 15. The EMT can safeguard his or her well-being by:
   A. understanding and dealing with job stress.
   B. ensuring scene safety.
   C. practicing body substance isolation.
   D. all of the above.

_____ 16. Each of the following is an example of a call that has a high potential for causing excess stress on EMS providers except:
   A. trauma to infants and children.
   B. an adult cardiac arrest.
   C. elder abuse.
   D. death or serious injury of a coworker.

_____ 17. Some warning signs that an EMT is being affected by stress include:
   A. overeating and ringing in the ears.
   B. rapid urination and sweating.
   C. indecisiveness and guilt.
   D. increased sexual activity and sleep.

_____ 18. All the following are recommended lifestyle changes an EMT may take to deal with job stress except:
   A. develop more healthful and positive dietary habits.
   B. devote time to relaxation.
   C. exercise.
   D. avoid talking about his or her feelings.

_____ 19. A meeting held by a team of peer counselors and mental health professionals within 24 to 72 hours after a major incident is a(n):
   A. incident critique.
   B. MCI.
   C. critical incident stress debriefing.
   D. quality circle.

_____ 20. It is thought by some psychologists that for CISM to be effective:
   A. it must not be an investigation of the events of the call.
   B. information discussed must remain confidential.
   C. an EMT must feel open to discuss feelings, fears, and reactions.
   D. all of the above.

_____ 21. According to some psychologists, which of the following statements is correct regarding a CISM?
   A. The debriefing can be combined with an incident critique.
   B. Pressure from peers is provided.
   C. It helps participants to suppress their feelings.
   D. It can accelerate the recovery process.

_____ 22. When a patient finds out that he is dying, he may go through which of the following emotional stages?
   A. Anger and laughter
   B. Denial and empathy
   C. Depression and acceptance
   D. Bargaining and elation

_____ 23. A dying patient may go through emotional stages in the following order:
  A. acceptance, rage, depression, acceptance, bargaining.
  B. denial, anger, bargaining, depression, acceptance.
  C. bargaining, acceptance, denial, anger, depression.
  D. depression, bargaining, denial, acceptance, anger.

_____ 24. An EMT will occasionally need to assist the patient who has a terminal illness. Experts suggest all of the following except:
  A. listen empathetically to the patient.
  B. tell the patient that everything will be fine.
  C. be tolerant of angry reactions from the patient or family members.
  D. try to recognize the patient's needs.

_____ 25. All of the following are part of the three Rs of reacting to danger except:
  A. retreat.   C. radio.
  B. respond.   D. reevaluate.

_____ 26. Stressors affecting the EMT may include:
  A. unpleasant dealings with people.   C. performance expectations.
  B. environmental factors.   D. all of the above.

_____ 27. The body's response to stress was studied by Dr. Hans Selye, who found there is a(n):
  A. resistance syndrome.   C. general adaptation syndrome.
  B. excess of the chemical cortisone. D. exhaustion syndrome.

_____ 28. The phases of adaption to stress include alarm, exhaustion, and:
  A. reaction.   C. resistance.
  B. distress.   D. rest.

_____ 29. A stress reaction that involves either physical or psychological behavior manifested days or weeks after an incident is called a(n):
  A. acute stress reaction.
  B. post-traumatic stress disorder.
  C. cumulative stress reaction.
  D. burnout.

_____ 30. The Centers for Disease Control and Prevention recommends the use of _____ when soap and water are not immediately available to help kill microorganisms on a rescuer's hands.
  A. liquid Cydex II solution
  B. hydrogen peroxide solution
  C. dry powder application
  D. alcohol-based hand cleaners

_____ 31. The normal mode of transmission of the disease chicken pox (varicella) is thought to be:
  A. blood or stool.   C. airborne droplets.
  B. accidental needlesticks.   D. ventilation systems.

_____ 32. Each of the following diseases is thought to be spread by respiratory secretions or oral or nasal secretions, except:
  A. hepatitis.   C. pneumonia.
  B. bacterial meningitis.   D. tuberculosis.

_____ 33. A disease that mothers are thought to be able to pass to their unborn child is:
  A. chicken pox (varicella).   C. tuberculosis.
  B. AIDS.   D. mumps.

©2009 Pearson Education, Inc.
Emergency Care, 11th Ed.

COMPLETE THE FOLLOWING

1. List five types of calls with a high potential of stress for EMS personnel.

   A. _____

   B. _____

   C. _____

   D. _____

   E. _____

2. List five signs or symptoms of stress.

   A. _____

   B. _____

   C. _____

   D. _____

   E. _____

3. List at least five of the critical elements of the infection control plan required by Title 29 Code of Federal Regulation 1910.1030.

   A. _____

   B. _____

   C. _____

   D. _____

   E. _____

STREET SCENES DISCUSSION

Review the Street Scene on p. 46 in the textbook. Then answer the questions below.

1. Because the EMT had an open cut on his hands and was exposed to the patient's blood from the facial laceration, what are some of the diseases he may have been exposed to?

2. Due to the potential exposure to HIV, what medication, tests, and instructions would you expect the ED physician to prescribe for the EMT?

3. Aside from wearing PPE, could the EMT have prevented contracting any of these bloodborne diseases? Explain your answer.

4. Of the diseases the EMT may have been exposed to, which one would he have the greatest chance of catching and how serious is the disease?

ON THE WEB

To help you review and practice basic skills, visit the *Emergency Care 11th Ed. Companion Website* at www.prenhall.com/limmer. For Online Test Preparation, visit www.prenhall.com/emtachieve.

EMT SKILLS PERFORMANCE CHECKLIST

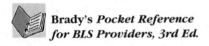 **Brady's** *Pocket Reference for BLS Providers, 3rd Ed.*

▶ **HAND-WASHING PROCEDURE (PP. 24–25)**

❑ Remove watch and rings. Roll up sleeves.

❑ Adjust water flow and temperature.

❑ Wet hands and distal forearms.

❑ Dispense soap into hands.

❑ Scrub lower arms and hands. Clean around and under the nails.

❑ Rinse thoroughly under running water to remove all soap. Do not touch the sink!

❑ Use a paper towel to shut off the faucet to avoid recontaminating hands.

NOTE: Even though you wear protective gloves with your patients, hand washing must still be performed immediately after each call.

CHAPTER

Medical/Legal and Ethical Issues

MATCH TERMINOLOGY/ DEFINITIONS

A. Permission to treat an unconscious patient until he or she becomes conscious

B. A written order given by the physician based upon a decision by a patient prior to his or her demise; instructions written in advance of an event

C. Being held legally responsible

D. An obligation to provide care to a patient

E. Permission given by adults who are of legal age and mentally competent to make a rational decision in regard to their medical well-being

F. Permission from the patient to treat him or her

G. A series of laws, varying in each state, designed to provide limited legal protection for citizens and some health care personnel who are administering emergency care

H. The collective medical, legal, and ethical guidelines that govern the EMT

I. Not providing the standard of care

J. A finding of failure to act properly in a situation in which there was a duty to act

K. A legal document, usually signed by the patient and his or her physician, which states that the patient does not wish to prolong life through resuscitative efforts

_____ **1.** Abandonment

_____ **2.** Advance directive

_____ **3.** Battery

_____ **4.** Breach of duty

_____ **5.** Confidentiality

_____ **6.** Consent

_____ **7.** DNR order

_____ **8.** Duty to act

_____ **9.** Emancipated minor

_____ **10.** Expressed consent

_____ **11.** Good Samaritan laws

_____ **12.** Implied consent

_____ **13.** Liability

_____ **14.** Negligence

_____ **15.** Scope of practice

_____ **16.** HIPAA

L. The obligation not to reveal information obtained about a patient except to other health care professionals involved in the patient's care, or under subpoena, or in a court of law

M. Leaving a patient after care has been initiated and before the patient has been transferred to someone with equal or greater medical training

N. Child who is married or of a specific age who, in certain states, can make legal decisions

O. Subjecting a patient to unwanted care and transport may be considered this in a court of law

P. A federal law protecting the privacy of patient-specific health care information

MULTIPLE-CHOICE REVIEW

_____ 1. The collective set of regulations and ethical considerations governing the EMT is called:
    A. duty to act.
    B. scope of practice.
    C. advance directives.
    D. Good Samaritan laws.

_____ 2. Legislation that governs the skills and medical interventions that may be performed by an EMT is:
    A. uniform throughout the country.
    B. different from state to state.
    C. uniform for regions within a state.
    D. governed by the U.S. Department of Transportation.

_____ 3. When the EMT makes the physical/emotional needs of the patient a priority, this is considered a(n) _____ of the EMT.
    A. advance directive
    B. protocol
    C. ethical responsibility
    D. legal responsibility

_____ 4. Which one of the following is <u>not</u> a type of consent required for any treatment or action by an EMT?
    A. Child and mentally incompetent adult
    B. Implied
    C. Applied
    D. Expressed

_____ 5. When you inform the adult patient of a procedure you are about to perform and its associated risks, you are looking for:
    A. expressed consent.
    B. negligence.
    C. implied consent.
    D. applied consent.

_____ 6. Consent that is based on the assumption that an unconscious patient would approve the EMT's life-saving interventions is called:
    A. expressed.
    B. negligence.
    C. implied consent.
    D. applied consent.

_____ 7. Your record of a patient's refusal of medical aid or transport should include all of the following <u>except</u>:
    A. informing the patient of the risks and consequences of refusal.
    B. documenting the steps you took.
    C. signing of the form by the Medical Director.
    D. obtaining a release form with the patient's witnessed signature.

©2009 Pearson Education, Inc.
Emergency Care, 11th Ed.

_____ **8.** Forcing a competent adult patient to go to the hospital against his or her will may result in _____ charges against the EMT.
    A. abandonment
    B. assault and battery
    C. implied consent
    D. negligence

_____ **9.** Which one of the following is an action you should <u>not</u> take if a patient refuses care?
    A. Leave phone stickers with emergency numbers.
    B. Recommend that a relative call the family physician to report the incident.
    C. Tell the patient to call his or her family physician if the problem reoccurs.
    D. Call a relative or neighbor who can stay with the patient.

_____ **10.** Another name for a DNR order is:
    A. deviated nervous response.
    B. duty not to react.
    C. refusal of treatment.
    D. advance directive.

_____ **11.** There are varying degrees of DNR orders, expressed through a variety of detailed instructions that may be part of the order, such as:
    A. allowing for CPR only if cardiac or respiratory arrest was observed.
    B. allowing comfort care measures such as intravenous feeding.
    C. disallowing the use of long-term life-support measures.
    D. specifying that only five minutes of artificial respiration will be attempted.

_____ **12.** In a hospital, long-term life-support and comfort care measures would consist of intravenous feeding and:
    A. routine inoculations.
    B. the use of a respirator.
    C. infection control by the health care providers.
    D. hourly patient documentation.

_____ **13.** If an EMT with a duty to act fails to provide the standard of care, and if this failure causes harm or injury to the patient, the EMT may be accused of:
    A. breach of promise.
    B. negligence.
    C. abandonment.
    D. assault.

_____ **14.** Termination of care of the patient without assuring the continuation of care at the same level or higher is called:
    A. liability infraction.
    B. battery.
    C. abandonment.
    D. breach of duty.

_____ **15.** The EMT should not discuss information about a patient outside of relaying pertinent information to the physician at the emergency department. Information considered confidential includes:
    A. patient history gained through interview.
    B. assessment findings.
    C. treatment rendered.
    D. all of the above.

_____ **16.** The EMT can release confidential patient information in all of the following circumstances <u>except</u> to:
    A. inform other health care professionals who need to know information to continue care.
    B. report incidents required by state law, such as rape or abuse.
    C. comply with a legal subpoena.
    D. protect the other victims of a motor vehicle collision.

_____ **17.** Medical identification insignia that indicate serious patient medical conditions come in the form of all of the following <u>except</u>:
    A. bracelets.
    B. necklaces.
    C. cards.
    D. patches.

_____ **18.** When treating a critical patient who has an organ donor card, the EMT should:

    A. transport without delay and document a DNR.

    B. treat the patient the same as any other patient and inform the ED physician.

    C. withhold oxygen therapy from the patient to keep the organ hypoxic.

    D. all of the above.

_____ **19.** At a crime scene, the EMT should:

    A. avoid disturbing any evidence at the scene unless emergency care requires.

    B. immediately remove the patient from the scene.

    C. move all obstacles from around the patient to make more room to work.

    D. search the house for clues to the cause of the crime.

_____ **20.** Commonly required reporting situations include all of the following <u>except</u>:

    A. child and elder abuse.   **C.** sexual assault.

    B. crimes in public places.   **D.** domestic abuse.

_____ **21.** The extent of limits of the EMT's job is called the:

    A. ethical dilemma.   **C.** scope of practice.

    B. national curriculum.   **D.** regional protocol.

_____ **22.** You were called to the scene of an incident where a 21-year-old male was knocked out in a bar fight. Upon your arrival, the patient is awake and has a broken nose but no life-threats. He admits to drinking six beers in the last hour. He wants to refuse medical attention. Why should you discourage an RMA?

    A. He is not legally old enough to consent.

    B. He may not be mentally competent at this time.

    C. Patients die from broken noses all the time.

    D. He is unable to actually sign the release.

_____ **23.** The federal law designed to protect the patient's private medical information is the:

    A. NHTSA.   **C.** HIPAA.

    B. ANSI.   **D.** OSHA.

_____ **24.** An agency privacy officer is required by the:

    A. Health Insurance Portability and Accountability Act.

    B. Ryan-White Law.

    C. National Fire Protection Association Standards.

    D. Privacy Control Act of 2002.

_____ **25.** Examples of microscopic evidence at a crime scene include:

    A. the position of the patient.

    B. dirt and carpet fibers.

    C. fingerprints.

    D. the condition of the scene.

COMPLETE THE FOLLOWING

1. In order for a patient to refuse care or transport, what are four conditions that must be fulfilled?

    A. _____

    B. _____

    C. _____

    D. _____

2. A finding of negligence, or failure to act properly, requires that all of the following circumstances be proven:

A. _____

B. _____

C. _____

3. Four examples of conditions that may be listed on a medical identification device (such as a necklace, bracelet, or card) include:

A. _____

B. _____

C. _____

D. _____

STREET SCENES DISCUSSION

Review the Street Scene on pp. 63–64 in the textbook. Then answer the questions below.

1. Suppose you observed that the patient's home was filthy. Would it be a violation of patient confidentiality to discuss the "roach house" with fellow workers? Explain.

2. Is it appropriate to write that the patient has AIDS on the prehospital care report? Explain your answer.

3. Is a patient's vomitus a hazard to your health? If so, what BSI equipment would be appropriate?

ON THE WEB

To help you review and practice basic skills, visit the *Emergency Care 11th Ed. Companion Website* at www.prenhall.com/limmer. For Online Test Preparation, visit www.prenhall.com/emtachieve.

EMT SKILLS PERFORMANCE CHECKLIST

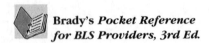
Brady's *Pocket Reference for BLS Providers, 3rd Ed.*

▶ **PATIENT REFUSAL PROCEDURE (PP. 50–52)**

❑ Spend time effectively communicating with the patient (includes reasoning, persistence, and strategies to convince the patient to go to the hospital).

❑ Clearly inform the patient of the consequences of not going to the hospital.

❑ Consult with medical direction.

❑ Contact family to help convince the patient.

❑ Call law enforcement who may be able to order or "arrest" the serious patient in order to force the patient to go to the hospital.

❑ Try to determine why the patient is refusing care.

❑ Complete thorough documentation of the refusal. Have both the patient and a witness (e.g., bystander, police officer) sign the refusal release.

NOTE: Procedure may differ by state and jurisdiction. Always follow your Medical Director's advice.

CASE STUDY

▶ **A WITNESSED COLLISION: FIRST ON THE SCENE**

It's a summer morning and you are traveling on the interstate highway with your family to the lake. Although the speed is posted at 55 mph, traffic has been moving along at least 10 mph faster. All of a sudden, you observe the station wagon a few cars in front of you going from the center lane to the passing lane, cutting off a car, and then veering off the center of the road down a ravine and rolling over numerous times. The vehicle comes to rest on its roof.

1. If you are an off-duty EMT, must you legally stop to offer assistance?

2. Are you protected from a lawsuit? Explain your answer.

3. Are you protected from a liability suit provided your treatment is appropriate?

As you secure your vehicle off the shoulder and assign another helper to set out some flares, your spouse uses a cellular phone to call for emergency assistance.

4. In most communities, what is the universal emergency phone number?

5. What types of questions would you expect the dispatcher to ask about the collision?

6. What emergency response agencies would you expect to be sent?

As you carefully climb down through the brush to the car, you notice there are two patients who were ejected from the vehicle. Another citizen arrives and she identifies herself as an EMT. You ask her to check out the two ejected patients while you check the car for additional patients. She reports that one ejected patient is dead, and the other is unconscious and has an obvious head injury.

7. As additional help arrives, how can they help with this patient?

8. What types of injuries could the patient have?

9. Do you need permission to treat the patient?

Inside the car there is a conscious male patient approximately 40 years old who appears to have been injured by the steering wheel in the left upper quadrant of his abdomen. He also has a broken upper left leg. You also notice that the car continues to leak gasoline from the dented fuel tank. After obtaining some additional help, you decide to carefully move this patient out of the car.

10. What potential injuries might this patient have?

11. How can you help minimize further injury to the leg?

12. Do you need permission to treat this patient? Explain.

Once the patient is out of the car, two ambulances arrive as well as the fire department with a paramedic engine and a heavy rescue truck. Meanwhile the police have arrived and are dealing with the traffic congestion that has developed.

13. Since there is now plenty of help, can you leave?

14. What would be the problem if you left prior to help arriving?

©2009 Pearson Education, Inc.
Emergency Care, 11th Ed.

The Human Body

MATCH TERMINOLOGY/ DEFINITIONS

▶ **PART A**

A. Main branch of the respiratory system that enters each of the lungs

B. Two upper chambers of the heart

C. Muscle that divides the chest cavity from the abdominal cavity

D. The carotid and this pulse are considered central pulses

E. Tiny blood vessels

F. Pulse in the neck at the side of the larynx

G. Body system that transports blood throughout the body

H. Area directly posterior to the mouth

I. Pulse in the arm used to take a blood pressure

J. Area directly posterior to nose

K. Ring-shaped structure that forms the lower larynx

L. Structure that contains the vocal cords

M. Leaf-shaped structure that closes to prevent food from going into the trachea

N. Pulse on the top of the foot lateral to the large tendon of the big toe

O. Vessels that carry blood away from the heart

_____ **1.** Arteries

_____ **2.** Atria

_____ **3.** Brachial pulse

_____ **4.** Bronchi

_____ **5.** Capillaries

_____ **6.** Cardiovascular system

_____ **7.** Carotid pulse

_____ **8.** Cricoid cartilage

_____ **9.** Diaphragm

_____ **10.** Dorsalis pedis pulse

_____ **11.** Epiglottis

_____ **12.** Femoral pulse

_____ **13.** Larynx

_____ **14.** Nasopharynx

_____ **15.** Oropharynx

A. Area posterior to the mouth and nose that includes the oropharynx and nasopharynx

B. Parts of the blood needed to form blood clots

C. Watery, salty fluid that makes up over half of the blood's volume

D. Pulse that may be palpated on the posterior aspect of the medial malleolus

E. Structure that carries inhaled air from the larynx to the lungs; also called the windpipe

F. Vessels that carry blood from the capillaries back to the heart

G. Blood pressure created in the arteries when the left ventricle contracts and forces blood out into circulation

H. Body system that takes in oxygen and eliminates carbon dioxide

I. Socket that holds the ball of the proximal femur to form the hip

J. The two lower chambers of the heart

K. Muscle type that responds automatically without the patient thinking about its operation

L. Two large veins that return blood to the heart

M. Long bone of the thigh

N. Pulse on the thumb side of the wrist

O. The smaller bone of the lower leg

_____ **1.** Acetabulum

_____ **2.** Femur

_____ **3.** Fibula

_____ **4.** Involuntary muscle

_____ **5.** Pharynx

_____ **6.** Platelets

_____ **7.** Plasma

_____ **8.** Posterior tibial pulse

_____ **9.** Radial pulse

_____ **10.** Respiratory system

_____ **11.** Systolic

_____ **12.** Trachea

_____ **13.** Veins

_____ **14.** Venae cavae

_____ **15.** Ventricles

▶ **PART C**

A. Medial anterior portion of the pelvis

B. Vertebrae that form the back of the pelvis

C. Standing face forward with palms forward

D. Inferior-most division of the spine that is referred to as the tailbone

E. Toward or closer to the midline

F. Lower jaw bone

G. Round ball of bone on the inside of the ankle

H. Wide bony ring that can be felt near the waist

I. System that consists of sensory and motor nerves

J. Round ball of bone on the outside of the ankle

K. Facial bone that surrounds each of the eyes

L. Breastbone

M. Seven vertebrae in the neck

N. Bones of the ankle

O. Medial and larger of the two bones of the lower leg

_____ **1.** Anatomical position

_____ **2.** Cervical spine

_____ **3.** Coccyx

_____ **4.** Iliac crest

_____ **5.** Lateral malleolus

_____ **6.** Mandible

_____ **7.** Medial

_____ **8.** Medial malleolus

_____ **9.** Orbit

_____ **10.** Peripheral nervous system

_____ **11.** Pubis

_____ **12.** Sacral spine

_____ **13.** Sternum

_____ **14.** Tarsals

_____ **15.** Tibia

A. Inferior tip of the sternum

B. Upper arm bone

C. Away from the midline

D. Nerves that transmit information from the body to the spinal cord and brain

E. When two points on the extremities are compared, the point closer to the torso

F. Outermost layer of the skin

G. When two points on the extremities are compared, the point farther away from the torso

H. Nerves that carry messages from the brain to the body

I. Above or toward the head end of the torso

J. Inner layer of the skin in which blood vessels and nerves are located

K. Bones in the fingers and toes

L. Joint where three bones of upper arm and forearm are connected

M. Front side of the body or body part

N. Heel bone

O. Back side of the body or body part

_____ 1. Anterior

_____ 2. Calcaneus

_____ 3. Dermis

_____ 4. Distal

_____ 5. Elbow

_____ 6. Epidermis

_____ 7. Humerus

_____ 8. Lateral

_____ 9. Motor nerves

_____ 10. Phalanges

_____ 11. Posterior

_____ 12. Proximal

_____ 13. Sensory nerves

_____ 14. Superior

_____ 15. Xiphoid process

▶ PART E

A. Body system that regulates metabolic functions such as sugar absorption by the cells

B. Body system that governs sensations, movement, and thought

C. Lateral bone of the forearm aligned with the thumb

D. Bones that make up the hand

E. Highest portion of the shoulder

F. Medial bone of the forearm

G. Bones that make up the wrist

H. Shoulder blade

I. Bone in the front of the shoulder or collarbone

J. The body less the extremities and the head

K. Lying on the back

L. An imaginary line drawn vertically from the center of the clavicle to the nipple below

M. The sitting position

N. Similar on both sides of the body

O. Lying supine with the legs elevated a few inches

_____ 1. Acromion process

_____ 2. Bilaterally

_____ 3. Carpals

_____ 4. Clavicle

_____ 5. Endocrine system

_____ 6. Fowler's

_____ 7. Metacarpals

_____ 8. Mid-clavicular

_____ 9. Nervous system

_____ 10. Radius

_____ 11. Scapula

_____ 12. Supine

_____ 13. Torso

_____ 14. Trendelenburg

_____ 15. Ulna

A. Muscle under conscious control of the brain

B. Four divisions of the abdomen used to pinpoint the location of pain

C. Referring to the sole of the foot

D. Blood vessels that supply the muscle of the heart

E. Referring to the back of the body

F. Upper jaw bone

G. Body system that provides protection and movement

H. Blood pressure in the arteries when the left ventricle is refilling

I. Kneecap

J. Vertebrae of the lower back

K. Rib area of the spinal column

L. Imaginary line drawn vertically through the middle of the body

M. Anatomical term for the armpit

N. Patient's left side

O. Lying on the stomach or face down

_____ **1.** Abdominal quadrants

_____ **2.** Axilla

_____ **3.** Coronary arteries

_____ **4.** Diastolic

_____ **5.** Dorsal

_____ **6.** Left side

_____ **7.** Lumbar spine

_____ **8.** Maxilla

_____ **9.** Midline

_____ **10.** Musculoskeletal system

_____ **11.** Patella

_____ **12.** Plantar

_____ **13.** Prone

_____ **14.** Thoracic spine

_____ **15.** Voluntary muscle

MULTIPLE-CHOICE REVIEW

_____ **1.** All the following are body systems <u>except</u>:
   A. respiratory.
   B. cardiovascular.
   C. abdominal.
   D. musculoskeletal.

_____ **2.** If a patient is lying on his or her left side, this position is called the _____ position:
   A. Fowler's
   B. recovery
   C. left supine
   D. left prone

_____ **3.** When a patient is placed in a sitting-up position on a stretcher, this position is called:
   A. prone.
   B. supine.
   C. Fowler's.
   D. Trendelenburg.

_____ **4.** When a patient is lying flat with head lower than legs, this position is called:
   A. prone.
   B. supine.
   C. Fowler's.
   D. Trendelenburg.

_____ **5.** The musculoskeletal system has three main functions. It gives the body shape, provides for body movements, and:
   A. gives the body sensation.
   B. protects vital internal organs.
   C. provides for the body's outer covering.
   D. allows transport of oxygen into the cells.

_____ **6.** The upper jaw is also called the:
   A. mandible.
   B. orbit.
   C. maxillae.
   D. nasal bone.

_____ **7.** The spinal column includes the _____ vertebrae.
  A. thoracic and coccyx   **C.** lumbar and sternal
  B. cervical and orbit   **D.** sacrum and pelvic

_____ **8.** An injury to the spinal cord at the _____ level may be fatal because control of the muscles of breathing arise from the spinal cord at this level.
  A. lumbar   **C.** cervical
  B. sacral   **D.** thoracic

_____ **9.** Bones in the lower extremities include the:
  A. femur, calcaneus, and phalanges.
  B. ischium, tibia, and ulna.
  C. orbit, lumbar, and shin.
  D. radius, fibula, and metatarsals.

_____ **10.** Bones in the upper extremities include the:
  A. humerus and radius.   **C.** phalanges and tibia.
  B. humerus and calcaneus.   **D.** ulna and cervical.

_____ **11.** The types of muscle tissue include:
  A. voluntary.   **C.** cardiac automaticity.
  B. involuntary.   **D.** all of the above.

_____ **12.** The type of muscle that allows body movement such as walking is called:
  A. voluntary.   **C.** cardiac.
  B. involuntary.   **D.** smooth.

_____ **13.** Involuntary, or smooth, muscle is found in the:
  A. trachea.
  B. walls of the blood vessels.
  C. heart.
  D. quadriceps and biceps.

_____ **14.** The structure in the throat that is described as the voicebox is called the:
  A. pharynx.   **C.** trachea.
  B. larynx.   **D.** sternum.

_____ **15.** A leaf-shaped valve that prevents food and foreign objects from entering the trachea is called the:
  A. pharynx.   **C.** larynx.
  B. epiglottis.   **D.** bronchi.

_____ **16.** Oxygen passes from the environment to the lungs in what order?
  A. Nose, bronchi, larynx, trachea, lung
  B. Larynx, esophagus, trachea, bronchi, alveoli
  C. Mouth, pharynx, trachea, bronchi, alveoli
  D. Epiglottis, trachea, cricoid, bronchi, alveoli

_____ **17.** When the diaphragm and intercostal muscles relax, the size of the chest cavity:
  A. increases, causing inhalation.   **C.** decreases, causing exhalation.
  B. increases, causing exhalation.   **D.** decreases, causing inhalation.

_____ **18.** The difference between the adult airway and the pediatric airway is that:
  A. the adult's tongue takes up proportionately more space in the mouth than the child's.
  B. the trachea is softer and more flexible in an adult.
  C. the cricoid cartilage is softer in an adult.
  D. all structures are smaller and more easily obstructed in a child.

_____ **19.** The body system that is responsible for the breakdown of food into absorbable forms is called the _____ system.
  A. nervous   **C.** endocrine
  B. digestive   **D.** integumentary

_____ **20.** An organ containing acidic gastric juices that begin the breakdown of food into components that the body will be able to convert to energy is the:
 A. large intestine.　　　　　　　**C.** stomach.
 B. small intestine.　　　　　　　**D.** liver.

_____ **21.** The major artery in the thigh is called the:
 A. carotid.　　　　　　　　　　**C.** radial.
 B. femoral.　　　　　　　　　　**D.** brachial.

_____ **22.** The vessel that carries oxygen-poor blood from the portions of the body below the heart and back to the right atrium is called the:
 A. posterior tibial.　　　　　　　**C.** inferior vena cava.
 B. internal jugular.　　　　　　　**D.** aorta.

_____ **23.** The left atrium:
 A. receives blood from the veins of the body.
 B. receives blood from the pulmonary veins.
 C. pumps blood to the lungs.
 D. pumps blood to the body.

_____ **24.** The fluid that carries the blood cells and nutrients is called:
 A. platelets.　　　　　　　　　　**C.** plasma.
 B. urine.　　　　　　　　　　　**D.** none of the above.

_____ **25.** The blood component that is essential to the formation of blood clots is called:
 A. plasma.　　　　　　　　　　**C.** white blood cells.
 B. platelets.　　　　　　　　　　**D.** red blood cells.

_____ **26.** The pressure on the walls of an artery when the left ventricle contracts is called the _____ pressure.
 A. systolic　　　　　　　　　　**C.** diastolic
 B. arterial　　　　　　　　　　**D.** residual

_____ **27.** The two main divisions of the nervous system are:
 A. central and peripheral.
 B. bones and muscles.
 C. brain and skin.
 D. spinal cord and brain.

_____ **28.** Nerves that carry information from throughout the body to the brain are _____ nerves.
 A. motor　　　　　　　　　　　**C.** spinal
 B. cardiac　　　　　　　　　　　**D.** sensory

_____ **29.** One of the functions of the skin is to:
 A. eliminate excess oxygen into the atmosphere.
 B. regulate the diameter of the blood vessels in the circulation.
 C. protect the body from the environment, bacteria, and other organisms.
 D. allow environmental water to carefully enter the body.

_____ **30.** The system that secretes hormones, such as insulin and adrenaline, and which is responsible for regulating many body activities, is called the _____ system.
 A. integumentary (skin)　　　　　**C.** endocrine
 B. nervous　　　　　　　　　　　**D.** gastrointestinal

©2009 Pearson Education, Inc.
Emergency Care, 11th Ed.

COMPLETE THE FOLLOWING

1. List the names of nine arteries in the body.

A. _____   F. _____

B. _____   G. _____

C. _____   H. _____

D. _____   I. _____

E. _____

2. List five functions of the skin.

A. _____

B. _____

C. _____

D. _____

E. _____

LABEL THE DIAGRAMS

Fill in the name of each anatomical position on the line provided.

▶ ANATOMICAL POSTURES

1. _____

2. _____

3. _____

Fill in the appropriate directional term or landmark on the line provided.

▶ **ANATOMICAL POSITION**

Diagram 1

Diagram 2

3.

4.

2.

5. (Toward)

1.

6. (Away from)

7.

(Left / Right) 10.

8. (Left / Right)
9.

12. ← → 11.

13.

14.

15.

1. _____

2. _____

3. _____

4. _____

5. _____

6. _____

7. _____

8. _____

9. _____

10. _____

11. _____

12. _____

13. _____

14. _____

15. _____

Fill in the name of each body region or structure on the line provided.

▶ TOPOGRAPHY OF THE TORSO

1. _____	8. _____
2. _____	9. _____
3. _____	10. _____
4. _____	11. _____
5. _____	12. _____
6. _____	13. _____
7. _____	

STREET SCENES DISCUSSION

Review the Street Scene on p. 103 of the textbook. Then answer the questions below.

1. Why was it necessary to stabilize the patient's head and neck when you got into the car?

2. Since the driver of the truck was walking around, was he still a patient in need of evaluation? Explain your answer.

ON THE WEB

To help you review and practice basic skills, visit the *Emergency Care 11th Ed. Companion Website* at www.prenhall.com/limmer. For Online Test Preparation, visit www.prenhall.com/emtachieve.

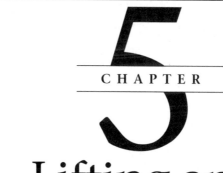

CHAPTER

Lifting and Moving Patients

MATCH TERMINOLOGY/ DEFINITIONS

A. Stretcher, made of a steel wire mesh and tubular steel rim or plastic and steel rim, used to transport patients from one level to another or over rough terrain

B. Portable folding chair with wheels used to transport the patient in a sitting position up or down stairs

C. Stretcher that splits in halves, which can be pushed together under the patient

D. Method of transferring a patient from bed to stretcher during which two or more rescuers curl the patient to their chests, then reverse the process to lower the patient to the stretcher

E. Patient move that may be made if speed is not a priority

F. Method of lifting and carrying a patient in which one rescuer slips hands under the patient's armpits and grasps the wrists, while another rescuer grasps the patient's knees

G. Made from a squatting position with weight to be lifted close to the body, feet apart and flat on ground, body weight on or just behind balls of feet, back locked in

H. Proper use of the body to facilitate lifting and moving and to prevent injury

I. Gripping with as much hand surface as possible the object being lifted, with all fingers bent at the same angle

J. Patient move that should be done quickly yet without any compromise of spinal integrity

_____ **1.** Basket stretcher

_____ **2.** Body mechanics

_____ **3.** Direct carry

_____ **4.** Direct ground lift

_____ **5.** Draw-sheet method

_____ **6.** Emergency move

_____ **7.** Extremity lift

_____ **8.** Log roll

_____ **9.** Long axis

_____ **10.** Non-urgent move

_____ **11.** Power grip

_____ **12.** Power lift

_____ **13.** Scoop (orthopedic) stretcher

_____ **14.** Stair chair

_____ **15.** Urgent move

K. Method of transferring a patient from bed to stretcher by grasping and pulling the loosened bottom sheet of the bed

L. Line that runs down the center of the body from the top of the head and along the spine

M. Method of lifting and carrying a patient from ground level to a stretcher in which two or more rescuers kneel, curl the patient to their chests, stand, then reverse the process to lower the patient to the stretcher

N. Removal of a patient from a hazardous environment in which safety is the first priority and spinal integrity is the second priority

O. Procedure done by three or four rescuers that is designed to move a supine patient onto a long backboard without compromising spinal integrity

MULTIPLE-CHOICE REVIEW

_____ **1.** To assure your own safety when lifting a patient, it is important to:
   A. always wear a back brace.
   B. keep the weight as far away from your body as possible.
   C. use your legs, not your back, to lift.
   D. avoid lifting a patient who weighs more than you do.

_____ **2.** When lifting a patient, you should do all of the following <u>except</u>:
   A. communicate clearly with your partner.
   B. twist while you lift the patient.
   C. know your physical ability and limitations.
   D. communicate frequently with your partner.

_____ **3.** When lifting a cot or stretcher,
   A. use an even number of people so that balance is maintained.
   B. keep both of your feet together and flat on the ground.
   C. use a third person positioned on the heaviest side.
   D. if you must use one hand only, compensate by using your back.

_____ **4.** When placing all fingers and the palm in contact with the object being lifted, you are using a:
   A. power grip.   **C.** lock grip.
   B. power lift.   **D.** grip lift.

_____ **5.** When you must push an object:
   A. keep the line of pull through the center of your body by bending your knees.
   B. push from an overhead position, keeping your knees locked.
   C. keep the weight you are pushing at least 20 inches away from your body.
   D. keep the elbows straight with arms close to your sides.

_____ **6.** The situations in which an emergency move would be used include all of the following <u>except</u>:
   A. fire or danger of fire.
   B. explosives or other hazardous chemicals.
   C. inability to protect the patient from other hazards at the scene.
   D. dispatcher is holding another, more serious call.

_____ **7.** If the patient is on the floor or ground and the EMT has decided that an emergency move is appropriate, the patient can be moved by:
   A. rolling her like a log.
   B. using a spine board and strapping her down.
   C. pulling on her clothing in the neck and shoulder area.
   D. using one rescuer on each extremity.

_____ **8.** If the patient has an altered mental status, the EMT should consider a(n) _____ move.
   A. emergency
   B. urgent
   C. non-urgent
   D. immediate

_____ **9.** When doing a log roll, lean from your hips and:
   A. keep your back curved only while leaning over the patient.
   B. position yourself at least 10 inches from the patient.
   C. use your shoulder muscles to help with the roll.
   D. roll the patient as fast as possible.

_____ **10.** The final step in packaging a patient on a wheeled stretcher is:
   A. securing the patient to the stretcher.
   B. placing a towel under the patient's head.
   C. covering the patient with a top sheet.
   D. adjusting the position of the back rest.

_____ **11.** If you are carrying a patient down stairs, when possible:
   A. flex at the waist with bent knees.
   B. keep your lower back muscles loose.
   C. place one hand on the railing for balance.
   D. use a stair chair instead of a stretcher.

_____ **12.** Which of the following is <u>not</u> recommended for moving a patient with a suspected spinal injury?
   A. Wheeled stretcher
   B. Scoop stretcher
   C. Short spine board
   D. Long spine board

_____ **13.** You have a patient positioned on a scoop-style stretcher and wish to lower the patient from a rooftop. You should:
   A. place the stretcher and patient in a plastic basket stretcher.
   B. transfer the patient to a wire basket stretcher.
   C. place the patient in a short spine board.
   D. lower the patient in the scoop stretcher.

_____ **14.** To avoid trauma to a patient with an injured spine, the best patient-carrying device would be the:
   A. long spine board.
   B. wheeled stretcher.
   C. Stokes basket.
   D. portable ambulance stretcher.

_____ **15.** The direct ground lift is an example of a(n) _____ move for a patient who has no spine injury.
   A. emergency
   B. urgent
   C. immediate
   D. non-urgent

_____ **16.** Another name for the squat-lift used by weight lifters and EMTs is:
   A. leg lift.
   B. power lift.
   C. thigh thrust.
   D. power grip.

_____ **17.** How should the EMT's feet be positioned when lifting?
   A. Shoulder width apart
   B. On firm ground
   C. On flat ground
   D. All of the above

_____ **18.** When the EMT has to lift with one hand, as in a litter carry, he must be careful <u>not</u> to:

    A. lift with the legs.

    B. compensate by leaning.

    C. lift with the weight close to the body.

    D. take breaks if they are needed.

_____ **19.** A comfortable new device that can be used to transport a supine patient who has sustained a spinal injury is a:

    A. scoop stretcher.

    B. stair chair with tracks.

    C. vacuum mattress.

    D. KED.

_____ **20.** When using an air mattress (vacuum mattress) the patient is placed on the device and the air is _____ by a pump. The mattress will then form a _____ and conforming surface around the patient.

    A. inflated, rigid

    B. withdrawn, rigid

    C. inflated, soft

    D. withdrawn, soft

COMPLETE THE FOLLOWING

1. List seven patient-carrying devices.

    A. _____

    B. _____

    C. _____

    D. _____

    E. _____

    F. _____

    G. _____

2. List four principles that will help you lift efficiently and prevent injury.

    A. _____

    B. _____

    C. _____

    D. _____

©2009 Pearson Education, Inc.
Emergency Care, 11th Ed.

LABEL THE PHOTOGRAPHS

Fill in the name of each lift, move, or drag on the line provided.

1. _____

2. _____

3. _____

4. _____

5. _____

6. _____

7.

8. _____

9. _____

10. _____

11. _____

12. _____

STREET SCENES DISCUSSION

Review the Street Scene on p. 130 in the textbook. Then answer the questions below.

1. In the call, the patient's weight was not discussed. Suppose the patient weighed 300 lb. Should you consider using a different device to immobilize her?

2. Suppose when it is time to remove the patient from the automobile, the vest-type immobilization device does not go entirely around her and the leg straps are too short. What should you do?

3. After getting the patient out of the car with some extra help, she lies supine in the vest-type immobilization device on a long backboard. She complains that the vest is making it difficult for her to breathe. What can you do?

ON THE WEB

To help you review and practice basic skills, visit the *Emergency Care 11th Ed. Companion Website* at www.prenhall.com/limmer. For Online Test Preparation, visit www.prenhall.com/emtachieve.

EMT SKILL PERFORMANCE CHECKLISTS

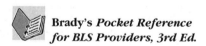

Brady's *Pocket Reference for BLS Providers, 3rd Ed.*

▶ FIREFIGHTER'S DRAG (P. 110)

❑ Place the patient in the supine position.

❑ Tie the patient's hands together with something that will not cut into the skin.

❑ Straddle the patient, facing his head.

❑ Crouch and pass your head through the patient's trussed arms and then raise your body to raise the patient's head, neck, and upper trunk.

❑ Crawl on your hands and knees, dragging the patient and keeping the patient's head low to the ground.

▶ Blanket Drag (p. 110)

❑ Gather half of the blanket up against the patient's side.

❑ Roll the patient toward your knees.

❑ Gently roll the patient back onto the blanket.

❑ Roll up the blanket by the patient's head, neck, and shoulders and drag this rolled material, keeping the patient's head as low to the ground as possible.

▶ One-Rescuer Assist (p. 111)

❑ Place the patient's arm around your neck.

❑ Grasp the patient's hand in your hand.

❑ Place your other arm around the patient's waist.

❑ Help the patient walk to safety, communicating with him about obstacles or uneven terrain.

▶ Cradle Carry (p. 111)

❑ Place one arm across the patient's back with your hand under his arm.

❑ Place your other arm under his knees and lift.

❑ If the patient is conscious, have him place nearest arm over your shoulder.

▶ Pack Strap Carry (p. 111)

❑ Have the patient stand.

❑ Turn your back to the patient, bringing his arms over your shoulders to cross your chest.

❑ Keep the patient's arms as straight as possible and armpits over your shoulders.

❑ Hold the patient's wrists, bend, and pull the patient onto your back.

▶ Piggyback Carry (p. 111)

❑ Assist the patient to a standing position.

❑ Turn your back to the patient, placing the patient's arms over your shoulders so the arms cross your chest.

❑ While the patient holds on with his arms, crouch and grasp the patient's thighs.

❑ Use a lifting motion to move the patient onto your back.

❑ Pass your forearms under the patient's knees and grasp his wrists.

©2009 Pearson Education, Inc.
Emergency Care, 11th Ed.

▶ FIREFIGHTER'S CARRY (P. 111)

❑ Place your toes against the patient's toes and pull the patient toward you.

❑ Bend at the waist and flex your knees.

❑ Duck and pull the patient across your shoulder, keeping hold of one of his wrists.

❑ Use your free arm to reach between his legs and grasp his thigh.

❑ Let the weight of the patient fall onto your shoulders.

❑ Stand up, transferring your grip on the patient's thigh to his wrist.

▶ TWO-RESCUER ASSIST (P. 112)

❑ An EMT stands at each side of the patient.

❑ Each places a patient's arm around his shoulder and grips the patient's hand.

❑ Each EMT then places his own free arm around the patient's waist.

❑ They both then help the patient walk to safety.

▶ LOADING THE WHEELED STRETCHER INTO THE AMBULANCE (PP. 115–116)

❑ Lift the rear step of the ambulance if necessary.

❑ Move the stretcher as close to the ambulance as possible.

❑ Make sure the stretcher is locked in its lowest level before lifting (depends on local procedure and type of stretcher).

❑ Position EMTs on opposite sides of the stretcher, bend at the knees, and grasp the lower bar of the stretcher frame.

❑ Both EMTs should come to a full standing position with their backs straight.

❑ Use sideways stepping movements to move the stretcher to the ambulance.

❑ Secure the stretcher into the ambulance, using the appropriate securing device.

❑ Engage both forward and rear catches to hold the stretcher in place.

▶ EXTREMITY CARRY (P. 124)

❑ EMT #1 places the patient on his back with his knees flexed.

❑ EMT #1 kneels at the patient's head and places his hands under the patient's shoulders.

❑ EMT #2 kneels at the patient's feet and grasps the patient's wrists.

❑ EMT #2 lifts patient forward while EMT #1 slips his arms under the patient's armpits and grasps the patient's wrists.

❑ EMT #2 grasps the patient's knees while facing him or turns and grasps the patient's knees while facing away from him.

❑ EMT #1 and EMT #2 both crouch, then stand at the same time and move as a unit when carrying the patient.

▶ Direct Ground Lift (p. 125)

❑ Set the stretcher in its lowest position and place opposite the patient.

❑ Two EMTs get in position along one side of the patient. EMT #1 is at the head, and EMT #2 is at the foot.

❑ The EMTs drop to one knee facing the patient.

❑ Place the patient's arms on his chest.

❑ EMT #1 at the head-end cradles the patient's head and neck by sliding one arm under the patient's neck to grasp shoulder; the other arm is placed under the patient's lower back.

❑ EMT #2 at the foot-end slides one arm under the patient's knees and the other under the patient above the buttocks.

❑ If a third rescuer is available, he should place both arms under the patient's waist while the two EMTs slide their arms up to the mid-back or down to the buttocks.

❑ On a signal, the crew lifts the patient to their knees.

❑ On a signal, the crew stands and carries the patient to the stretcher. They drop to one knee and roll forward to place the patient onto the mattress.

▶ Draw-Sheet Method (p. 124)

❑ Loosen the bottom sheet of the bed and roll it from both sides toward the patient.

❑ Assure the stretcher is at the same height as the bed and the side rail is down.

❑ Push the stretcher and the bed tightly together.

❑ Firmly grasp the rolled sheet, holding it taut, with an underhand grasp in the area of the head/chest and hip/knee.

❑ On the count of three, EMTs carefully slide the patient onto the stretcher.

▶ Direct Carry (p. 126)

❑ EMT #1 and #2: Get in position along one side of patient. EMT #1 is at the head-end; EMT #2 is at the foot-end.

❑ EMT #1 cradles the patient's head and neck by sliding one arm under the patient's neck to grasp the shoulder.

❑ EMT #2 slides a hand under the patient's hip and lifts slightly.

❑ EMT #1 slides his other arm under the patient's back.

❑ EMT #2 places his arms under the patient's hips and calves.

❑ Both EMTs slide the patient to the edge of the bed and bend toward him with their knees slightly bent.

❑ They lift and curl the patient to their chests and return to a standing position.

❑ They rotate and then slide the patient gently onto the stretcher.

©2009 Pearson Education, Inc.
Emergency Care, 11th Ed.

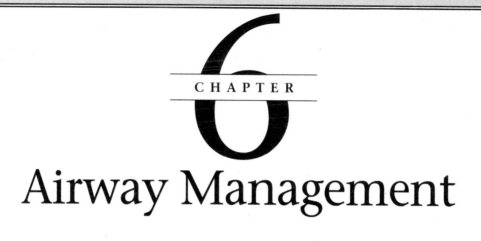

Airway Management

MATCH TERMINOLOGY/ DEFINITIONS

▶ **PART A**

A. The flap of tissue that caps the trachea as you swallow

B. A means of correcting blockage of the airway by the tongue by tilting the head back and lifting the chin

C. The area inside the mouth joining the nasal passageways and the throat

D. The two large tubes that bring air to and from the lungs

E. The voicebox, which contains the epiglottis and vocal cords

F. The ring-shaped structure that forms the lower portion of the larynx

G. The process of breathing in

H. The muscle of breathing that separates the abdomen from the thorax

I. The process of breathing out

J. A means of correcting blockage of the airway by moving the jaw forward without tilting the head or neck

_____ **1.** Bronchi

_____ **2.** Cricoid cartilage

_____ **3.** Diaphragm

_____ **4.** Epiglottis

_____ **5.** Exhalation

_____ **6.** Head-tilt, chin-lift maneuver

_____ **7.** Inhalation

_____ **8.** Jaw-thrust maneuver

_____ **9.** Larynx

_____ **10.** Pharynx

PART B

A. A device that uses oxygen under pressure to deliver artificial ventilations

B. A handheld device with a face mask and self-refilling bag that can be squeezed to provide artificial ventilations to a patient

C. Expansion of the stomach caused by too forceful ventilation pressures, which cause excess air to enter the stomach instead of the lungs

D. Another word for breathing

E. A permanent surgical opening in the neck through which the patient breathes

F. A device connected to the flowmeter to add moisture to the dry oxygen coming from an oxygen cylinder

G. The passageway by which air enters or leaves the body

H. Forcing air or oxygen into the lungs when a patient has stopped breathing or has inadequate breathing

I. A blue or gray skin color resulting from lack of oxygen in the body

J. The breathing in of air or oxygen

_____ **1.** Airway

_____ **2.** Artificial ventilation

_____ **3.** Bag-valve mask

_____ **4.** Cyanosis

_____ **5.** Flow-restricted, oxygen-powered ventilation device

_____ **6.** Gastric distention

_____ **7.** Humidifier

_____ **8.** Respiration

_____ **9.** Stoma

_____ **10.** Ventilation

PART C

A. A flexible breathing tube inserted through the patient's nose into the pharynx to help maintain an open airway

B. A face mask and reservoir bag device that delivers high concentrations of oxygen. The patient's exhaled air escapes through a valve.

C. A device that delivers low concentrations of oxygen through two prongs that rest in the patient's nostrils

D. A device connected to an oxygen cylinder to reduce cylinder pressure to a safe pressure for delivery of oxygen to a patient

E. A device, usually with a one-way valve, to aid in artificial ventilation. A rescuer breathes through the valve when the device is placed over the patient's face. It also acts as a barrier to prevent contact with a patient's breath or body fluids and can be used with supplemental oxygen when fitted with an oxygen inlet.

F. An open and clean passageway for air into the lungs

G. To provide ventilations at a higher rate to compensate for oxygen not delivered during suctioning

H. Container filled with oxygen under pressure

I. Use of a vacuum device to remove blood, vomitus, and other secretions or foreign materials from the airway

J. A rigid curved device inserted through the patient's mouth into the pharynx to help maintain an open airway

K. Vomiting or retching that results when something is placed in the pharynx

_____ **1.** Flowmeter

_____ **2.** Gag reflex

_____ **3.** Ventilate

_____ **4.** Hypoxia

_____ **5.** Nasal cannula

_____ **6.** Nasopharyngeal airway

_____ **7.** Nonrebreather mask

_____ **8.** Oropharyngeal airway

_____ **9.** Oxygen cylinder

_____ **10.** Pocket face mask

_____ **11.** Pop-off valve

_____ **12.** Pressure regulator

_____ **13.** Respiratory arrest

_____ **14.** Respiratory failure

_____ **15.** Suctioning

_____ **16.** Patent airway

L. The reduction of breathing to the point where not enough oxygen is being taken in to sustain life

M. An insufficiency of oxygen in the body's tissues

N. A valve that indicates the flow of oxygen in liters per minute

O. A valve on a BVM designed to blow off excessive pressure; this valve is no longer allowed per AHA standards on any BVM due to the danger of underinflation of the lungs.

P. When breathing completely stops

MULTIPLE-CHOICE REVIEW

_____ **1.** During respiration:
   A. oxygen enters the body during each inspiration.
   B. carbon dioxide enters the body during each expiration.
   C. oxygen does not exit the body on expiration.
   D. carbon dioxide does not enter the body.

_____ **2.** Respiratory failure is:
   A. the cessation of breathing.
   B. the reduction of breathing to a point where oxygen intake is not sufficient to support life.
   C. the same as respiratory arrest.
   D. caused by electrocution.

_____ **3.** Which of the following is <u>not</u> a sign of adequate breathing?
   A. air moving out of the nose and mouth
   B. equal expansion of both sides of the chest
   C. breathing limited to abdominal movement
   D. absence of blue or gray skin coloration

_____ **4.** Signs of inadequate breathing in children may include:
   A. cyanotic skin, lips, tongue, or earlobes.
   B. retractions between the ribs.
   C. nasal flaring.
   D. all of the above.

_____ **5.** Each of the following are signs of inadequate breathing <u>except</u>:
   A. inspirations or expirations that are prolonged.
   B. breathing rate in an adult of 14–18 breaths per minute.
   C. breathing is very shallow, very deep, or appears labored.
   D. the patient is unable to speak in full sentences.

_____ **6.** Additional signs of inadequate breathing include all of the following <u>except</u>:
   A. absent chest movement.
   B. air that can be felt at the nose or mouth.
   C. diminished breath sounds.
   D. noises such as wheezing or crowing.

_____ **7.** Inadequate breathing in a child is defined as:
   A. less than 15 breaths per minute.
   B. more than 30 breaths per minute.
   C. both of the above.
   D. neither of the above.

_____ **8.** When at rest, the normal adequate breathing rate for an adult is _____ times per minute.
   A. 12 to 20
   B. 30 to 40
   C. 60 to 80
   D. 75 to 100

_____ **9.** Cyanosis can be checked by observing the patient's:
   A. tongue.
   B. earlobes.
   C. nail beds.
   D. tongue, nail beds, and earlobes.

_____ **10.** One indication that a patient is experiencing inadequate breathing is that she:
   A. has a headache.
   B. complains of nausea.
   C. talks in short, choppy sentences.
   D. is dizzy when standing.

_____ **11.** The very first step to aid a patient who is not breathing is to:
   A. clear the mouth.
   B. administer oxygen.
   C. apply positive ventilation.
   D. open the airway.

_____ **12.** What is the importance of mechanism of injury to airway care?
   A. An injured patient will need more oxygen.
   B. The procedure for opening the patient's airway is different in trauma.
   C. Patients without a mechanism of injury will have an open airway.
   D. An injury can make airway care easier to manage than a medical emergency.

_____ **13.** To open the airway of a patient with no suspected head, neck, or spine injury, the EMT should use a _____ maneuver.
   A. jaw-thrust
   B. head-tilt, chin-lift
   C. head-tilt, neck-lift
   D. modified chin-thrust

_____ **14.** When performing the head-tilt, chin-lift maneuver, the EMT should:
   A. not allow the patient's mouth to close.
   B. position himself at the top of the patient's head.
   C. tilt the head by applying pressure to the patient's chin.
   D. use fingertips to lift the neck.

_____ **15.** When performing the jaw-thrust maneuver, the EMT should do each one of the following <u>except</u>:
   A. kneel at the top of the patient's head.
   B. stabilize the patient's head with forearms.
   C. use the index fingers to push the angles of the patient's lower jaw forward.
   D. tilt the head by applying gentle pressure to the patient's forehead.

_____ **16.** The main purpose of the jaw-thrust maneuver is to:
   A. open the mouth with only one hand.
   B. open the airway without moving the head or neck.
   C. create an airway for the medical patient.
   D. create an airway when it is not possible to jut the jaw.

_____ **17.** Various techniques the EMT can use to provide artificial ventilation are listed below.
   1) one-rescuer bag-valve mask
   2) flow-restricted, oxygen-powered ventilation device
   3) two-rescuer bag-valve mask with high-concentration supplemental oxygen at 15 lpm
   4) mouth-to-mask with high-concentration supplemental oxygen at 15 lpm

   What is the order of preference of these techniques?
   A. 1, 2, 3, 4
   B. 2, 4, 1, 3
   C. 4, 3, 2, 1
   D. 4, 1, 2, 3

_____ **18.** All the following are signs of inadequate artificial ventilations <u>except</u>:
   A. chest does not rise and fall with ventilation.
   B. rate of ventilation is too slow or too fast.
   C. patient's color changes from cyanotic to pink.
   D. patient's heart rate does not return to normal with ventilations.

_____ **19.** When performing mouth-to-mask ventilation on an adult patient, ventilations should be delivered over _____ seconds.
- **A.** 1¹/₂ to 2
- **B.** 2¹/₂ to 3
- **C.** 5 or 6
- **D.** 10

_____ **20.** The bag-valve mask on your ambulance should have:
- **A.** a non-refilling shell that is easily cleaned.
- **B.** a non-jam valve with an oxygen inlet.
- **C.** a standard 9/12-mm fitting.
- **D.** manual disabling pop-off valve.

_____ **21.** The bag-valve mask should be capable of:
- **A.** withstanding cold temperatures.
- **B.** providing a high pressure in the chest and airway.
- **C.** blowing off at pressures above 40 mm of water pressure.
- **D.** receiving an oxygen inlet flow of 25 liters per minute.

_____ **22.** When ventilating a suspected trauma patient with a bag-valve mask, it is most effective to do all of the following except:
- **A.** use a device with a volume of 1,000–1,600 mL.
- **B.** use two EMTs to perform the procedure.
- **C.** position the EMT who is maintaining the mask seal at the patient's head.
- **D.** maintain the head-tilt, chin-lift maneuver.

_____ **23.** When ventilating an unconscious patient, a bag-valve mask is complete if it is used with:
- **A.** a reservoir bag.
- **B.** an oral airway.
- **C.** an oxygen tank and liter flow regulator.
- **D.** all of the above.

_____ **24.** If the patient's chest does not rise and fall when using a bag-valve mask, the EMT should do all of the following except:
- **A.** reposition the head and reattempt ventilations.
- **B.** check for escape of air around the mask.
- **C.** use an alternative method of artificial ventilation.
- **D.** increase the rate at which the bag is squeezed.

_____ **25.** If the patient has a _____ and needs ventilatory assistance, the best device to use is a _____ .
- **A.** stoma, pocket mask
- **B.** tracheotomy, positive-pressure ventilator
- **C.** stoma, bag-valve mask
- **D.** tracheotomy, nasal airway

_____ **26.** The flow-restricted, oxygen-powered ventilation device should:
- **A.** operate in both ordinary and extreme environmental conditions.
- **B.** have an audible alarm when the relief valve is activated.
- **C.** have a trigger so two hands can be used to seal the mask.
- **D.** do all of the above.

_____ **27.** An oral or nasal airway should be:
- **A.** cleaned for reuse after the call.
- **B.** inserted in all critically injured patients.
- **C.** used to keep the tongue from blocking the airway.
- **D.** used in order to prevent the need for suctioning.

_____ **28.** If something is placed in the patient's throat, the gag reflex causes the patient to:
- **A.** take deep breaths.
- **B.** pass out.
- **C.** vomit or retch.
- **D.** all of the above.

_____ 29. An oropharyngeal airway of proper size will extend from the:
   A. corner of the patient's mouth to the tip of the earlobe.
   B. lips to the larynx.
   C. nose to the angle of the jaw.
   D. none of the above.

_____ 30. An oral airway should be inserted:
   A. upside down, with the tip toward the roof of the mouth, then flipped 180 degrees over the tongue.
   B. right side up, using a tongue depressor to press the tongue down and forward to keep it from obstructing the airway.
   C. either of the above.
   D. neither of the above.

_____ 31. A nasopharyngeal airway should be:
   A. inserted with the bevel on the lateral side of the nostril.
   B. measured from the patient's nostril to the earlobe.
   C. inserted in the left nostril when possible.
   D. turned 180 degrees with the tip facing the roof of the mouth.

_____ 32. When inserting a nasopharyngeal airway, lubricate the outside of the tube with a(n):
   A. petroleum jelly.   C. silicone-based gel.
   B. oil-based lubricant.   D. water-based lubricant.

_____ 33. The purposes of suctioning include removal of:
   A. teeth and large pieces of solid material.
   B. excess oxygen from the patient.
   C. blood, vomitus, and other secretions.
   D. all of the above.

_____ 34. When a patient begins to vomit, it is essential that you have a(n) _____ ready to go at the patient's side.
   A. suction unit   C. blood pressure cuff
   B. oxygen tank   D. pocket mask

_____ 35. Which of the following is <u>not</u> true of the Yankauer suction tip?
   A. It has a rigid tip.
   B. It allows for excellent control over the distal end of the device.
   C. It is most successfully used with responsive patients.
   D. It has a larger bore than flexible catheters.

_____ 36. When using a soft, flexible-tip catheter,
   A. measure so that it is inserted only as far as the base of the tongue.
   B. never pass the catheter through a nasal tube.
   C. insert the device with the suction turned on.
   D. do none of the above.

_____ 37. When suctioning an adult patient who is unconscious, avoid suctioning for longer than _____ seconds at a time.
   A. 5   C. 15
   B. 10   D. 20

_____ 38. When inserting a rigid-tip suction catheter,
   A. insert the device only as far as you can see.
   B. measure from the nose to the earlobe.
   C. slide the device along the palate in children.
   D. insert the device with the suction on.

_____ 39. Atmospheric air contains _____ oxygen.
   A. 10%   C. 21%
   B. 16%   D. 25%

©2009 Pearson Education, Inc.
Emergency Care, 11th Ed.

_____ **40.** A fully pressurized oxygen tank should have approximately _____ psi.
    A. 1,000   **C.** 2,000
    B. 1,500   **D.** 2,500

_____ **41.** Which <u>portable</u> oxygen cylinder, when full, will last the longest when delivering oxygen?
    A. D   **C.** A
    B. E   **D.** M

_____ **42.** Before connecting a regulator to an oxygen supply cylinder, the EMT should:
    A. remove the protective seal and then open the valve.
    B. stand to the side of the main valve opening and crack the cylinder valve slightly.
    C. attach the nonrebreather mask to the flowmeter; then attach to the tank.
    D. do all of the above.

_____ **43.** Humidified oxygen is:
    A. not possible in an ambulance.
    B. not used for patients on chronic oxygen therapy.
    C. not needed in adult patients being transported for short distances.
    D. habit forming.

_____ **44.** Concerns about the dangers of giving too much oxygen to patients with COPD:
    A. are invalid in the prehospital setting.
    B. have been understated and proven with research.
    C. are invalid when the patient is over the age of 60.
    D. are dealt with by using a nonrebreather mask at low flow rates.

_____ **45.** The best method for EMTs to use when giving a high concentration of oxygen to breathing patients is a:
    A. nasal cannula.   **C.** simple face mask.
    B. Venturi mask.   **D.** nonrebreather mask.

_____ **46.** The oxygen concentration of a nonrebreather mask is between:
    A. 20% and 40%.   **C.** 60% and 80%.
    B. 40% and 60%.   **D.** 80% and 100%.

_____ **47.** The flow rate of a nonrebreather mask should be:
    A. adjusted so that when the patient inhales, the bag deflates by two-thirds.
    B. 12 to 15 liters per minute.
    C. adjusted to 6 liters per minute.
    D. all of the above.

_____ **48.** The oxygen concentration of a nasal cannula is between:
    A. 4% and 6%.   **C.** 24% and 44%.
    B. 8% and 20%.   **D.** 50% and 65%.

_____ **49.** When an elderly patient, who fell and injured her ribs, is found breathing very rapidly at a rate of 40 and shallow, how can this be a serious life threat?
    A. She is inhaling too much oxygen.
    B. Her minute volume may be diminished.
    C. Her minute volume is excessive.
    D. She is exceeding her dead space.

_____ **50.** What is meant by anatomical dead space?
    A. the maximum amount of room for dying cells in the body
    B. the compartment where tissue swells like edema
    C. hollow chambers like the sinus
    D. the area in the lungs outside the alveoli

COMPLETE THE FOLLOWING

1. List at least six signs of inadequate breathing.

   A. _____

   B. _____

   C. _____

   D. _____

   E. _____

   F. _____

2. List in order of preference the four techniques available to the EMT to provide artificial ventilations.

   A. _____

   B. _____

   C. _____

   D. _____

3. **A.** Oxygen safety is of prime importance. List four practices the EMT should always do when working with oxygen cylinders.

   1. _____

   2. _____

   3. _____

   4. _____

3. **B.** List four practices the EMT should never do when working with oxygen cylinders.

   1. _____

   2. _____

   3. _____

   4. _____

©2009 Pearson Education, Inc.
Emergency Care, 11th Ed.

LABEL THE DIAGRAM

Write the name of each part of the respiratory system on the line provided.

1. _____

2. _____

3. _____

4. _____

5. _____

6. _____

7. _____

8. _____

9. _____

10. _____

11. _____

12. _____

13. _____

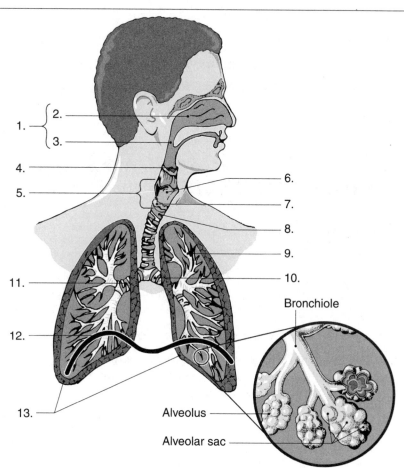

Bronchiole

Alveolus

Alveolar sac

STREET SCENES DISCUSSION

Review the Street Scene on p. 184 of your textbook. Then answer the questions below.

1. If the patient had no gag reflex, what airway adjunct would you consider using? How would you insert it?

2. If the patient vomits during BVM ventilation, what should you do?

3. If the patient's pulse had not increased so quickly, should you have called for an ALS intercept? Why or why not?

ON THE WEB

To help you review and practice basic skills, visit the *Emergency Care 11th Ed. Companion Website* at www.prenhall.com/limmer. For Online Test Preparation, visit www.prenhall.com/emtachieve.

EMT SKILL PERFORMANCE CHECKLISTS

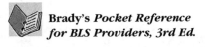 **Brady's *Pocket Reference for BLS Providers*, 3rd Ed.**

▶ HEAD-TILT, CHIN-LIFT MANEUVER (P. 145)

❏ Take Standard Precautions.

❏ Once patient is supine, place one hand on the forehead. Place the fingertips of your other hand under the bony area at the center of the patient's lower jaw.

❏ Tilt the head by applying gentle pressure to the patient's forehead.

❏ Use your fingertips to lift the chin and to support the lower jaw. Move the jaw forward to a point where the lower teeth are almost touching the upper teeth. Do not compress the soft tissues under the lower jaw.

❏ Do not close the patient's mouth. It is best to insert an oral airway if the patient has no gag reflex.

▶ JAW-THRUST MANEUVER (PP. 145–146)

❑ Take Standard Precautions.

❑ Carefully keep the patient's head, neck, and spine aligned, moving him as a unit as you place him in the supine position.

❑ Kneel approximately 18 inches above the head of the supine patient.

❑ Reach forward and gently place one hand on each side of the patient's lower jaw. Run your fingers along the jaw until you just pass the angle of the jaw.

❑ Stabilize the patient's head with your palms and forearms.

❑ Using your index fingers, push the angles of the patient's lower jaw forward.

❑ To keep the mouth open, use an oropharyngeal airway on a patient with no gag reflex.

❑ Do not tilt or rotate the patient's head.

NOTE: Remember the purpose of the jaw-thrust manuever is to open the airway without moving the head or neck from the neutral position.

▶ OROPHARYNGEAL (ORAL) AIRWAY INSERTION (OPA) (PP. 158–159)

❑ Take Standard Precautions.

❑ Select appropriate-size airway.

❑ Measure airway (center of mouth to angle of jaw, or corner of mouth to tip of earlobe).

❑ Insert airway without pushing the tongue back into throat. Insert upside down and flip 180 degrees over the tongue, or insert straight in with a tongue blade holding tongue forward.

❑ Remove oropharyngeal airway quickly if patient gags.

▶ NASOPHARYNGEAL (NASAL) AIRWAY INSERTION (NPA) (PP. 159–162)

❑ Take Standard Precautions.

❑ Select appropriate-size airway (diameter of patient's little finger). An alternative method is to measure length from patient's nostril to earlobe or to angle of jaw.

❑ Measure airway (nostril to earlobe).

❑ Lubricate nasopharyngeal airway with water-soluble gel.

❑ Fully insert the airway with the bevel facing the nasal septum.

▶ MOUTH-TO-MASK VENTILATION (P. 148)

❑ Take Standard Precautions.

❑ Connect one-way valve to mask.

❑ Connect oxygen to inlet on face mask. Oxygen should be run at 15 lpm.

❑ Kneel about 18 inches above the head of the supine patient.

❑ Open the airway (manually or with adjunct).

❑ Position mask on patient's face so that the apex is over bridge of nose and the base is between lower lip and prominence of chin.

(continued next page)

❑ Position thumbs over top half of mask, index and middle fingers over the bottom half.

❑ Use ring and middle fingers to bring patient's jaw up to mask and maintain head-tilt, chin-lift. *Tilt the head back as if you were trying to stand the patient on his or her head!*

❑ Ventilate over 1 second to achieve visible chest rise.

❑ Remove your mouth from the port to allow for passive exhalation.

NOTE: Do not delay mouth-to-mask ventilation if oxygen is not immediately available.

▶ OROPHARYNGEAL SUCTIONING (PP. 162–167)

❑ Take Standard Precautions.

❑ Position yourself at patient's head, and turn patient onto his or her side.*

❑ A rigid tip (Yankauer) is preferred. When inserting, never lose sight of the tip.

❑ Measure a flexible suction catheter (distance between patient's earlobe and corner or mouth, or center of mouth to angle of jaw).

❑ Turn suction unit on. Attach the catheter and test for suction.

❑ Open and clear the patient's mouth.

❑ Place the rigid pharyngeal tip so that the convex (bulging-out) side is against roof of patient's mouth. Insert tip just to the base of the tongue. Do not push tip down into the throat or larynx.

❑ Apply suction only after the tip of the catheter or rigid tip is in place, suctioning on the way out, moving tip from side to side. Suction for no longer than 15 seconds. (As per U.S. DOT, suction toddlers for no longer than 10 seconds and infants for no longer than 5 seconds.**) If the patient continues to vomit, you must still continue to suction.

❑ Ventilate the patient with 100% oxygen.

NOTES: *If trauma is suspected, leave the patient supine.
**AHA Guidelines say limit any interruptions in chest compressions during CPR to 10 seconds.

▶ TWO-RESCUER BAG-VALVE MASK VENTILATION (PP. 151–153)

❑ Take Standard Precautions.

❑ Open the medical patient's airway using head-tilt, chin-lift maneuver.

❑ Suction and insert an oropharyngeal airway.

❑ Select correct bag-valve-mask size (adult, child, or infant). A pop-off valve is not acceptable!

❑ Kneel approximately 18 inches above the head of the supine patient.

❑ Position mask on patient's face so that the apex is over bridge of nose and the base is between the lower lip and prominence of chin.

❑ Position thumbs over top half of mask, index and middle fingers over bottom half.

❑ Use ring and middle fingers to bring patient's jaw up to mask and maintain head-tilt, chin-lift. *Tilt the head back as if you were trying to stand patient on his or her head!*

©2009 Pearson Education, Inc.
Emergency Care, 11th Ed.

- ❑ The second rescuer should connect bag to mask, if not already done. While you maintain mask seal, the second rescuer should squeeze the bag with two hands, providing a ventilation over 1 second to achieve visible chest rise.

- ❑ The second rescuer should release pressure on the bag and let the patient exhale passively. While this occurs, the oxygen reservoir is refilling.

NOTE: This technique may be used for a trauma patient by combining a jaw-thrust maneuver with manual stabilization of the head and neck.

▶ PREPARING THE OXYGEN DELIVERY SYSTEM (PP. 174–176)

- ❑ Select desired cylinder. Check label and hydrostat date.
- ❑ Place the cylinder in an upright position and stand to one side.
- ❑ Remove the plastic wrapper or cap protecting the cylinder outlet.
- ❑ Keep the plastic washer (some setups).
- ❑ Crack the main valve for 1 second to clean it out.
- ❑ Select the correct pressure regulator and flowmeter.
- ❑ Place cylinder valve gasket on regulator oxygen port.
- ❑ Make certain that the pressure regulator is closed.
- ❑ Align pins or thread by hand.
- ❑ Tighten T-screw for pin yoke.
- ❑ Tighten with a wrench for a threaded outlet.
- ❑ Attach tubing and delivery device.

▶ OXYGEN ADMINISTRATION—NONREBREATHER MASK (PP. 178–179)

- ❑ Take Standard Precautions.
- ❑ Assemble regulator onto tank.
- ❑ Open main valve on tank.
- ❑ Check for leaks.
- ❑ Check tank pressure.
- ❑ Attach nonrebreather mask.
- ❑ Adjust liter flow to 12 to 15 liters per minute.
- ❑ Prefill reservoir.
- ❑ Apply and adjust mask to the patient's face, explaining the need for oxygen.
- ❑ Secure tank during transport.

▶ OXYGEN ADMINISTRATION—NASAL CANNULA (PP. 179–180)

- ❑ Take Standard Precautions.
- ❑ Assemble regulator onto tank.
- ❑ Open main valve on tank.
- ❑ Check for leaks.
- ❑ Check tank pressure.

(continued next page)

❑ Attach nasal cannula to regulator.

❑ Place nasal prongs into the patient's nose, and adjust tubing for comfort.

❑ Adjust liter flow to 1 to 6 liters per minute.

❑ Secure tank during transport.

▶ DISCONTINUING OXYGEN ADMINISTRATION (PP. 178–179)

❑ Remove delivery device from patient.

❑ Turn off the liter flow rate.

❑ Close the main valve.

❑ Remove the delivery tubing.

❑ Bleed the flowmeter.

❑ Change the tank before the volume reaches 200 psi or less (or your service policy).

▶ POSITIONING THE ADULT PATIENT FOR BASIC LIFE SUPPORT (P. 144)

❑ Take Standard Precautions.

❑ Straighten the patient's legs and position arm closest to you above his head.

❑ Cradle the patient's head and neck. Grasp under the distant armpit.

❑ Move the patient as a unit onto his side.

❑ Move the patient onto back and reposition the extended arm.

NOTE: This maneuver is used to initiate airway evaluation, artificial ventilation, or CPR when the EMT must act alone. When trauma is suspected, the four-rescuer log roll is the preferred technique.

CASE STUDY

▶ THE COMPLICATED AIRWAY: THE SELF-INFLICTED SHOOTING

Your unit and the police are dispatched to the scene of an attempted suicide with shots fired. Apparently the call was received by a family member who was called by the patient threatening to do harm to himself with a handgun. The police arrive before you and advise that the scene is secure (safe) and that you should respond directly to the scene, which is a private home in a suburban community. Upon arrival, you find a 45-year-old male lying with his face covered with blood. He is moaning, and his chest and abdomen appear to be moving as he breathes. After donning protective gloves, mask, and goggles, both you and your partners carefully provide manual stabilization of the neck and log roll the patient onto a long backboard.

What you reveal is a mandible and tongue that are severely lacerated, and the mouth and nose are bubbling with blood as the patient attempts to breathe.

1. How should you open the airway of this patient?

©2009 Pearson Education, Inc.
Emergency Care, 11th Ed.

2. A) Does this patient need to be suctioned? **B)** If so, what is the maximum amount of time to accomplish this procedure?

A. _____

B. _____

3. Should an airway adjunct be used on this patient?

Once the patient's airway is opened and cleared, you need to oxygenate this patient. He has no other obvious injuries, yet you are treating him for a possible spinal injury due to the impact of the bullet and his backward fall from his desk chair during the incident. The police think that this is why he shot his chin instead of his brain during the suicide attempt. You evaluate the patient's breathing rate as 28, shallow and labored, and his pulse as 120, weak and regular.

4. What device should be used to administer oxygen to this patient?

5. A. What is the proper liter flow to set the regulator for the device you chose in question number 4?

5. B. If your unit has a pulse oximeter, should it be used?

6. Your portable D cylinder was full at the beginning of the shift and this is your first call. **A)** How many liters are in the tank? **B)** How much pressure is in it? **C)** How much time can you expect to get out of the tank, considering your service's policy is to refill tanks at 200 psi?

A. _____

B. _____

C. _____

7. As you prepare to transport the patient, you continue to suction him, making sure not to exceed **A)** _____ seconds per attempt because as you suction you are also removing **B)** _____ . **C)** Which would be better to use, a rigid-tip or a flexible catheter?

A. _____

B. _____

C. _____

8. The patient has a blood pressure of 100/70 mmHg and his oxygen saturation is 95%, so you decide his priority is **A)** [high, low]. The major problem with this patient is his **B)** _____ . He should be transported **C)** [right away, in a few minutes] to the **D)** [local hospital, trauma center].

A. _____

B. _____

C. _____

D. _____

9. From your knowledge of your EMS system, what ALS (advanced life support) treatment might be helpful to this patient if you can arrange for an ALS intercept?

10. What should you do if you hear hissing or bubbling around the mask as you ventilate?

©2009 Pearson Education, Inc.
Emergency Care, 11th Ed.

Interim Exam 1

Use the answer sheet on pages 64–65 to complete this exam. It is perforated so it can be easily removed from this workbook.

1. Most EMT training programs are based on standards developed by the:
   A. American Red Cross (ARC).
   B. American Heart Association (AHA).
   C. United States Department of Transportation (DOT).
   D. National Institute of Health (NIH).

2. An EMT can inspire patient confidence and cooperation by:
   A. transporting the patient from the scene to a hospital.
   B. providing patient care without regard for her own personal safety.
   C. telling the patient that everything will be all right.
   D. being pleasant, cooperative, sincere, and a good listener.

3. If an on-duty EMT fails to provide the standard of care and if this failure causes harm or injury to the patient, the EMT may be accused of:
   A. assault.
   B. abandonment.
   C. negligence.
   D. breach of promise.

4. A conscious and mentally competent adult patient has the right to refuse care. This refusal must be _____ and documented.
   A. implied
   B. actual
   C. involuntary
   D. informed

5. The EMT can treat and transport an unconscious patient because of the legal consideration known as _____ consent.
   A. applied
   B. implied
   C. triage
   D. immunity

6. A child falls off a trampoline at an elementary school and twists her ankle. Since the parents are not present, the child's consent is:
   A. not needed.
   B. actual.
   C. implied.
   D. meaningless.

7. _____ help protect the off-duty EMT from lawsuits when stopping at the scene of a collision to offer assistance.
   A. Professional associations
   B. Blanket insurance policies
   C. Good Samaritan laws
   D. Abandonment laws

8. Each of the following is the responsibility of an EMT at a hazardous-materials (hazmat) incident except:
   A. entering hazmat scenes with SCBA.
   B. protecting yourself and others.
   C. recognizing potential problems.
   D. notifying hazardous-materials response team.

9. The form of infection control that assumes that all body fluids should be considered potentially infectious is:
   A. infectious disease.
   B. body substance isolation/standard precautions.
   C. immunity.
   D. universal precautions.

10. When planning to lift, all the following are important considerations except:
    A. the weight of the object.
    B. one's physical characteristics.
    C. communicating with one's partner.
    D. the distance the object is to be carried.

11. When lifting, the EMT should:
    A. keep the back loose and knees locked.
    B. twist or attempt to make moves other than the lift.
    C. use the leg muscles to do the lift.
    D. try not to talk to his partner.

12. When carrying a conscious patient on the stairs, the EMT should:
    A. keep the stretcher as level as possible.
    B. use a long backboard at all times.
    C. use a stair chair whenever possible.
    D. do all of the above.

13. Ways an EMT can avoid a potential back injury include all the following except:
    A. push, rather than pull, a load.
    B. keep back locked in while lifting.
    C. keep arms straight when pulling.
    D. push or pull from a kneeling position if the weight is below waist level.

14. An emergency move is required in each of the following situations except when:
    A. the scene is hazardous.
    B. care of life-threatening conditions requires repositioning.
    C. other patients must be reached who have life threats.
    D. the patient is unconscious.

15. Which of the following is the greatest danger to the patient in an emergency move?
    A. A spinal injury may be aggravated.
    B. Bleeding may increase after movement.
    C. The airway may become obstructed.
    D. There is no danger associated with an emergency move.

16. A method of lifting and carrying a patient in which one EMT slips hands under the patient's armpits and grasps the wrists while another EMT grasps the patient's knees is called the:
    A. direct ground lift.
    B. extremity lift.
    C. draw-sheet method.
    D. direct carry method.

17. When moving a patient from the ambulance stretcher to the hospital stretcher, you probably will use the:
    A. cradle carry.
    B. modified draw-sheet method.
    C. direct ground lift.
    D. extremity lift.

18. To load the wheeled ambulance stretcher into the ambulance, the two EMTs should position themselves on _____ of the stretcher.
    A. opposite sides
    B. opposite ends
    C. the same side
    D. one end and one side

19. Move a patient who has no broken bones or spinal injury from the floor to a stair chair using the:
    A. indirect carry.
    B. extremity lift.
    C. slide transfer.
    D. chair lift.

20. Drags are used only in emergencies because they:
    A. do not protect the patient's neck and spine.
    B. require excessive energy from the EMT.
    C. may injure the EMT's back.
    D. provide full immobilization.

21. In order to maintain balance when lifting a patient-carrying device, it is best to use _____ rescuers to carry the device.
    A. three
    B. an even number of
    C. an odd number of
    D. bystanders and

22. The driver of a vehicle involved in a collision requires immediate airway and bleeding control. You are unable to provide this treatment in the vehicle. You should:
    A. check the patient's vital signs.
    B. make an urgent move.
    C. remove the patient on a short backboard.
    D. do all of the above.

23. Which carry is considered very difficult to use with an unconscious person?
    A. cradle   C. shoulder
    B. three-rescuer   D. piggyback

24. The _____ carry must be performed in one unbroken sweep.
    A. pack strap
    B. front piggyback
    C. firefighter's
    D. four-rescuer

25. A canvas or rubberized stretcher that can be used to move a patient through a narrow hallway or restricted area is called a _____ stretcher.
    A. basket
    B. portable
    C. flexible
    D. wheeled-ambulance

26. A victim with obvious spinal injuries is found on the floor of a burning building. The EMT rates the situation hazardous, but not yet dire. Alone and without special equipment, the EMT should use the:
    A. cradle carry.
    B. clothes drag.
    C. firefighter's carry.
    D. pack-strap method.

27. The patient-carrying device of choice for the uninjured patient is the _____ stretcher.
    A. portable ambulance
    B. wire basket
    C. wheeled ambulance
    D. slat

28. If you are an EMT with a service that does not provide the appropriate personal protective equipment, why should you serve as an advocate for this equipment?
    A. Your crew members could be injured unnecessarily.
    B. You could be seriously injured.
    C. An injured EMT is of little help to the patient.
    D. All of the above.

©2009 Pearson Education, Inc.
Emergency Care, 11th Ed.

29. During an EMS call, a lethal threat is recognized. The EMT should first:
    A. retreat to a safe area.
    B. radio for assistance.
    C. reevaluate the situation.
    D. remedy the situation.

30. Of the different types of stress, which is a positive form that helps the EMT work under pressure and respond effectively?
    A. cumulative stress
    B. eustress
    C. distress
    D. critical incident stress

31. When responding to a violent situation, observation begins when you:
    A. enter the scene.
    B. exit the ambulance.
    C. enter the neighborhood.
    D. arrive at the patient's side.

32. To ensure crew safety, one member of the crew should always:
    A. remain in the ambulance.
    B. carry a portable radio.
    C. wear a bulletproof vest.
    D. carry a canister of "pepper gas."

33. While you are treating a patient with a severely bleeding forearm, the patient's pet dog appears. The patient states, "He won't hurt you. He's very friendly." Your best course of action would be to:
    A. have your partner observe the dog closely while you treat the patient.
    B. quickly control the bleeding; then have the dog locked in another room.
    C. ignore the dog since the patient assures it is friendly and will not harm you.
    D. do all of the above.

34. If a patient refuses care and then becomes unconscious, it is best for the EMT to:
    A. refuse to treat or transport the patient.
    B. ask a family member for permission to treat.
    C. treat life-threatening problems and transport.
    D. contact medical direction for advice.

35. An advantage of the "advance directive" is that:
    A. the patient is not involved in making a decision about her treatment.
    B. the patient's expressed wishes may be followed.
    C. no matter what the family says, CPR is not given.
    D. it protects the EMT from charges of negligence.

36. In most cases, the oral wishes of the patient's family to withhold care are:
    A. all that is needed to stop CPR from being initiated.
    B. all that is needed to stop CPR once it is initiated.
    C. not a reason to withhold medical care.
    D. not sufficient unless they are given in writing.

37. You can prevent most lawsuits if you:
    A. provide care within the scope of your practice.
    B. properly document your care.
    C. are courteous and respectful to all your patients.
    D. do all of the above.

38. The negligent EMT may be required to pay for all of the following except the patient's:
    A. lost wages.
    B. medical expenses.
    C. pain and suffering.
    D. health insurance costs.

39. Which of the following is not a function of the musculoskeletal system?
    A. It gives the body shape.
    B. It protects the internal organs.
    C. It provides for body movement.
    D. It regulates body temperature.

40. The superior portion of the sternum is called the:
    A. xiphoid process.   C. manubrium.
    B. sternal body.   D. clavicle.

41. A young girl fell while ice skating, injuring the protrusion on the inside of the ankle. The medical term for this location is the:
    A. acromion.   C. lateral malleolus.
    B. medial malleolus.   D. calcaneus.

42. The heart muscle has a property called _____ . This means that the heart has the ability to generate and conduct electrical impulses on its own.
    A. contractility
    B. automaticity
    C. involuntary contraction
    D. conductibility

43. A division of the peripheral nervous system that controls involuntary motor functions is called the _____ nervous system.
    A. autonomic   C. sensory
    B. central   D. motor

44. When in the anatomical position, the person will be facing:
    A. away from you.   C. face down.
    B. the observer.   D. face up.

45. In the anatomical position, the person's palms will be facing:
  A. forward.
  B. backward.
  C. upward.
  D. downward.

46. An anatomical term that is occasionally used to refer to the sole of the foot is:
  A. calcaneus.
  B. ventral.
  C. dorsal.
  D. plantar.

47. The bones of the cheek are called the _____ bones.
  A. orbit
  B. maxillae
  C. zygomatic
  D. mandible

48. The heart is _____ to the stomach.
  A. distal
  B. medial
  C. proximal
  D. superior

49. When comparing body structure positions, the knees are said to be _____ to the toes, and the toes are _____ to the knees.
  A. inferior, superior
  B. proximal, distal
  C. distal, dorsal
  D. anterior, posterior

50. A patient found lying on her back is in the _____ position.
  A. anatomical
  B. prone
  C. supine
  D. lateral recumbent

51. To assist in describing the location of abdominal organs, we divide the abdomen into _____ parts.
  A. two
  B. three
  C. four
  D. five

52. The torso of the body is composed of the abdomen, pelvis, and:
  A. thorax.
  B. upper arms and legs.
  C. extremities.
  D. head.

53. The heart is located in the center of the _____ cavity.
  A. thoracic
  B. cranial
  C. pelvic
  D. cardiac

54. The structure that divides the chest cavity from the abdominal cavity is the:
  A. meninges.
  B. duodenum.
  C. diaphragm.
  D. spinal column.

55. The anatomical name for the kneecap is the:
  A. ilium.
  B. malleolus.
  C. patella.
  D. phalange.

56. The cranium consists of the:
  A. facial bones.
  B. mandible and maxillae.
  C. top, back, and sides of the skull.
  D. zygomatic bones.

57. The highest point in the shoulder is the:
  A. acromion process.
  B. humerus.
  C. metatarsal.
  D. clavicle.

58. At the scene of a collision, an off-duty EMT provides care to the patient, acting in good faith and to the best of her abilities. In many states, this EMT is protected from care-related lawsuits by _____ laws.
  A. applied consent
  B. total immunity
  C. Good Samaritan
  D. jeopardy

59. When confronted with an unconscious minor without parents or a legal guardian present, the EMT should:
  A. seek a physician's approval before beginning care.
  B. consider consent for care to be implied and begin care.
  C. ask the child for consent and begin care.
  D. consider consent to be applied and begin care.

60. The legal concept of negligence requires that three circumstances must be demonstrated. Which of the following is not one of the three circumstances?
  A. The EMT had a duty to act.
  B. The EMT committed a breach of duty.
  C. The EMT had a local duty.
  D. The breach of duty caused harm.

61. A person lying on his stomach with his face down is in the _____ position.
  A. supine
  B. prone
  C. coma
  D. recovery

62. In a trauma center, surgery teams are:
  A. on call 12 hours a day.
  B. available most of the time.
  C. available 24 hours a day.
  D. supervised by the Medical Director.

63. In 1970, the _____ was founded to establish professional standards for EMS personnel.
  A. American Medical Association
  B. National Registry of Emergency Medical Technicians
  C. National Highway Traffic Safety Administration
  D. U.S. Department of Transportation

64. Safe, reliable transportation is a critical component of an EMS system. Most patients can be effectively transported by:
  A. airplane.
  B. helicopter.
  C. rescue vehicle.
  D. ambulance.

©2009 Pearson Education, Inc.
Emergency Care, 11th Ed.

65. An _____ is a national-level EMT who has been trained to start IVs, perform advanced airway techniques, and administer some medicines beyond the EMT.
    A. EMT-First Responder
    B. EMT-Intermediate
    C. EMT-Critical Care
    D. EMT-Paramedic

66. A continuous self-review with the purpose of identifying and correcting aspects of the EMS system that require improvement is called:
    A. standing orders.
    B. quality improvement.
    C. protocols.
    D. medical direction.

67. A physician who assumes the ultimate responsibility for the patient care aspects of the EMS system is called the:
    A. Designated Agent.
    B. Medical Director.
    C. Off-line Director.
    D. Primary Care Physician.

68. A common cause of lawsuits against EMS agencies is:
    A. patients who refuse care.
    B. on-scene deaths.
    C. cardiac arrest cases.
    D. pedestrians struck by cars.

69. The legal extent or limits of the EMT's job are formally defined by the:
    A. patient.
    B. DOT curriculum.
    C. state.
    D. scope of practice.

70. Which is not generally considered a sign or symptom of stress?
    A. decisiveness
    B. guilt
    C. loss of interest in work
    D. difficulty sleeping

71. All the following are types of calls that have a high potential for causing excessive stress except:
    A. calls involving infants and children.
    B. patients with severe injuries.
    C. cases of abuse and neglect.
    D. motor vehicle collisions.

72. Lifestyle changes that can help the EMT deal with stress include all the following except:
    A. exercise to burn off tension.
    B. increase consumption of fatty foods.
    C. decrease caffeine consumption.
    D. decrease consumption of alcohol.

73. Changes in your professional life to reduce and prevent stress could include:
    A. requesting a change of shift or location.
    B. taking on another part-time position.
    C. working additional overtime shifts.
    D. requesting a busier location.

74. After CISM:
    A. management investigates the call.
    B. performance appraisals are initiated.
    C. the peer team writes a detailed critique.
    D. the peer team offers support.

75. Stress after a major EMS incident is:
    A. unusual and unexpected.
    B. a sign of weakness.
    C. normal and to be expected.
    D. part of the grieving process.

76. Retreating to a world of one's own after hearing one is going to die is a result of the stage of grief called:
    A. bargaining.   C. denial.
    B. depression.   D. anxiety.

77. All of the following communicable diseases should be of particular concern to the EMT except:
    A. hepatitis B.   C. HIV/AIDS.
    B. tuberculosis.   D. PPD.

78. A disease that is spread by exposure to an open wound or sore of an infected individual is caused by a(n) _____ pathogen.
    A. universal   C. bloodborne
    B. airborne   D. infectious

79. An infection that causes inflammation of the liver is called:
    A. meningitis.   C. typhoid.
    B. tuberculosis.   D. hepatitis.

80. A disease spread by inhaling or absorbing droplets from the air through the eyes, nose, or mouth is considered:
    A. bloodborne.
    B. noncommunicable.
    C. airborne.
    D. viral.

81. The communicable disease that kills the most health workers every year in the United States is:
    A. tuberculosis.   C. meningitis.
    B. HIV/AIDS.   D. hepatitis B virus.

82. Always assume that any patient with a:
    A. cold has a bloodborne disease.
    B. productive cough has TB.
    C. fever has typhoid.
    D. rash has measles.

83. Which of the following is <u>not</u> true about the human immunodeficiency virus (HIV)?
- **A.** It attacks the immune system.
- **B.** It doesn't survive well outside the human body.
- **C.** It can be introduced through puncture wounds.
- **D.** It is an airborne pathogen.

84. Your patient has hepatitis B. You are accidentally stuck with a needle that has some of this patient's infected blood on it. Your chance of contracting the disease is about:
- **A.** 10%.
- **B.** 20%.
- **C.** 30%.
- **D.** 40%.

85. Your patient has HIV. You are accidentally stuck with a needle that has some infected blood on it. Your chance of contracting the disease is about:
- **A.** 0.5%.
- **B.** 5%.
- **C.** 10%.
- **D.** 15%.

86. If you think your patient has TB, you should wear the usual personal protective equipment plus a:
- **A.** surgeon's mask.
- **B.** gown.
- **C.** HEPA respirator.
- **D.** Tyvek suit.

87. When alone, instead of providing mouth-to-mouth ventilations on the nonbreathing patient, the EMT should use a(n):
- **A.** pocket mask with a one-way valve.
- **B.** one-way valve.
- **C.** bag-valve mask.
- **D.** endotracheal tube.

88. Which method of infection control will reduce exposure to yourself, your crew, and your next patient?
- **A.** wearing a HEPA respirator
- **B.** taking universal precautions
- **C.** hand washing after each patient contact
- **D.** none of the above

89. An act that establishes procedures through which emergency response workers can find out if they have been exposed to life-threatening infectious diseases is called:
- **A.** OSHA 1910.1030.
- **B.** Ryan White CARE Act.
- **C.** AIDS Protection Act.
- **D.** OSHA 1910.120.

90. Each emergency response employer must develop a plan that identifies and documents job classifications and tasks in which there is the possibility of exposure to potentially infectious body fluids. This is required by:
- **A.** OSHA 1910.1030.
- **B.** Ryan White CARE Act.
- **C.** AIDS Protection Act.
- **D.** OSHA 1910.120.

91. Every employer of EMTs must provide free of charge:
- **A.** a yearly physical examination.
- **B.** a life insurance policy.
- **C.** universal health insurance.
- **D.** hepatitis B vaccination.

92. Engineering controls that prevent the spread of bloodborne diseases include:
- **A.** pocket masks.
- **B.** needle containers.
- **C.** disposable airway equipment.
- **D.** all of the above.

93. Which of the following is <u>not</u> required by the OSHA bloodborne pathogen standard?
- **A.** postexposure evaluation and follow-up
- **B.** personal protective equipment
- **C.** HEPA respirator
- **D.** housekeeping controls and labeling

94. Which of the following is <u>not</u> considered a high risk area for TB?
- **A.** correctional facilities
- **B.** day care centers
- **C.** homeless shelters
- **D.** nursing homes

95. As you near an emergency scene, you should:
- **A.** sound your siren to broadcast your arrival.
- **B.** go straight to the front door.
- **C.** secure the scene as quickly as possible.
- **D.** turn off your lights and siren.

96. If anyone at the scene is in possession of a weapon, the EMT should:
- **A.** notify the police immediately.
- **B.** ask the person to give it to you.
- **C.** ignore the person with the weapon.
- **D.** advise the person to leave the scene.

97. The reduction of breathing to the point where oxygen intake is not sufficient to support life is called:
- **A.** respiratory failure.
- **B.** anoxic metabolism.
- **C.** respiratory arrest.
- **D.** respiratory support.

98. Adequate signs of breathing include all the following except:
   A. equal expansion of both sides of the chest.
   B. air moving in and out of the nose.
   C. blue or gray skin coloration.
   D. present and equal breath sounds.

99. The widening of the nostrils of the nose with respirations is called:
   A. hyperventilating.
   B. nasal flaring.
   C. nasal gurgling.
   D. wheezing.

100. The condition in which a patient's skin or lips are blue or gray is called:
   A. stridor.
   B. cyanosis.
   C. pallor.
   D. anemia.

101. If a patient is unable to speak in full sentences, this could be a sign of:
   A. complete airway blockage.
   B. snoring.
   C. shortness of breath.
   D. respiratory arrest.

102. The procedures by which life-threatening respiratory problems are initially treated by the EMT include all of the following except:
   A. opening and maintaining the airway.
   B. inserting an endotracheal tube immediately.
   C. providing supplemental oxygen to the breathing patient.
   D. assuring a clear airway with frequent suctioning.

103. Most airway problems are caused by:
   A. the tongue.
   B. asthma.
   C. shock.
   D. the epiglottis.

104. Which maneuver is most appropriate for an unconscious patient found lying at the bottom of a stairwell?
   A. head-tilt, chin-lift
   B. head-tilt, neck-lift
   C. jaw-pull lift
   D. jaw-thrust

105. When choosing a means of ventilating a patient, your last choice would be:
   A. flow-restricted, oxygen-powered ventilation device.
   B. one-rescuer bag-valve mask.
   C. two-rescuer bag-valve mask.
   D. mouth-to-mask with high-flow supplemental oxygen.

106. Artificial ventilation may be inadequate if the:
   A. chest rises with each ventilation.
   B. heart rate returns to normal.
   C. rate of ventilation is too fast or too slow.
   D. skin becomes warm and dry.

107. The standard respiratory fitting on a bag-valve mask that ensures a proper fit with other respiratory equipment is:
   A. 15/22 mm.   C. 5/20 mm.
   B. 10/14 mm.   D. 20/26 mm.

108. A bag-valve mask should have all of the following except:
   A. self-refilling shell.
   B. a clear face mask.
   C. be easily cleaned and sterilized.
   D. a pop-off valve.

109. The proper oxygen flow rate when ventilating a patient with a BVM is _____ liters per minute.
   A. 5   C. 15
   B. 10   D. 20

110. According to the American Heart Association guidelines, when ventilating a patient with a bag mask that has supplementary oxygen the volume administered should be:
   A. 400 milliliters.
   B. sufficient to achieve visible chest rise.
   C. 800 milliliters.
   D. as much as possible during the 1-second time frame.

111. The first step in providing artificial ventilation of a stoma breather is to:
   A. leave the head and neck in a neutral position.
   B. ventilate at the appropriate rate for the patient's age.
   C. clear any mucus or secretions obstructing the stoma.
   D. establish a seal using a pediatric-sized mask.

112. A flow-restricted, oxygen-powered ventilation device should have all of the following features except:
   A. an audible alarm when ventilation is activated.
   B. a trigger that enables the rescuer to use both hands.
   C. a peak flow rate of up to 40 liters per minute.
   D. a rugged design and construction.

©2009 Pearson Education, Inc.
Emergency Care, 11th Ed.

113. The two most common airway adjuncts for the EMT to use are the oropharyngeal airway and the:
   A. nasal cannula.
   B. nasopharyngeal airway.
   C. endotracheal tube.
   D. Yankauer.

114. An oropharyngeal airway should be inserted in:
   A. all patients with inadequate breathing.
   B. trauma patients with a gag reflex.
   C. medical patients with a gag reflex.
   D. all unconscious patients with no gag reflex.

115. When suctioning a patient, the EMT should:
   A. suction on the way in and way out.
   B. avoid using eyewear or a mask.
   C. never suction for longer than 15 seconds.
   D. hypoventilate prior to suctioning.

116. The emergency situation in which there is a failure of the cardiovascular system to provide sufficient blood to all the vital tissues is called:
   A. respiratory arrest.
   B. respiratory failure.
   C. shock.
   D. cardiac arrest.

117. An insufficiency in the supply of oxygen to the body's tissues is called:
   A. anoxia.
   B. no-oxia.
   C. hypoxia.
   D. cyanosis.

118. Before the oxygen cylinder's pressure gauge reads a minimum of _____ psi, you must switch to a fresh cylinder.
   A. 200   C. 800
   B. 400   D. 1,000

119. When handling oxygen cylinders, the EMT should do all of the following except:
   A. have the cylinders hydrostatically tested every 5 years.
   B. ensure that valve seat inserts and gaskets are in good condition.
   C. store reserve cylinders in a warm, humid room.
   D. use medical-grade oxygen in all cylinders.

120. The best way to deliver high-concentration oxygen to a breathing patient is to use a:
   A. nonrebreather mask.
   B. partial rebreather mask.
   C. bag-valve mask.
   D. nasal cannula.

121. A nasal cannula provides between _____ % and _____ % oxygen concentrations.
   A. 10, 21   C. 36, 58
   B. 24, 44   D. 72, 96

122. If the patient has dentures, during airway procedures the EMT should:
   A. remove them right away.
   B. leave them in unless they are loose.
   C. remove the teeth one at a time.
   D. hold them in place with a free hand.

123. When managing the airway of a child, an airway consideration you should remember is that the:
   A. mouth and nose are smaller and more easily obstructed.
   B. chest wall is firmer in a child.
   C. trachea is wider and less easily obstructed.
   D. all of the above.

124. When breathing stops completely, the patient is in:
   A. respiratory arrest.
   B. ventilatory reduction.
   C. artificial ventilation.
   D. respiratory failure.

125. Which ventilation device is contraindicated in infants and children?
   A. bag-valve mask
   B. pediatric pocket mask
   C. flow-restricted, oxygen-powered ventilation device
   D. nonrebreather mask

126. A device that allows the control of oxygen in liters per minute is called a:
   A. flowmeter.   C. humidifier.
   B. G tank.   D. reservoir.

127. A type of flowmeter that has no gauge and allows for the adjustment of flow in liters per minute in stepped increments is called a:
   A. Bourdon gauge flowmeter.
   B. constant flow selector valve.
   C. humidifier.
   D. pressure compensated flowmeter.

©2009 Pearson Education, Inc.
Emergency Care, 11th Ed.

128. Why do some systems use humidified oxygen?
  A. Lack of humidity can dry out the patient's mucous membranes.
  B. It provides a reservoir for the oxygen.
  C. It limits the risk of infection.
  D. It is helpful when transporting patients short distances.

129. A patient in the end stage of a respiratory disease may have switched over to:
  A. hyperventilation syndrome.
  B. hyperbaric therapy.
  C. hypoxic drive.
  D. carbon dioxide drive.

130. What is COPD?
  A. type of shock
  B. type of ventilation
  C. mechanism of breathing
  D. chronic pulmonary disease

131. When using an air mattress the patient is placed on the device and the air is _____ by a pump. The mattress will then form a _____ and conforming surface around the patient.
  A. inflated, rigid
  B. withdrawn, soft
  C. inflated, soft
  D. withdrawn, rigid

132. The body system that is responsible for the breakdown of food into absorbable forms is called the _____ system.
  A. urinary
  B. nervous
  C. digestive
  D. integumentary

133. A stress reaction that involves either physical or psychological behavior manifested days or weeks after an incident is called a(n):
  A. cumulative stress disorder.
  B. burnout.
  C. post-traumatic stress disorder.
  D. acute stress reaction.

134. An agency privacy officer is required by the:
  A. Ryan White Law.
  B. Health Insurance Portability and Accountability Act.
  C. National Fire Protection Association Standards.
  D. Privacy Control Act of 2002.

135. When an adult patient is breathing at a respiratory rate of 12 times a minute, you would expect that the minute volume would be approximately _____ mL per minute.
  A. 3,000   **C.** 5,000
  B. 4,500   **D.** 6,000

Interim Exam 1 Answer Sheet

Fill in the correct answer for each item. When scoring, note there are 135 questions valued at 0.747 points each.

1. [ ] A	[ ] B	[ ] C	[ ] D		36. [ ] A	[ ] B	[ ] C	[ ] D
2. [ ] A	[ ] B	[ ] C	[ ] D		37. [ ] A	[ ] B	[ ] C	[ ] D
3. [ ] A	[ ] B	[ ] C	[ ] D		38. [ ] A	[ ] B	[ ] C	[ ] D
4. [ ] A	[ ] B	[ ] C	[ ] D		39. [ ] A	[ ] B	[ ] C	[ ] D
5. [ ] A	[ ] B	[ ] C	[ ] D		40. [ ] A	[ ] B	[ ] C	[ ] D
6. [ ] A	[ ] B	[ ] C	[ ] D		41. [ ] A	[ ] B	[ ] C	[ ] D
7. [ ] A	[ ] B	[ ] C	[ ] D		42. [ ] A	[ ] B	[ ] C	[ ] D
8. [ ] A	[ ] B	[ ] C	[ ] D		43. [ ] A	[ ] B	[ ] C	[ ] D
9. [ ] A	[ ] B	[ ] C	[ ] D		44. [ ] A	[ ] B	[ ] C	[ ] D
10. [ ] A	[ ] B	[ ] C	[ ] D		45. [ ] A	[ ] B	[ ] C	[ ] D
11. [ ] A	[ ] B	[ ] C	[ ] D		46. [ ] A	[ ] B	[ ] C	[ ] D
12. [ ] A	[ ] B	[ ] C	[ ] D		47. [ ] A	[ ] B	[ ] C	[ ] D
13. [ ] A	[ ] B	[ ] C	[ ] D		48. [ ] A	[ ] B	[ ] C	[ ] D
14. [ ] A	[ ] B	[ ] C	[ ] D		49. [ ] A	[ ] B	[ ] C	[ ] D
15. [ ] A	[ ] B	[ ] C	[ ] D		50. [ ] A	[ ] B	[ ] C	[ ] D
16. [ ] A	[ ] B	[ ] C	[ ] D		51. [ ] A	[ ] B	[ ] C	[ ] D
17. [ ] A	[ ] B	[ ] C	[ ] D		52. [ ] A	[ ] B	[ ] C	[ ] D
18. [ ] A	[ ] B	[ ] C	[ ] D		53. [ ] A	[ ] B	[ ] C	[ ] D
19. [ ] A	[ ] B	[ ] C	[ ] D		54. [ ] A	[ ] B	[ ] C	[ ] D
20. [ ] A	[ ] B	[ ] C	[ ] D		55. [ ] A	[ ] B	[ ] C	[ ] D
21. [ ] A	[ ] B	[ ] C	[ ] D		56. [ ] A	[ ] B	[ ] C	[ ] D
22. [ ] A	[ ] B	[ ] C	[ ] D		57. [ ] A	[ ] B	[ ] C	[ ] D
23. [ ] A	[ ] B	[ ] C	[ ] D		58. [ ] A	[ ] B	[ ] C	[ ] D
24. [ ] A	[ ] B	[ ] C	[ ] D		59. [ ] A	[ ] B	[ ] C	[ ] D
25. [ ] A	[ ] B	[ ] C	[ ] D		60. [ ] A	[ ] B	[ ] C	[ ] D
26. [ ] A	[ ] B	[ ] C	[ ] D		61. [ ] A	[ ] B	[ ] C	[ ] D
27. [ ] A	[ ] B	[ ] C	[ ] D		62. [ ] A	[ ] B	[ ] C	[ ] D
28. [ ] A	[ ] B	[ ] C	[ ] D		63. [ ] A	[ ] B	[ ] C	[ ] D
29. [ ] A	[ ] B	[ ] C	[ ] D		64. [ ] A	[ ] B	[ ] C	[ ] D
30. [ ] A	[ ] B	[ ] C	[ ] D		65. [ ] A	[ ] B	[ ] C	[ ] D
31. [ ] A	[ ] B	[ ] C	[ ] D		66. [ ] A	[ ] B	[ ] C	[ ] D
32. [ ] A	[ ] B	[ ] C	[ ] D		67. [ ] A	[ ] B	[ ] C	[ ] D
33. [ ] A	[ ] B	[ ] C	[ ] D		68. [ ] A	[ ] B	[ ] C	[ ] D
34. [ ] A	[ ] B	[ ] C	[ ] D		69. [ ] A	[ ] B	[ ] C	[ ] D
35. [ ] A	[ ] B	[ ] C	[ ] D		70. [ ] A	[ ] B	[ ] C	[ ] D

©2009 Pearson Education, Inc.
Emergency Care, 11th Ed.

71.	[ ] A	[ ] B	[ ] C	[ ] D
72.	[ ] A	[ ] B	[ ] C	[ ] D
73.	[ ] A	[ ] B	[ ] C	[ ] D
74.	[ ] A	[ ] B	[ ] C	[ ] D
75.	[ ] A	[ ] B	[ ] C	[ ] D
76.	[ ] A	[ ] B	[ ] C	[ ] D
77.	[ ] A	[ ] B	[ ] C	[ ] D
78.	[ ] A	[ ] B	[ ] C	[ ] D
79.	[ ] A	[ ] B	[ ] C	[ ] D
80.	[ ] A	[ ] B	[ ] C	[ ] D
81.	[ ] A	[ ] B	[ ] C	[ ] D
82.	[ ] A	[ ] B	[ ] C	[ ] D
83.	[ ] A	[ ] B	[ ] C	[ ] D
84.	[ ] A	[ ] B	[ ] C	[ ] D
85.	[ ] A	[ ] B	[ ] C	[ ] D
86.	[ ] A	[ ] B	[ ] C	[ ] D
87.	[ ] A	[ ] B	[ ] C	[ ] D
88.	[ ] A	[ ] B	[ ] C	[ ] D
89.	[ ] A	[ ] B	[ ] C	[ ] D
90.	[ ] A	[ ] B	[ ] C	[ ] D
91.	[ ] A	[ ] B	[ ] C	[ ] D
92.	[ ] A	[ ] B	[ ] C	[ ] D
93.	[ ] A	[ ] B	[ ] C	[ ] D
94.	[ ] A	[ ] B	[ ] C	[ ] D
95.	[ ] A	[ ] B	[ ] C	[ ] D
96.	[ ] A	[ ] B	[ ] C	[ ] D
97.	[ ] A	[ ] B	[ ] C	[ ] D
98.	[ ] A	[ ] B	[ ] C	[ ] D
99.	[ ] A	[ ] B	[ ] C	[ ] D
100.	[ ] A	[ ] B	[ ] C	[ ] D
101.	[ ] A	[ ] B	[ ] C	[ ] D
102.	[ ] A	[ ] B	[ ] C	[ ] D
103.	[ ] A	[ ] B	[ ] C	[ ] D

104.	[ ] A	[ ] B	[ ] C	[ ] D
105.	[ ] A	[ ] B	[ ] C	[ ] D
106.	[ ] A	[ ] B	[ ] C	[ ] D
107.	[ ] A	[ ] B	[ ] C	[ ] D
108.	[ ] A	[ ] B	[ ] C	[ ] D
109.	[ ] A	[ ] B	[ ] C	[ ] D
110.	[ ] A	[ ] B	[ ] C	[ ] D
111.	[ ] A	[ ] B	[ ] C	[ ] D
112.	[ ] A	[ ] B	[ ] C	[ ] D
113.	[ ] A	[ ] B	[ ] C	[ ] D
114.	[ ] A	[ ] B	[ ] C	[ ] D
115.	[ ] A	[ ] B	[ ] C	[ ] D
116.	[ ] A	[ ] B	[ ] C	[ ] D
117.	[ ] A	[ ] B	[ ] C	[ ] D
118.	[ ] A	[ ] B	[ ] C	[ ] D
119.	[ ] A	[ ] B	[ ] C	[ ] D
120.	[ ] A	[ ] B	[ ] C	[ ] D
121.	[ ] A	[ ] B	[ ] C	[ ] D
122.	[ ] A	[ ] B	[ ] C	[ ] D
123.	[ ] A	[ ] B	[ ] C	[ ] D
124.	[ ] A	[ ] B	[ ] C	[ ] D
125.	[ ] A	[ ] B	[ ] C	[ ] D
126.	[ ] A	[ ] B	[ ] C	[ ] D
127.	[ ] A	[ ] B	[ ] C	[ ] D
128.	[ ] A	[ ] B	[ ] C	[ ] D
129.	[ ] A	[ ] B	[ ] C	[ ] D
130.	[ ] A	[ ] B	[ ] C	[ ] D
131.	[ ] A	[ ] B	[ ] C	[ ] D
132.	[ ] A	[ ] B	[ ] C	[ ] D
133.	[ ] A	[ ] B	[ ] C	[ ] D
134.	[ ] A	[ ] B	[ ] C	[ ] D
135.	[ ] A	[ ] B	[ ] C	[ ] D

7

Scene Size-up

MATCH TERMINOLOGY/ DEFINITIONS

A. Force or forces that may have caused injury

B. Injury caused by an object that passes through the skin and other body tissues

C. Steps taken by EMS providers when approaching, arriving, and attending at the scene of an emergency call to ensure the safety of the crew, the patient, and bystanders

D. Area around the wreckage of a vehicle collision or other incident within which special safety precautions should be taken

E. Principle that a body in motion will remain in motion unless acted on by an outside force

F. Keen awareness that a person may have injuries

G. Agency that provides advice on hazardous materials via a hotline

H. Injury caused by a blow that does not penetrate through the skin or other body tissues

I. Material available for rescuers to obtain quick information about hazardous materials

J. Violence in the home

_____ **1.** Blunt-force trauma

_____ **2.** CHEMTREC

_____ **3.** Danger zone

_____ **4.** Domestic violence

_____ **5.** High index of suspicion

_____ **6.** Law of inertia

_____ **7.** Mechanism of injury

_____ **8.** North American Emergency Response Guidebook

_____ **9.** Penetrating trauma

_____ **10.** Scene size-up

MULTIPLE-CHOICE REVIEW

_____ 1. Your top priority when conducting a scene size-up is determining:
  A. patient safety.   **C.** number of injured.
  B. personal safety.   **D.** mechanism of injury.

_____ 2. Which of the following is the most accurate statement about scene size-up?
  A. It takes place as you are approaching the scene.
  B. It is replaced by patient care once you arrive at the scene.
  C. It is confined to the first part of the assessment process.
  D. It is an ongoing process throughout the call.

_____ 3. If you arrive at a collision scene where there are police, fire vehicles, and other ambulances already present, you should:
  A. immediately begin patient care.
  B. conduct your own scene size-up.
  C. ensure that no bystanders are injured.
  D. all of the above.

_____ 4. Which of the following is <u>not</u> an appropriate action when you near the scene of a traffic collision?
  A. Look and listen for other EMS units as you near intersections.
  B. Look for signs of collision-related power outages.
  C. Observe traffic flow to anticipate blockage at the scene.
  D. Attempt to park your vehicle downhill from the scene.

_____ 5. When you are in sight of the collision scene, you should watch for the signals of police officers and other emergency service personnel because:
  A. they may have information about hazards or the location of injured persons.
  B. the first ones on the scene are considered to be in charge.
  C. federal law requires you to follow the command of other responders.
  D. they are considered the medical-care experts on the scene.

_____ 6. When there are no apparent hazards, consider the danger zone to extend _____ feet in all directions from the wreckage.
  A. 25   **C.** 100
  B. 50   **D.** 200

_____ 7. When a collision vehicle is on fire, consider the danger zone to extend at least _____ feet in all directions, even if the fire appears small and limited to the engine compartment.
  A. 25   **C.** 100
  B. 50   **D.** 200

_____ 8. A good scene size-up should identify:
  A. the potential for a violent situation.
  B. the name and amount of toxic substances.
  C. the number of patients and their diagnoses.
  D. all of the above.

_____ 9. The EMT's Standard Precautions equipment during the scene size-up may include all of the following <u>except</u>:
  A. eye protection.   **C.** mask.
  B. disposable gloves.   **D.** oxygen mask.

_____ 10. The key element of BSI or Standard Precautions is to:
  A. always wear all the protective clothing.
  B. always have personal protective equipment readily available.
  C. place equipment on the patient as well as the rescuer.
  D. determine which body fluids are a danger to the EMT.

_____ 11. Injuries to bones and joints are usually associated with:
  A. fights and drug usage.   C. fires and explosions.
  B. falls and vehicle collisions.   D. bullet wounds.

_____ 12. Knowing the mechanism of injury assists the EMT in:
  A. immobilizing the patient's spine.
  B. determining which Standard Precautions to use.
  C. predicting various injury patterns.
  D. all of the above.

_____ 13. The law of inertia states that:
  A. the faster you enter a turn, the more your vehicle will be pulled straight.
  B. the slower the speed, the greater is the energy loss.
  C. a body in motion will remain in motion unless acted upon by
     an outside force.
  D. the mass or weight of an object is the most important contributor
     to an injury.

_____ 14. An unrestrained driver involved in a head-on, up-and-over collision is likely
     to sustain injuries to the:
  A. skull.   C. knees.
  B. fibula.   D. femur.

_____ 15. Which of the following is least likely to be considered a mechanism of injury
     in up-and-over and down-and-under head-on collisions?
  A. steering wheel   C. brake pedal
  B. windshield   D. dashboard

_____ 16. Knee, leg, and hip injuries are common in a _____ collision.
  A. head-on, up-and-over   C. head-on, down-and-under
  B. rear-end   D. rotational impact

_____ 17. Which type of collision is most serious because it has the potential for
     multiple impacts?
  A. side impact   C. head-on, up-and-over
  B. rear-end impact   D. roll-over

_____ 18. All of the following are examples of mechanisms of injury <u>except</u> a:
  A. patient who fell three times her height.
  B. spiderweb crack in the windshield.
  C. broken steering column in a collision.
  D. flat rear tire.

_____ 19. A severe fall for an adult is:
  A. over 15 feet.
  B. often accompanied by an amputation.
  C. less than 10 feet.
  D. always fatal.

_____ 20. A penetrating injury that is usually limited to the penetrated area is called
     a _____ injury.
  A. low-velocity   C. high-velocity
  B. medium-velocity   D. super-velocity

_____ 21. The pressure wave around the bullet's tract through the body is called:
  A. exsanguination.   C. cavitation.
  B. gas penetration.   D. pressure damage.

_____ 22. An injury caused by a blow that strikes the body but does not penetrate
     the skin is called:
  A. inertia trauma.   C. blunt-force trauma.
  B. cavitation.   D. rotational impact.

©2009 Pearson Education, Inc.
Emergency Care, 11th Ed.

_____ **23.** In which of the following situations would it be necessary for you and your partner to call for additional assistance?

A. You are treating a patient who has flulike symptoms who also has a toddler with similar symptoms.

B. Your patient is a 350-pound male who fell down the stairs and has a broken leg.

C. You are treating a patient with a deep laceration in his right forearm.

D. Your patient loses consciousness while you are carrying her to the ambulance.

_____ **24.** While in the living room of a private house treating a patient for nausea, headache, and general body weakness, your eyes begin to tear. Three family members have the same symptoms. You should immediately:

A. evacuate all people from the building.

B. call for three additional ambulances.

C. notify the police department.

D. begin to flush out everyone's eyes.

_____ **25.** If the number of patients is more than the responding units can effectively handle, the EMT should:

A. involve bystanders in care of the injured.

B. call for additional EMS resources immediately.

C. advise medical direction that assistance is needed.

D. do all of the above.

COMPLETE THE FOLLOWING

1. List the four parts of the scene size-up.

A. _____

B. _____

C. _____

D. _____

2. List five signs of danger from violence that you may observe as you approach the scene.

A. _____

B. _____

C. _____

D. _____

E. _____

3. List five types of motor vehicle collisions.

A. _____

B. _____

C. _____

D. _____

E. _____

4. List three sources of information about the nature of illness.

A. _____

B. _____

C. _____

STREET SCENES DISCUSSION

Review the Street Scene on p. 207 of the textbook. Then answer the questions below.

1. Suppose the situation played out in a different way. On arrival at the scene, the driver of the truck comes running up to your ambulance and says, "My truck is overturned and leaking toxic chemicals all over the place." What should you do next?

2. Instead of a hazardous-materials incident, suppose upon arrival you find the driver of the truck is acting as if he is intoxicated. He also is holding a rifle in his lap with his right hand in position for firing. What should you do?

ON THE WEB

To help you review and practice basic skills, visit the *Emergency Care 11th Ed. Companion Website* at www.prenhall.com/limmer. For Online Test Preparation, visit www.prenhall.com/emtachieve.

CHAPTER

The Initial Assessment

MATCH TERMINOLOGY/ DEFINITIONS

A. Steps taken by the EMT for the purpose of discovering and dealing with a patient's life-threatening problems

B. Level of a patient's responsiveness

C. Method of assessing circulation in a pediatric patient

D. Reason EMS was called

E. Part of the EMT's evaluation that includes assessment of the environment and the patient's chief complaint and appearance

F. Memory aid for classifying the levels of responsiveness or mental status

G. Actions taken to correct a patient's problems

H. Awake and oriented

I. Lack of response to any stimuli

J. Ability to respond to stimuli

_____ **1.** Alert

_____ **2.** AVPU

_____ **3.** Capillary refill

_____ **4.** Chief complaint

_____ **5.** General impression

_____ **6.** Initial assessment

_____ **7.** Interventions

_____ **8.** Mental status

_____ **9.** Responsive

_____ **10.** Unresponsive

MULTIPLE-CHOICE REVIEW

_____ **1.** Which of the following steps is <u>not</u> a part of the initial assessment or primary survey of a responsive patient with a medical problem?
 A. Assess the patient's mental status.
 B. Assess the adequacy of breathing.
 C. Determine the patient's priority.
 D. Obtain the blood pressure.

_____ **2.** The general impression is an evaluation of all of the following <u>except</u>:
 A. chief complaint.   **C.** environment.
 B. appearance.   **D.** past medical history.

_____ 3. An example of a patient's environment providing information about the patient's condition is:
  A. a bruise on the patient's chest.
  B. an alleyway that is not well lit.
  C. drug-use paraphernalia.
  D. a medical history of asthma.

_____ 4. Clinical judgment is also referred to as a(n):
  A. license to diagnose what is wrong with the patient.
  B. sixth sense that provides clues to the severity of a patient's condition.
  C. reliance on medical direction to recommend treatment.
  D. ability to judge the patient's mental status without using AVPU.

_____ 5. During the general impression, the EMT should:
  A. look.
  B. listen.
  C. smell.
  D. do all of the above.

_____ 6. One way to determine the patient's level of responsiveness is to:
  A. put ammonia inhalants into each nostril.
  B. rub the patient's sternum briskly.
  C. place the patient's hands in water.
  D. press on the patient's nail beds.

_____ 7. The "A" in AVPU stands for:
  A. action.
  B. airway.
  C. assess.
  D. alert.

_____ 8. The "V" in AVPU stands for:
  A. violent.
  B. very painful.
  C. verbal.
  D. venous.

_____ 9. The "P" in AVPU stands for:
  A. priority.
  B. painful.
  C. position.
  D. patient.

_____ 10. One major difference between the initial assessment of a responsive trauma patient and the initial assessment of an unresponsive trauma patient is:
  A. the initial assessment is done more quickly on the responsive patient.
  B. the unresponsive patient is a higher priority for immediate transport.
  C. there is no difference between the two assessments.
  D. a jaw-thrust maneuver should always be used on the responsive patient.

_____ 11. If a patient is not alert and his breathing rate is slower than 8, the EMT should:
  A. give high-concentration oxygen via nonrebreather mask.
  B. quickly evaluate the circulation and treat for shock.
  C. suction the patient and perform rescue breathing.
  D. provide positive pressure ventilations with 100% oxygen.

_____ 12. During the initial assessment, if the patient is alert and the breathing rate is faster than 24, provide the patient with:
  A. positive pressure ventilations with 100% oxygen.
  B. high-concentration oxygen via nonrebreather mask.
  C. low-concentration oxygen via bag-valve mask.
  D. medium-concentration oxygen via nasal cannula.

_____ 13. In the initial assessment or primary survey, the circulation assessment includes evaluating all of the following except:
  A. pulse.
  B. skin.
  C. severity of bleeding.
  D. blood pressure.

_____ 14. If a patient's skin is warm, dry, and a normal color, it indicates:
  A. a serious sunburn.
  B. heat exposure.
  C. alcohol abuse.
  D. good circulation.

©2009 Pearson Education, Inc.
Emergency Care, 11th Ed.

_____ **15.** If a patient's skin is cool, pale, and moist, it indicates:
   A. increased perfusion. **C.** poor circulation.
   B. high blood pressure. **D.** cold exposure.

_____ **16.** In order to evaluate skin color in a dark-skinned patient, the EMT should also:
   A. evaluate the tissues of the lips or nail beds.
   B. evaluate the tissues of the heels of the feet.
   C. check the pupils of the eyes.
   D. do all of the above.

_____ **17.** When assessing the circulation, you should check for and control severe bleeding because:
   A. open wounds can become infected.
   B. it may lead to long-term complications.
   C. a patient can bleed to death in minutes.
   D. the blood pressure may drop over time.

_____ **18.** When a life threat is observed in the initial assessment, the EMT should:
   A. complete the assessment, then treat.
   B. treat it immediately.
   C. determine the patient's priority, then treat.
   D. package the patient for transport.

_____ **19.** High-priority conditions include:
   A. poor general impression. **C.** shock (hypoperfusion).
   B. unresponsiveness. **D.** all of the above.

_____ **20.** All of the following would be considered high-priority conditions <u>except</u>:
   A. difficulty breathing.
   B. responsive but not following commands.
   C. an uncomplicated childbirth.
   D. chest pain with systolic pressure less than 100.

_____ **21.** During the initial assessment of an adult medical patient you note the breathing rate is 28. You should consider:
   A. oxygen by a nasal cannula.
   B. providing bag-valve mask ventilations.
   C. administering oxygen by nonrebreather mask.
   D. using a paper bag to slow down the rate.

_____ **22.** If the adult trauma patient you are assessing has inadequate breathing with a rate greater than _____, you should provide pressure ventilations and high-concentration oxygen.
   A. 20 **C.** 28
   B. 24 **D.** 32

_____ **23.** Another phrase used to describe the initial assessment of the patient is the:
   A. ongoing assessment. **C.** vital signs check.
   B. primary survey. **D.** expanded assessment.

COMPLETE THE FOLLOWING

1. List the six steps of the initial assessment.

A. _____   D. _____

B. _____   E. _____

C. _____   F. _____

2. State what the letters in AVPU stand for.

A _____

V _____

P _____

U _____

3. List five high-priority conditions.

A. _____

B. _____

C. _____

D. _____

E. _____

EMT SKILL PERFORMANCE CHECKLIST

Brady's *Pocket Reference for BLS Providers, 3rd Ed.*

▶ INITIAL ASSESSMENT (PP. 210–213)

❑ Take Standard Precautions.

❑ Form a general impression based on assessment of the environment and the patient's chief complaint and appearance.

❑ Assess mental status. Determine level of responsiveness using AVPU (alert, verbal, painful, unresponsive).

❑ Assess the airway. If it is not open or if it is endangered, take measures to open it.

❑ Assess breathing. If needed, initiate any appropriate oxygen therapy and assure adequate ventilation.

❑ Assess circulation (assess for and control major bleeding; assess pulse; assess skin color, temperature, and condition).

❑ Determine patient's treatment priority (high/low, stable/unstable) and make a transport decision.

NOTE: Apply manual stabilization upon first contact with any patient who you suspect may have an injury to the spine.

STREET SCENES DISCUSSION

Review the Street Scene on p. 223 of the textbook. Then answer the questions below.

1. Imagine that your 78-year-old patient, who fell to the floor, does not wake up and his respirations continue with gurgling sounds due to blood in the back of his throat. What should you do?

2. What priority would this patient be? Would ALS be appropriate to call for?

3. Look again at the third patient encounter. Is it necessary to take this patient to the hospital? Explain.

ON THE WEB

To help you review and practice basic skills, visit the *Emergency Care 11th Ed. Companion Website* at www.prenhall.com/limmer. For Online Test Preparation, visit www.prenhall.com/emtachieve.

CHAPTER

Vital Signs and SAMPLE History

MATCH TERMINOLOGY/ DEFINITIONS

▶ **PART A**

A. Pressure remaining in the arteries when the left ventricle of the heart is relaxed and refilling

B. Slow pulse; any pulse rate below 60 beats per minute in an adult

C. Force of blood against the walls of the blood vessels

D. Pulse felt along the large artery on either side of the neck

E. Feeling with the fingertips

F. Number of pulse beats per minute

G. Reacting to light by changing size such as occurs in the pupils of the eyes

H. Rhythmic beats felt as the heart pumps blood through the arteries

I. Rhythm (regular or irregular) and force (strong or weak) of the pulse

J. Major artery of the arm

K. Black center of the eye

L. When a stethoscope is used to listen for characteristic sounds

M. To get larger

N. To get smaller

O. Pulse felt at the wrist on the lateral (thumb) side

_____ **1.** Auscultation

_____ **2.** Blood pressure

_____ **3.** Brachial artery

_____ **4.** Bradycardia

_____ **5.** Carotid pulse

_____ **6.** Constrict

_____ **7.** Dilate

_____ **8.** Diastolic blood pressure

_____ **9.** Palpation

_____ **10.** Pulse

_____ **11.** Pulse quality

_____ **12.** Pulse rate

_____ **13.** Pupil

_____ **14.** Radial pulse

_____ **15.** Reactivity

A. Normal or abnormal (shallow, labored, noisy) character of breathing

B. Number of breaths taken in 1 minute

C. Rapid pulse; any pulse rate above 100 beats per minute in an adult

D. Pressure created when the heart contracts and forces blood into the arteries

E. Regular or irregular spacing of breaths

F. Information about the present problem (signs and symptoms) and past medical history of the patient

G. An indication of a patient's condition that is objective or that you see, hear, feel, or smell

H. An indication of a patient's condition that cannot be observed by another person but rather is subjective or something felt and reported by the patient

I. Cuff and gauge used to measure blood pressure

J. Outward signs of what is going on inside the body, including respiration; pulse; skin color, temperature, and condition; pupils; and blood pressure

_____ 1. Respiratory quality

_____ 2. Respiratory rate

_____ 3. Respiratory rhythm

_____ 4. SAMPLE history

_____ 5. Sign

_____ 6. Sphygmomanometer

_____ 7. Symptom

_____ 8. Systolic pressure

_____ 9. Tachycardia

_____ 10. Vital signs

MULTIPLE-CHOICE REVIEW

_____ 1. The assessed components of the vital signs include all of the following except:
   A. respiratory rate and quality.
   B. skin color and condition.
   C. pulse rate and quality.
   D. pulse oximetry.

_____ 2. A sign that gives important information about the patient's condition but is not considered a vital sign is:
   A. blood pressure.
   B. mental status.
   C. pulse rate.
   D. respiratory rhythm.

_____ 3. Why is it essential that vital signs be recorded as they are obtained?
   A. To avoid having to take them more than once
   B. To prevent forgetting them and to note the time they were taken
   C. To give the patient a chance to calm down
   D. Because they will always change quickly

_____ 4. When an adult patient's pulse rate exceeds 100 beats per minute, this is called:
   A. normal.
   B. regular.
   C. bradycardia.
   D. tachycardia.

_____ 5. Based upon the pulse alone, a sign that something may be seriously wrong with a patient could be:
   A. a sustained rate below 50 beats per minute.
   B. a sustained rate above 120 beats per minute.
   C. a rate above 150 beats per minute.
   D. all of the above.

_____ 6. In addition to the answer to question 5, another serious indicator found in the pulse may be a(n):
   A. regular strong rhythm.
   B. irregular rhythm.
   C. athlete with a pulse of 50.
   D. increase in rate after exercise.

_____ 7. The quality of the pulse includes determining the:
A. rhythm and rate.
B. rate and force.
C. rhythm and force.
D. presence and balance.

_____ 8. A patient described as having a "thready" pulse has a(n) _____ pulse.
A. strong
B. irregular
C. weak
D. infrequent

_____ 9. The normal pulse rate for a school-age child (6–10 years) is:
A. 120 to 160.
B. 60 to 100.
C. 70 to 110.
D. 80 to 120.

_____ 10. The normal pulse rate for an adult is:
A. 60 to 100.
B. 70 to 110.
C. 80 to 120.
D. 90 to 140.

_____ 11. The pulse at the thumb side of the wrist is referred to as the _____ pulse.
A. femoral
B. radial
C. carotid
D. brachial

_____ 12. When assessing the carotid pulse, the EMT should:
A. palpate the artery as hard as he can.
B. assess both sides at exactly the same time.
C. be aware that excessive pressure can slow the heart.
D. apply pressure until he feels the pulse rate rise.

_____ 13. The number of breaths a patient takes in 1 minute is called the:
A. minute volume.
B. minute pressure.
C. respiratory rate.
D. quality of breathing.

_____ 14. The respiratory rate is classified as:
A. normal, slow, or rapid.
B. noisy, shallow, or normal.
C. labored, quick, or noisy.
D. weak, thready, or full.

_____ 15. If the EMT is treating a patient with a sustained respiratory rate above _____ or below _____ breaths per minute, high-concentration oxygen must be administered.
A. 20, 10
B. 20, 12
C. 24, 8
D. 24, 10

_____ 16. The normal respiration rate for an adult at rest is:
A. 12 to 24.
B. 12 to 20.
C. 20 to 30.
D. 20 to 40.

_____ 17. The normal respiration rate for a toddler (1–3 years) is:
A. 12 to 24.
B. 12 to 20.
C. 20 to 30.
D. 20 to 40.

_____ 18. Shallow breathing occurs when:
A. there is only slight movement of the chest or abdomen.
B. there is stridor or grunting on expiration.
C. there is a complete obstruction.
D. the chest muscles fully expand with each breath.

_____ 19. Many resting people breathe more with their _____ than with their _____ muscles.
A. diaphragm, pelvic
B. diaphragm, chest
C. chest, abdominal
D. chest, pelvic

_____ 20. Signs of labored breathing include all of the following except:
A. increase in the work of breathing.
B. use of accessory muscles.
C. retractions above the collarbones.
D. delayed capillary refill.

©2009 Pearson Education, Inc.
Emergency Care, 11th Ed.

21. A harsh, high-pitched sound heard on inspiration when a patient has labored breathing is called:
  A. nasal flaring.   **C.** stridor.
  B. grunting.   **D.** gurgling.

22. When the quality of a patient's respirations is abnormal due to something blocking the flow of air, this is referred to as _____ breathing.
  A. normal   **C.** noisy
  B. shallow   **D.** labored

23. A sound made by the patient that usually indicates the need to suction the airway is called:
  A. gurgling.   **C.** stridor.
  B. crowing.   **D.** wheezing.

24. The best places to assess skin color in adults are:
  A. under the chin and the nostrils.
  B. the inside of the cheek and the nail beds.
  C. the nail beds and the upper chest.
  D. the toes and the earlobes.

25. Blood loss, shock, hypotension, or emotional distress may result in skin that is:
  A. flushed.   **C.** pale.
  B. gray.   **D.** jaundiced.

26. A patient with a lack of oxygen in the red blood cells resulting from inadequate breathing or inadequate heart function will exhibit _____ skin.
  A. pink   **C.** flushed
  B. pale   **D.** cyanotic

27. The skin of a patient who has liver abnormalities will appear:
  A. flushed.   **C.** pale.
  B. mottled.   **D.** jaundiced.

28. Cold, dry skin is frequently associated with:
  A. high fever and/or heat exposure.
  B. exposure to cold.
  C. shock and anxiety.
  D. a body that is losing heat.

29. Hot, dry skin is frequently associated with:
  A. high fever, heat exposure.   **C.** shock and anxiety.
  B. exposure to cold.   **D.** heat loss.

30. You notice that the patient's right arm is much cooler than the rest of the patient's body. This should lead you to consider a _____ system problem.
  A. nervous   **C.** circulatory
  B. respiratory   **D.** endocrine

31. If you press on a child's nail bed and watch how long it takes for the normal pink color to return, you are testing for:
  A. reflexes.   **C.** pain response.
  B. capillary refill. **D.** nail bed temperature.

32. If a patient is in direct sunlight or very bright conditions, the EMT should test the pupils by:
  A. using a very bright light that is similar to the environmental light.
  B. covering the patient's eyes for a few moments, then uncovering one eye at a time.
  C. applying a cold towel to the patient's eyelids for 10 seconds.
  D. moving the patient indoors to an area that has dimmer light.

_____ 33. The pupils may be unequal due to any of the following conditions except:
   A. stroke.   C. eye injury.
   B. head injury.   D. shock.

_____ 34. Fright, blood loss, drugs, and treatment with eyedrops may cause the patient's pupils to become:
   A. constricted.   C. unequal.
   B. dilated.   D. unreactive.

_____ 35. When the left ventricle of the heart relaxes and refills, the pressure in the arteries is called the _____ pressure.
   A. diastolic   C. ventricular
   B. carotid   D. systolic

_____ 36. The pulse oximeter should be used with:
   A. patients who have carbon monoxide poisoning.
   B. patients complaining of respiratory problems.
   C. any patient who is hypothermic.
   D. any patient suffering from severe shock.

_____ 37. The pulse oximeter is helpful because it:
   A. encourages you to be more aggressive with oxygen therapy.
   B. helps you decide when you should withhold oxygen.
   C. indicates when a patient is about to become hypothermic.
   D. gives an indication that the patient is a heavy smoker.

_____ 38. The oximeter will produce falsely high readings in patients with:
   A. hypoxia.
   B. barbiturate poisoning.
   C. carbon monoxide poisoning.
   D. croup.

_____ 39. Chronic smokers may have a pulse oximeter reading that is:
   A. lower than normal.   C. 20% to 25% off.
   B. higher than normal.   D. difficult to read.

_____ 40. In a normal healthy person, one would expect the oximeter reading to be:
   A. 86% to 90%.   C. 95% to 99%.
   B. 91% to 94%.   D. none of the above.

_____ 41. To determine a patient's skin temperature, the EMT should:
   A. hold a thermometer in the axilla for 30 seconds.
   B. have the patient exhale onto a warming device.
   C. feel the patient's skin with the back of the hand.
   D. listen carefully with a stethoscope.

_____ 42. The presence of "goose pimples" is associated with:
   A. head injury.   C. shock.
   B. the chills.   D. heat stress.

_____ 43. The systolic blood pressure is:
   A. created when the heart contracts.
   B. listed as the lower number in the BP fraction.
   C. created when the heart relaxes.
   D. seldom used in prehospital care.

_____ 44. An EMT was in a noisy environment so he chose to take the patient's BP by _____, revealing only the _____ pressure.
   A. auscultation, systolic
   B. auscultation, diastolic
   C. palpation, systolic
   D. palpation, diastolic

©2009 Pearson Education, Inc.
Emergency Care, 11th Ed.

_____ **45.** Serious hypotension in an adult patient is normally defined as a systolic
below _____ mmHg.
  A. 200
  B. 140
  C. 90
  D. 60

_____ **46.** When obtaining the SAMPLE history, the "M" can include questioning the
patient about:
  A. prescribed medications.
  B. recreational drugs.
  C. herbal supplements.
  D. all of the above.

COMPLETE THE FOLLOWING

1. List five vital signs.

  A. _____

  B. _____

  C. _____

  D. _____

  E. _____

2. List the components of the SAMPLE history.

  S _____

  A _____

  M _____

  P _____

  L _____

  E _____

LABEL THE DIAGRAM

Fill in the name of the pulse that can be found at each numbered location on the line provided.

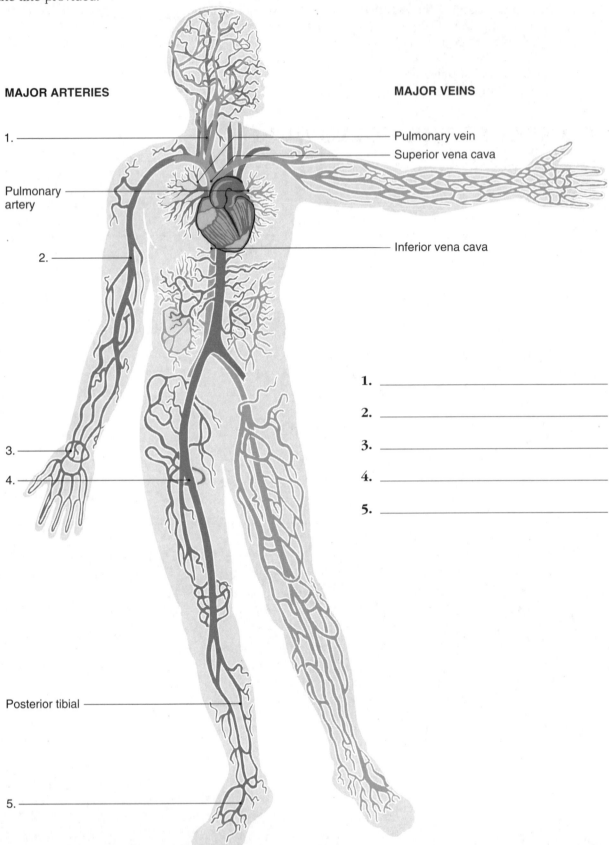

MAJOR ARTERIES

1. —————

Pulmonary artery

2. —————

3. —————

4. —————

Posterior tibial —————

5. —————

MAJOR VEINS

————— Pulmonary vein
————— Superior vena cava

————— Inferior vena cava

1. _____

2. _____

3. _____

4. _____

5. _____

STREET SCENES DISCUSSION

Review the Street Scene on pp. 246–247 of the textbook. Then answer the questions below.

1. This patient's vital signs were not normal, which helped make it clear that she should go to the hospital. If her vital signs had been normal, would a refusal of transport have been acceptable? (HINT: Review Table 8–1.)

2. What would be considered the "normal" range of vital signs for this patient? Would an SpO_2 of 97% be acceptable?

3. Would you include in your prehospital care report the fact that the patient was having "black, tarry stools." Why or why not?

ON THE WEB

To help you review and practice basic skills, visit the *Emergency Care 11th Ed. Companion Website* at www.prenhall.com/limmer. For Online Test Preparation, visit www.prenhall.com/emtachieve.

EMT SKILLS PERFORMANCE CHECKLISTS

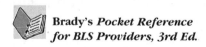 **Brady's** *Pocket Reference for BLS Providers, 3rd Ed.*

▶ **BLOOD PRESSURE BY AUSCULTATION (PP. 237–238)**

❑ Place the stethoscope around your neck.

❑ The patient should be seated or lying down.

❑ If the patient has not been injured, support his arm at the level of his heart.

❑ Place the cuff snugly around the upper arm so that the bottom of the cuff is about 1 inch above the crease of the elbow.

❑ With your fingertips, palpate the brachial artery at the crease of the elbow.

(continued on next page)

- ❑ Place the tips of the stethoscope arms in your ears.
- ❑ Position the diaphragm of the stethoscope directly over the brachial pulse or over the medial anterior elbow (front of the elbow) if no brachial pulse can be felt. Listen for the brachial pulse.
- ❑ Inflate the cuff with the bulb valve closed.
- ❑ Once you no longer hear the brachial pulse, continue to inflate the cuff until the gauge reads 30 mmHg higher than the point where the sound of the pulse disappeared.
- ❑ Slowly release air from the cuff by opening the bulb valve, allowing the pressure to fall smoothly at the rate of approximately 10 mm per second.
- ❑ When you hear the first clicking or tapping sounds, note the reading on the gauge. This is the systolic pressure.
- ❑ Continue to deflate the cuff and listen for the point at which these distinctive sounds fade. When the sounds turn to dull, muffled thuds, the reading on the gauge is the diastolic pressure.
- ❑ After obtaining the diastolic pressure, let the cuff deflate rapidly.

▶ BLOOD PRESSURE BY PALPATION (P. 238)

- ❑ Find the radial pulse on the arm to which the blood pressure cuff is applied.
- ❑ With the bulb valve closed, inflate the cuff to a point where you can no longer feel the radial pulse.
- ❑ Note this point on the gauge and continue to inflate the cuff until the gauge reads 30 mmHg higher than the point where the pulse disappeared.
- ❑ Slowly deflate the cuff, noting the reading at which the radial pulse returns. This reading is the systolic pressure.
- ❑ After obtaining the systolic reading, let the cuff deflate.

NOTE: You cannot determine a diastolic reading by palpation.

▶ USING THE PULSE OXIMETER (PP. 239–242)

- ❑ Review the manufacturer's instruction manual for the specific unit you are using.
- ❑ Properly assemble finger-clip sensor and extension to pulse oximeter.
- ❑ Properly affix finger-clip sensor to finger. (It may be necessary to quickly remove patient's fingernail polish.)
- ❑ Turn on pulse oximeter, and record heart and oxygen readings.
- ❑ When done using oximeter, shut off the unit. After each use, disassemble and store wiring and accessories in pouch provided.
- ❑ Review operation of all display indicators, pulse amplitude, low battery, pulse search, oxygen saturation, and pulse rate.
- ❑ Review all controls (i.e., measure button, battery check button, printer on/off, printer paper advance).
- ❑ Change battery and paper printout as needed.

CHAPTER 10

Assessment of the Trauma Patient

MATCH TERMINOLOGY/ DEFINITIONS

A. Found upon palpation of a body part

B. Movement of part of the chest in the opposite direction from the rest of the chest during respiration

C. Persistent erection of the penis that can result from spinal cord injury or certain medical problems

D. Quick assessment of the head, neck, chest, abdomen, pelvis, extremities, and posterior body to detect signs of injury

E. Surgical opening in the wall of the abdomen with a bag in place to collect excretions from the digestive system

F. Memory aid, the initials of which stand for deformities, contusions, abrasions, punctures/penetrations, burns, tenderness, lacerations, and swelling

G. Surgical incision in the neck held open by a metal or plastic tube

H. Bulging of the neck veins

I. Step of patient assessment that follows the initial assessment

J. A cut

K. Condition of being stretched, inflated, or larger than normal

L. An assessment of the head (including face, ears, eyes, nose, and mouth), neck, chest, abdomen, pelvis, extremities, and posterior of the body to detect signs and symptoms of injury

M. Permanent surgical opening in the neck through which the patient breathes

N. A bruise

O. Grating sensation or sound made when fractured bones rub against each other

_____ **1.** Colostomy

_____ **2.** Contusion

_____ **3.** Crepitation

_____ **4.** DCAP-BTLS

_____ **5.** Detailed physical exam

_____ **6.** Distention

_____ **7.** Focused history and physical exam

_____ **8.** Jugular vein distention

_____ **9.** Laceration

_____ **10.** Paradoxical motion

_____ **11.** Priapism

_____ **12.** Rapid trauma assessment/exam

_____ **13.** Stoma

_____ **14.** Tenderness

_____ **15.** Tracheostomy

MULTIPLE-CHOICE REVIEW

_____ 1. When evaluating a patient during the focused physical exam, the EMT needs to _____ each body part.
   A. auscultate and visualize
   B. percuss and palpate
   C. inspect and palpate
   D. visualize and percuss

_____ 2. The memory aid for remembering what to look for when conducting a physical exam is:
   A. AVPU.
   B. PULSE.
   C. SAMPLE.
   D. DCAP-BTLS.

_____ 3. The "C" in DCAP-BTLS refers to:
   A. compound.
   B. contusions.
   C. cardiac.
   D. circulation.

_____ 4. The "A" in DCAP-BTLS refers to:
   A. alert.
   B. appearance.
   C. asthma.
   D. abrasions.

_____ 5. The "P" in DCAP-BTLS refers to:
   A. punctures/penetrations.
   B. palpation/pulse.
   C. priapism/penetrations.
   D. paradoxical motion/punctures.

_____ 6. The "S" in DCAP-BTLS refers to:
   A. soft tissue.
   B. stable.
   C. swelling.
   D. stomach.

_____ 7. When a body part no longer has its normal shape, this is referred to as a:
   A. hematoma.
   B. deformity.
   C. fracture.
   D. crepitation.

_____ 8. Reddened, blistered, or charred-looking areas are called:
   A. abrasions.
   B. burns.
   C. lacerations.
   D. contusions.

_____ 9. The difference between pain and tenderness is:
   A. pain only occurs when you squeeze an injury site, whereas tender areas hurt all the time.
   B. pain is considered unbearable, whereas tenderness is usually bearable.
   C. tenderness may not hurt unless the area is palpated, whereas pain is evident without palpation.
   D. pain only hurts for the first 10 minutes, whereas tenderness doesn't go away.

_____ 10. A common result of injured capillaries bleeding under the skin is called:
   A. swelling.
   B. puncture.
   C. laceration.
   D. abrasion.

_____ 11. When is it appropriate to apply a cervical collar?
   A. If the mechanism of injury exerts great force on the upper body
   B. If there is any pain in the abdomen
   C. If there is any burn injury to the neck
   D. If the patient has experienced any trauma

_____ 12. Any blow above the _____ may damage the cervical spine.
   A. clavicles
   B. diaphragm
   C. femur
   D. pelvis

_____ 13. The experienced EMT may refer to a soft cervical collar as a:
   A. device of choice for a neck injury.
   B. "neck warmer."
   C. requirement for all auto collision patients.
   D. preferred extrication collar.

©2009 Pearson Education, Inc.
Emergency Care, 11th Ed.

14. If a cervical collar is the wrong size, it may:
   A. cause additional injury to the spine.
   B. make breathing more difficult or obstruct the airway.
   C. prevent the patient from moving her neck.
   D. take too much time to adjust and apply correctly.

15. The need for cervical immobilization should be based upon:
   A. the trauma patient's level of responsiveness.
   B. the location of injuries to the patient.
   C. the mechanism of injury.
   D. all of the above.

16. Prior to applying the cervical collar, the EMT should:
   A. complete the rapid trauma assessment.
   B. complete the detailed physical exam.
   C. assess the patient's neck.
   D. obtain the baseline vital signs.

17. When reconsidering the mechanism of injury (MOI), which of the following would not be considered a significant mechanism of injury in an adult?
   A. High-speed motorcycle crash
   B. Vehicle-pedestrian collision
   C. A 10-foot fall
   D. Rollover vehicle collision

18. You are treating a patient who was in the front seat of an automobile involved in a collision. You observe that there is a spider-web crack in the windshield and the patient has facial lacerations. Most likely the patient:
   A. will have a life-threatening head injury.
   B. did not wear a seat belt or three-point harness.
   C. will also complain of leg injuries.
   D. was involved in a rollover collision.

19. The EMT should lift and look under the airbag after the patient has been removed from the vehicle in order to:
   A. obtain the serial number of the airbag.
   B. see if a hazardous chemical has been released.
   C. note any visible damage to the steering wheel.
   D. determine if it deployed properly.

20. When assessing the head of a critical trauma patient, in addition to DCAP-BTLS, the EMT should inspect/palpate for:
   A. hematoma.   **C.** crepitation.
   B. scalp lacerations.   **D.** abrasions.

21. When assessing the neck of a critical trauma patient, in addition to DCAP-BTLS, the EMT should inspect/palpate for:
   A. jugular vein distention.   **C.** lacerations.
   B. swelling.   **D.** burns.

22. The neck veins are usually not visible when the patient is:
   A. lying flat.   **C.** supine.
   B. sitting up.   **D.** prone.

23. When assessing the chest of a critical trauma patient, in addition to DCAP-BTLS, the EMT should inspect/palpate for:
   A. hematoma.   **C.** hemothorax.
   B. paradoxical motion.   **D.** jugular vein distention.

24. When assessing the abdomen of a critical trauma patient, in addition to DCAP-BTLS, the EMT should inspect/palpate for:
   A. distention of the kidneys.   **C.** crepitation.
   B. colostomy and/or ileostomy.   **D.** paradoxical motion.

_____ 25. When assessing the pelvis of a critical trauma patient, in addition to DCAP-BTLS, the EMT should inspect/palpate for:
A. paradoxical motion.
B. burns.
C. priapism.
D. bleeding.

_____ 26. The main difference between the rapid trauma assessment/exam and the detailed physical exam is that the:
A. rapid trauma assessment is less detailed.
B. detailed physical exam is only done on medical patients.
C. rapid trauma exam is done in the ambulance.
D. detailed physical exam is done more quickly.

_____ 27. If you are treating a severely injured patient, it may be appropriate to skip the:
A. initial physical exam.
B. detailed physical exam.
C. vital signs.
D. initial assessment.

_____ 28. Areas you will assess in the detailed physical exam that were not assessed in the rapid trauma assessment/exam are:
A. face, ears, eyes, nose, and mouth.
B. head, neck, chest, and abdomen.
C. chest, abdomen, pelvis, and extremities.
D. extremities and posterior of the body.

_____ 29. The final step of the detailed physical exam is to:
A. complete the head-to-toe exam.
B. reassess the vital signs.
C. conduct a rapid trauma assessment.
D. examine the posterior of the body.

_____ 30. A bruise behind the ear is called:
A. raccoon's eyes.
B. orbital hematoma.
C. Battle's sign.
D. Cushing reflex.

_____ 31. When performing the detailed physical exam, you note blood in the anterior chamber of the eye. This tells you that the:
A. patient was wearing contact lenses.
B. patient has a serious brain injury.
C. patient's eye is bleeding inside.
D. all of the above.

_____ 32. Clear fluid that may be draining from the ears and nose is called _____ fluid.
A. lymphatic
B. cerebrospinal
C. mucous
D. synovial

_____ 33. In addition to looking for DCAP-BTLS when examining the mouth, you should look for all of the following except:
A. possible airway obstructions.
B. loose or broken teeth.
C. tongue lacerations or swelling.
D. crepitation.

_____ 34. The detailed physical exam is not designed for the:
A. trauma patient with a significant mechanism of injury (MOI).
B. patient with an unclear mechanism of injury (MOI).
C. medical patient with few signs and symptoms.
D. patient who could be either medical or trauma.

_____ 35. If you are treating a patient who could be either medical or trauma, it is always best to assess for:
A. the medical problem first.
B. both problems at once.
C. the trauma problem first.
D. loss of consciousness.

©2009 Pearson Education, Inc.
Emergency Care, 11th Ed.

COMPLETE THE FOLLOWING

1. List the components of the focused history and physical exam for a trauma patient who is found with significant mechanism of injury.

A. _____

B. _____

C. _____

D. _____

E. _____

F. _____

G. _____

H. _____

2. List the components of the rapid trauma assessment/exam.

A. _____

B. _____

C. _____

D. _____

E. _____

F. _____

G. _____

3. List six examples of significant MOI.

A. _____

B. _____

C. _____

D. _____

E. _____

F. _____

LABEL THE PHOTOGRAPHS

Fill in the name of each injury assessed for in the focused physical exam of the trauma patient.

1. _____

5. _____

2. _____

6. _____

3. _____

7. _____

4. _____

8. _____

COMPLETE THE CHART

Fill in the additional things to assess in each area of the body during the rapid trauma assessment/exam.

Body Part	DCAP-BTLS	Plus
Head	Yes	1.
Neck	Yes	2. 3.
Chest	Yes	4. 5. 6.
Abdomen	Yes	7. 8. 9.
Pelvis	Yes	10. 11. 12.
Extremities	Yes	13. 14. 15.
Posterior	Yes	—

STREET SCENES DISCUSSION

Review the Street Scene on p. 288 of the textbook. Then answer the questions below.

1. This patient has a wound to the chest. At what point should you consider ventilating him?

2. Should ALS be called?

3. If the patient had lost consciousness, what would have been your priorities for emergency care?

4. If the patient is injured on the left side of the chest at the mid-clavicular line at nipple level, what organs may be injured?

ON THE WEB

To help you review and practice basic skills, visit the *Emergency Care 11th Ed. Companion Website* at www.prenhall.com/limmer. For Online Test Preparation, visit www.prenhall.com/emtachieve.

EMT SKILL PERFORMANCE CHECKLISTS

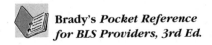 Brady's *Pocket Reference for BLS Providers, 3rd Ed.*

▶ **FOCUSED HISTORY AND PHYSICAL EXAM—TRAUMA PATIENT WITH NO SIGNIFICANT MOI (PP. 249–252)**

❑ Take Standard Precautions.

❑ Reconsider the MOI.

❑ Determine the patient's chief complaint.

❑ Conduct a focused physical exam focusing on the area the patient complains of plus areas of potential injury suggested by the MOI.

❑ Obtain baseline vital signs.

❑ Take a SAMPLE history.

❑ Perform interventions as needed.

❑ Transport.

▶ **FOCUSED HISTORY AND PHYSICAL EXAM—TRAUMA PATIENT WITH SIGNIFICANT MOI (PP. 249–255)**

❑ Take Standard Precautions.

❑ Reconsider the MOI.

❑ Continue manual stabilization of the head and neck.

❑ Consider requesting advanced life support.

(continued on next page)

- ❑ Reconsider your transport decision.
- ❑ Reassess mental status.
- ❑ Perform a rapid trauma assessment. After assessing the head and neck, apply a cervical collar and continue to maintain manual stabilization.
- ❑ Obtain baseline vital signs.
- ❑ Take a SAMPLE history.
- ❑ Perform a detailed physical exam on scene, if there is time, or en route to the hospital.
- ❑ Perform an ongoing assessment, including vital signs.
- ❑ Transport.

▶ RAPID TRAUMA ASSESSMENT/EXAM (PP. 260–262)

- ❑ Take Standard Precautions.
- ❑ Assess head: DCAP-BTLS + crepitation.
- ❑ Assess neck: DCAP-BTLS + jugular vein distention (JVD), crepitation.
- ❑ Assess chest: DCAP-BTLS + paradoxical motion, crepitation, breath sounds.
- ❑ Assess abdomen: DCAP-BTLS + firmness, softness, distention.
- ❑ Assess pelvis: DCAP-BTLS + pain, tenderness, distention.
- ❑ Assess extremities: DCAP-BTLS + distal pulse, motor function, sensation.
- ❑ Assess posterior: DCAP-BTLS.

▶ DETAILED PHYSICAL EXAM (PP. 275–277)

- ❑ Take Standard Precautions.
- ❑ Assess scalp and cranium: DCAP-BTLS + crepitation.
- ❑ Assess ears: DCAP-BTLS + drainage.
- ❑ Assess face: DCAP-BTLS.
- ❑ Assess eyes: DCAP-BTLS + discoloration, unequal pupils, foreign bodies, blood in anterior chamber.
- ❑ Assess nose: DCAP-BTLS + drainage, bleeding.
- ❑ Assess mouth: DCAP-BTLS + loose or broken teeth, objects that could cause obstruction, swelling or laceration of tongue, unusual breath odor, discoloration.
- ❑ Assess neck: DCAP-BTLS + jugular vein distention (JVD), crepitation.
- ❑ Assess chest: DCAP-BTLS + paradoxical motion, crepitation, breath sounds.
- ❑ Assess pelvis: DCAP-BTLS + pain, tenderness, motion.
- ❑ Assess extremities: DCAP-BTLS + distal pulse, motor function, sensation.
- ❑ Assess posterior: DCAP-BTLS.
- ❑ Reassess vital signs.

CASE STUDY

▶ **MOTORCYCLE MISHAP**

You are dispatched to a motorcycle collision in an intersection in your community. Apparently, a car made a right turn on red without stopping and the motorcycle, which had the green light, collided with the left side of the car. On arrival, you conduct a scene size-up.

What four things should you be concerned about in the scene size-up of this collision?

1. _____

2. _____

3. _____

4. _____

You find out from a witness who was standing on the corner at the bus stop that the vehicles were probably traveling 40 mph and the cyclist crashed into the rear left door of the car. He was thrown off the motorcycle onto the roof of the car and then landed on his back in the street. The witness immediately rushed to aid the cyclist and at the same time motioned people in another vehicle to stop traffic and to call 911. The witness stated that the patient was in a lot of pain but never hit his head or lost consciousness. The cyclist was wearing a helmet, which he removed after the collision.

5. How does forming a general impression help you provide emergency care to the patient? On what is the general impression based?

Your general impression reveals a 20-year-old responsive male trauma patient with severe external blood loss. The patient is able to talk with you, although he is experiencing considerable pain in both his thighs and lower back. He is able to describe what happened in the collision, knows the day of the week, and is concerned about his new Sportster. His name is Tony, and he was on his way to the beach, which explains why he was wearing shorts and a T-shirt.

6. As you question Tony, what should one of your partners be doing?

7. What is Tony's mental status on the AVPU scale?

Tony keeps crying out, "It's my legs!" They are obviously broken but no longer seriously bleeding. You proceed with the initial assessment beginning with an assessment of Tony's airway.

8. Explain why it would be wrong to be distracted by Tony's pain and begin to treat his broken legs.

9. What should your initial assessment of Tony consist of?

Based upon your initial assessment of Tony, you have determined he is a high-priority patient, and an ALS unit should be requested if it is not en route already. You found his airway was open and clear, his breathing was present and adequate, he was moving air into both sides of his chest equally, but he has a weak, rapid radial pulse and his skin is pale, cool, and clammy to touch—possible signs of shock. One of your crew members has controlled the bleeding from Tony's thighs.

10. Why is Tony a high-priority patient?

11. How long should you wait for an ALS unit to arrive before transporting Tony?

As one of your crew members attends to Tony's injured legs and then places him onto a long backboard, you continue with the focused history and physical exam. Since you have reconsidered the mechanism of injury (MOI), you have decided to provide early transport for Tony as soon as he is packaged.

12. What would you be looking for with DCAP-BTLS?

13. What would you be asking about for the SAMPLE history?

14. What vital signs should you assess?

En route to the hospital, you have time to conduct a detailed physical exam. Tony is immobilized, receiving oxygen via nonrebreather mask, the backboard is in the Trendelenburg position, and you are keeping him warm with a blanket. His vitals are a respiration rate of 20—good quality, a pulse rate of 120—weak and regular, a blood pressure of 110/70 mmHg, SpO_2 90%, and pale, cool, and clammy skin.

15. What would the detailed physical exam include?

©2009 Pearson Education, Inc.
Emergency Care, 11th Ed.

11

Assessment of the Medical Patient

MATCH TERMINOLOGY/ DEFINITIONS

A. Description of where pain is located and where it spreads to

B. Description of the pain, such as stabbing, crampy, dull, or sharp

C. Description of what makes the pain worse, such as sitting, standing, eating certain foods

D. Description of how bad the pain is, often described on a scale of 1 to 10

E. Memory jogger designed to remind the EMT of what questions to ask the patient about his chief complaint

F. Necklace or bracelet designed to notify emergency personnel that a patient has a specific medical history or condition

G. Medicine-like bottle kept in the patient's refrigerator that contains a listing of his past medical history

H. Description of how fast or slow the pain came on and what the patient was doing when the pain started

I. The reason why EMS was called, usually in the patient's own words

J. History relating to the patient's chief complaint

_____ **1.** Chief complaint

_____ **2.** Medical identification device

_____ **3.** Onset of pain

_____ **4.** OPQRST

_____ **5.** Pertinent past history

_____ **6.** Provocation of pain

_____ **7.** Quality of pain

_____ **8.** Radiation of pain

_____ **9.** Severity of pain

_____ **10.** Vial of Life®

MULTIPLE-CHOICE REVIEW

_____ 1. The components of the focused history and physical exam for a responsive medical patient include all of the following except:
   A. history of the present illness.
   B. SAMPLE history.
   C. baseline vital signs.
   D. rapid trauma exam.

_____ 2. OPQRST is a memory aid to help the EMT remember the:
   A. questions that ask about the past medical history.
   B. questions that expand on the history of the present illness.
   C. status of the patient's condition.
   D. mental status.

_____ 3. When you ask a patient "Can you think of anything that might have triggered or caused this pain?" you are questioning about:
   A. onset.
   B. provocation.
   C. quality.
   D. radiation.

_____ 4. When you ask a patient "How bad is the pain?", you are questioning about:
   A. quality.
   B. severity.
   C. time.
   D. radiation.

_____ 5. The "T" in "OPQRST" stands for:
   A. temperature.
   B. tibia.
   C. time.
   D. trembling.

_____ 6. When you ask a patient "Have you vomited?", you are questioning about:
   A. signs and symptoms.
   B. allergies.
   C. medication.
   D. pertinent past history.

_____ 7. The "P" in "SAMPLE" stands for:
   A. perforation.
   B. pertinent past history.
   C. puncture wound.
   D. prehospital care report.

_____ 8. When you ask a patient "How have you felt today?", you are asking about:
   A. pertinent past history.
   B. signs and symptoms.
   C. events leading to the illness.
   D. last oral intake.

_____ 9. A patient with a specific chief complaint and a known history may carry medication or other treatment with her. The EMT may need to request medical direction's permission to assist the patient with:
   A. an inhaler.
   B. nitroglycerin.
   C. epinephrine.
   D. any one of the above.

_____ 10. When a medical patient complains of difficulty breathing, but does not take any prescribed medication for this condition, you should generally:
   A. look for a medical identification device.
   B. consult with the patient's personal physician.
   C. transport the patient to the hospital.
   D. do all of the above.

_____ 11. In terms of the initial approach to the focused history and physical exam, the biggest difference between a responsive and an unresponsive patient would be that:
   A. the responsive patient gets the OPQRST questions last.
   B. the unresponsive patient will be given a rapid physical exam first.
   C. bystanders become more important if the patient is responsive.
   D. a rapid trauma exam is not done on an unconscious patient.

©2009 Pearson Education, Inc.
Emergency Care, 11th Ed.

_____ 12. In addition to DCAP-BTLS in the rapid physical exam on an unresponsive medical patient, you should include all of the following except:
   A. look for jugular vein distention.
   B. determine firmness or rigidity of abdomen.
   C. check for incontinence of urine or feces.
   D. ask the SAMPLE history questions.

_____ 13. When assessing a medical patient's extremities, be sure to check for:
   A. central cyanosis.
   B. sensation and motor function.
   C. pulmonary edema.
   D. capillary refill.

_____ 14. When conducting a physical exam, look for a necklace or bracelet. This is important because it may:
   A. reveal the patient's name.
   B. give clues to the patient's residence.
   C. be a medical identification device.
   D. be the cause of the emergency.

_____ 15. Why might it be important to check the refrigerator of a patient who is found unconscious at home?
   A. Last night's meal could be the cause.
   B. The patient may have a Vial of Life®.
   C. Most medications are kept in the refrigerator.
   D. The person's diet could be the cause of the problem.

COMPLETE THE FOLLOWING

1. List the components of a focused history and physical exam for an unresponsive medical patient.

   A. _____

   B. _____

   C. _____

   D. _____

2. List four questions to ask bystanders who witness a patient's medical emergency.

   A. _____

   B. _____

   C. _____

   D. _____

COMPLETE THE CHART

Complete the chart by writing the remainder of the word that follows each letter in the acronyms.

1.	S
2.	A
3.	M
4.	P
5.	L
6.	E
7.	O
8.	P
9.	Q
10.	R
11.	S
12.	T

STREET SCENES DISCUSSION

Review the Street Scene on p. 305 of the textbook. Then answer the questions below.

1. What would it have suggested to you if the patient had been talking in short, choppy sentences?

2. You found the patient's lung sounds "equal, but noisy, like a whistling sound." If you had found that this patient's chest was silent, would that have been a good thing?

3. What is the term for the lung sounds heard in this patient's chest?

4. If the patient had her Albuterol inhaler with her, would it have been appropriate to contact medical direction for permission to assist in the administration of the medication?

5. You assess the patient with a pulse oximeter. What does an SpO_2 of 96% mean?

ON THE WEB

To help you review and practice basic skills, visit the *Emergency Care 11th Ed. Companion Website* at www.prenhall.com/limmer. For Online Test Preparation, visit www.prenhall.com/emtachieve.

EMT SKILLS PERFORMANCE CHECKLIST

Brady's *Pocket Reference for BLS Providers, 3rd Ed.*

▶ **FOCUSED HISTORY AND PHYSICAL EXAM—RESPONSIVE MEDICAL PATIENT (PP. 291–292)**

❑ Take Standard Precautions.

❑ Gather a history of the present illness from patient by asking OPQRST questions.

❑ Gather a SAMPLE history from patient.

❑ Conduct a focused physical exam (focusing on the area patient complains of).

❑ Obtain baseline vital signs.

❑ Perform interventions and contact on-line medical direction as needed. Reassess vital signs.

❑ Transport. (Reevaluate transport decision.)

▶ Focused History and Physical Exam—Unresponsive Medical Patient (p. 297)

❑ Take Standard Precautions.

❑ Conduct a rapid physical exam by assessing:

- Head
- Neck
- Chest
- Abdomen
- Pelvis
- Extremities
- Posterior

❑ Obtain baseline vital signs.

❑ Consider request for advanced life support.

❑ Gather a history of the present illness by asking family or bystanders OPQRST questions.

❑ Gather a SAMPLE history from family or bystanders.

❑ Perform interventions. (Obtain medical direction as required locally.) Reassess vital signs.

❑ Transport. (Reevaluate transport decision.)

CHAPTER 12

Ongoing Assessment

MATCH TERMINOLOGY/ DEFINITIONS

A. Changes in a patient's condition over time that may show improvement or deterioration, and that can be shown by documenting repeated assessments

B. Actions taken to correct a patient's problems

C. Four-step procedure for detecting changes in a patient's condition

_____ 1. Interventions

_____ 2. Ongoing assessment

_____ 3. Trending

MULTIPLE-CHOICE REVIEW

_____ 1. Which one of the following best describes the purpose of performing the ongoing assessment?
A. To stabilize the patient's condition or to treat any life threats
B. To detect and treat life threats and to evaluate the EMS system's effectiveness
C. To evaluate the EMS system's effectiveness and to detect changes in patient condition
D. To repeat key elements of assessment procedures already performed in order to detect changes in patient condition

_____ 2. The ongoing assessment may be omitted if:
A. the patient care report is not completed.
B. you do not want to interrupt patient conversation.
C. life-saving interventions prevent doing it.
D. a short transport time prevents completion.

_____ 3. During the ongoing assessment of an infant or child patient:
A. avoid eye contact at all times.
B. stand above the patient.
C. speak in a loud voice.
D. use a reassuring voice.

_____ **4.** The ongoing assessment includes all the following steps <u>except</u>:
   A. reassess vital signs.
   B. repeat the initial assessment for life threats.
   C. repeat the focused assessment.
   D. repeat all interventions.

_____ **5.** Which of the following is the last step in the ongoing assessment?
   A. Reassess the vital signs.
   B. Check interventions.
   C. Repeat the initial assessment.
   D. Repeat the focused assessment.

_____ **6.** Which of the following is <u>not</u> a step when repeating the initial assessment?
   A. Reestablish patient priorities.
   B. Monitor skin color and temperature.
   C. Maintain an open airway.
   D. Apply a cervical collar.

_____ **7.** During your ongoing assessment, you note that the patient's pulse is rapid and his skin is cool and pale. This may indicate:
   A. deterioration in mental status.
   B. heat exhaustion.
   C. an occluded airway.
   D. the onset of shock.

_____ **8.** The mental status of an unresponsive child or infant can be checked by:
   A. a sternal rub.
   B. assessing the capillaries for refill.
   C. shouting or by flicking the feet.
   D. asking the parent to stick a pin in the child's foot.

_____ **9.** An example of checking interventions during the ongoing assessment of a medical patient is:
   A. taking an initial blood pressure.
   B. bandaging a severe laceration.
   C. applying a tourniquet.
   D. assuring adequacy of oxygen delivery.

_____ **10.** Frequently reassessing a patient establishes:
   A. a paper trail.
   B. legal evidence.
   C. trends.
   D. a reason for treating the patient.

_____ **11.** The best way to determine if the patient is improving or deteriorating is to:
   A. ask the hospital.
   B. contact medical direction.
   C. do frequent ongoing assessments.
   D. keep repeating the initial assessment.

_____ **12.** If the patient is considered stable, the recommended interval for reassessment is every _____ minutes.
   A. 5
   B. 10
   C. 15
   D. 20

_____ **13.** You are treating a patient with a head injury who is breathing adequately, yet has an altered mental status. The recommended interval for reassessment is every _____ minutes.
   A. 5
   B. 10
   C. 15
   D. 20

_____ **14.** You should repeat at least the initial assessment:
   A. after you have noticed and documented trends.
   B. whenever you or your partner have the time and opportunity to do so.
   C. whenever you believe there may have been a change in the patient's condition.
   D. when directed to do so by medical direction.

_____ **15.** During your ongoing assessment of an unresponsive patient, you hear gurgling sounds in her airway. What intervention should you take?

A. Sit the patient up.

B. Suction the patient.

C. Check oxygen tubing.

D. All of the above.

COMPLETE THE FOLLOWING

1. List the six steps involved in repeating the initial assessment.

A. _____

B. _____

C. _____

D. _____

E. _____

F. _____

2. List the three steps for checking interventions.

A. _____

B. _____

C. _____

STREET SCENES DISCUSSION

Review the Street Scene on pp. 316–317 of the textbook. Then answer the questions below.

1. Why do you think it is so important to monitor and maintain the airway of a stroke patient?

2. Many times a patient experiencing a stroke can hear but not speak. Why do you think this is something you should be aware of?

ON THE WEB

To help you review and practice basic skills, visit the *Emergency Care 11th Ed. Companion Website* at www.prenhall.com/limmer. For Online Test Preparation, visit www.prenhall.com/emtachieve.

EMT-BASIC SKILLS PERFORMANCE CHECKLIST

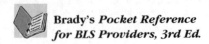 **Brady's *Pocket Reference for BLS Providers*, 3rd Ed.**

▶ **ONGOING ASSESSMENT (P. 308)**

❑ Take Standard Precautions.

❑ Repeat the initial assessment for life threats:

- Reassess mental status.
- Maintain an open airway.
- Monitor breathing rate and quality.
- Reassess pulse rate and quality.
- Monitor skin color, temperature, and condition.
- Reestablish patient treatment priorities.

❑ Reassess and record vital signs.

❑ Repeat focused assessment related to chief complaint or injuries.

❑ Check interventions.

- Assure adequacy of oxygen delivery and ventilation support.
- Assure management of bleeding.
- Assure adequacy of other interventions.

NOTE: Repeat the ongoing assessment every 15 minutes for a stable patient and every 5 minutes for an unstable patient.

CHAPTER 13
Communications

MATCH TERMINOLOGY/ DEFINITIONS

A. Federal agency that regulates radio communications

B. Device that picks up signals from lower-power radio units such as mobile and portable radios and retransmits them at a higher power

C. Unit used to measure the output power of a radio

D. Handheld two-way radio

E. Two-way radio at a fixed site such as a hospital or dispatch center

F. Update on the patient's condition given to hospital personnel either face to face or over a radio

G. Two-way radio that is used or affixed in a vehicle

H. Phone that transmits through the air instead of over wires so that the phone can be transported and used over a wide area

I. Equipment that permits transmission of standard messages in condensed form by punching a key

J. "Press to talk" button on the EMS radio

_____ 1. Base station

_____ 2. Cellular phone

_____ 3. Digital radio equipment

_____ 4. FCC

_____ 5. Mobile radio

_____ 6. Portable radio

_____ 7. PTT

_____ 8. Repeater

_____ 9. Verbal report

_____ 10. Watt

MULTIPLE-CHOICE REVIEW

_____ 1. The EMT's ability to communicate effectively is important because:
A. all EMTs are expected to be good public speakers.
B. little information about a patient's condition is obtained by talking to the patient, bystanders, or family members.
C. describing your assessment findings to the hospital may make a difference in the care the patient receives.
D. none of the above.

_____ **2.** One of the key contributions to improvement in EMS over the years has been:
  A. the type II, van-style ambulance vehicle.
  B. development of radio links among dispatcher, mobile units, and hospitals.
  C. the military antishock trousers.
  D. air conditioning in the transport vehicles.

_____ **3.** Components of a communications system include:
  A. base stations.
  B. mobile units.
  C. portable radios.
  D. all of the above.

_____ **4.** A device that picks up radio signals from lower-powered units and retransmits them at a higher power is called a:
  A. mobile.
  B. cellular.
  C. repeater.
  D. portable.

_____ **5.** The government agency that maintains order on the airwaves is called the:
  A. FCC.
  B. FAA.
  C. FEMA.
  D. DOT.

_____ **6.** The purposes of always following the general principles of radio transmission are to allow all persons to use the frequencies and to:
  A. avoid having to repeat orders from medical direction.
  B. enable the EMT to talk in code language.
  C. prevent delays.
  D. do all of the above.

_____ **7.** Of the following components of a radio report, which is the correct order?
  1) Major past illness
  2) Chief complaint
  3) Unit identification and level of provider
  4) Emergency medical care given
  A. 4, 1, 2, 3
  B. 3, 4, 1, 2
  C. 3, 2, 1, 4
  D. 1, 2, 4, 3

_____ **8.** The reason for the ambulance call is the:
  A. major past illness.
  B. chief complaint.
  C. presenting diagnosis.
  D. call type.

_____ **9.** During a radio report, when the EMT says "The patient's abdomen does not feel rigid," he or she is attempting to advise the hospital of:
  A. the baseline vital signs.
  B. the emergency medical care given.
  C. response of patient to the emergency medical care.
  D. pertinent findings of the physical exam.

_____ **10.** During a radio report, when the EMT says "The patient's mental status has not changed during our care," he or she is attempting to advise the hospital of the:
  A. baseline vital signs.
  B. emergency medical care given.
  C. response of patient to the emergency medical care.
  D. pertinent findings of the physical exam.

_____ **11.** Whenever the EMT is requesting an order for medical direction over the radio, it is a good practice to:
  A. repeat the physician's order word for word back to the physician.
  B. question all verbal orders that are given.
  C. speak quickly because the physician is busy.
  D. call the physician back again to verify.

12. If an order from the on-line physician appears to be inappropriate, then the EMT should:
    A. switch to another frequency to find another physician.
    B. question the physician about the order.
    C. follow the physician's order as stated.
    D. ignore the order and do what he or she thinks is correct.

13. When an EMT stands with arms crossed looking down at the patient, the nonverbal message is:
    A. "I am here to help you."
    B. "I am not really interested."
    C. "I can empathize with your problem."
    D. "I am afraid of catching your disease."

14. If it is obvious that a patient has a broken leg with a bone protruding, and the patient asks, "Is my leg broken?" what would be the most appropriate response?
    A. "Relax and stay calm, you will be all right."
    B. "I am not qualified to make that determination."
    C. "No, it's a bad cut, and I'll control the bleeding with a bandage."
    D. "Yes it is, and I will be as gentle as possible splinting it."

15. When treating a toddler, the best approach is to:
    A. kneel down so you are at the child's level.
    B. speak louder so the child can hear you above all the crying.
    C. stare directly into the child's eyes.
    D. tell the child you are a friend of his parents.

COMPLETE THE FOLLOWING

1. List five examples of components of a communications system.

    A. _____

    B. _____

    C. _____

    D. _____

    E. _____

2. List six interpersonal communications guidelines to use when dealing with patients, families, friends, and bystanders.

    A. _____

    B. _____

    C. _____

    D. _____

    E. _____

    F. _____

STREET SCENES DISCUSSION

Review the Street Scene on p. 330 of the textbook. Then answer the questions below.

1. Why was it important to call the hospital to alert them to a serious patient on the way?

2. If this call had occurred in your response area, who would have made the decision to call a helicopter?

3. In addition to radio communication, what other types of communication were involved in this call?

ON THE WEB

To help you review and practice basic skills, visit the *Emergency Care 11th Ed. Companion Website* at www.prenhall.com/limmer. For Online Test Preparation visit www.prenhall.com/emtachieve.

©2009 Pearson Education, Inc.
Emergency Care, 11th Ed.

EMT SKILLS
PERFORMANCE CHECKLIST

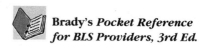 **Brady's *Pocket Reference*
*for BLS Providers, 3rd Ed.***

▶ RADIO REPORT (PP. 323–325)

Pick an ambulance call on which you were recently an observer or a patient whom you examined during the hospital observation portion of the EMT course. Without releasing any confidential information about the call, such as the patient's name and address, take a moment and organize your thoughts so you can provide a mock radio report to another crew member or your instructor.

❏ Unit identification (ambulance #_____).

❏ Level of provider.

❏ Estimated time of arrival (ETA).

❏ Patient's age and sex.

❏ Chief complaint (why the patient called ambulance).

❏ Brief, pertinent history of the present illness or injury.

❏ Major past illnesses.

❏ Mental status (AVPU).

❏ Baseline vital signs.

❏ Pertinent findings of the physical exam.

❏ Emergency medical care given.

❏ Response to emergency medical care.

❏ Does medical direction have any questions or orders?

NOTE: There are a number of local formats for radio reports that may differ somewhat, yet they all adhere to the same principles. They should follow a logical order, be concise, and paint a picture of the patient's problem and the priorities for the hospital personnel.

CHAPTER

14

Documentation

MATCH TERMINOLOGY/ DEFINITIONS

A. Information from an individual point of view

B. Report form used by EMS agencies to document prehospital assessment and care

C. Inaccurate entry or misrepresentation on a prehospital care report usually intended to cover up serious flaws in assessment or in care

D. Observable, measurable, and verifiable information

E. Exam finding that is not present or not true but is important to note (for example, patient denies any shortness of breath)

F. Report on unusual, complex, or involved situations that is completed according to your service's standard operating procedures

G. Each individual box on a prehospital care report

H. Minimum elements recommended by the U.S. Department of Transportation for inclusion in all prehospital care reports nationwide

I. Clipboard-format device that is able to recognize handwriting and convert it to computer text

J. Item affixed to a patient at a multiple-casualty incident used to record chief complaint and injuries, vital signs, and treatment given

_____ **1.** Data element

_____ **2.** Falsification

_____ **3.** Minimum data set

_____ **4.** Objective statement

_____ **5.** PCR

_____ **6.** Electronic clipboard

_____ **7.** Pertinent negative

_____ **8.** Special situation report

_____ **9.** Subjective information

_____ **10.** Triage tag

©2009 Pearson Education, Inc.
Emergency Care, 11th Ed.

MULTIPLE-CHOICE REVIEW

_____ 1. The prehospital care report (PCR) serves as a legal document as well as a(n):
    A. press release form for your EMS agency.
    B. receipt for the patient.
    C. aid to research, education, and administrative efforts.
    D. form to report all calls to the local police department.

_____ 2. Why is it necessary to complete a prehospital care report (PCR) if on each call you give the emergency department staff a good oral report?
    A. The QI committee needs something to hold you to.
    B. It provides a means for the emergency department staff to review the patient's prehospital care.
    C. They usually do not listen to oral reports.
    D. Duplication is helpful in emergency call documentation.

_____ 3. The copy of the prehospital care report left at the hospital:
    A. is returned to the state for quality review and follow-up.
    B. is thrown out once it is key punched and added to computer file.
    C. should become part of the patient's permanent hospital record.
    D. is sent to the regional Emergency Medical Services agency.

_____ 4. You are called to court to testify about a civil matter when a patient sues the city for an injury that occurred in a public place. Which of the following will best help you recall the events of the call?
    A. The questioning by the defense's attorney
    B. The questioning by the plaintiff's attorney
    C. A complete and accurate prehospital care report
    D. Your tape recording of the call dispatch

_____ 5. The person who completed a prehospital care report may be called to court to testify about:
    A. the call in a criminal proceeding.
    B. the care provided to the patient.
    C. the call in a civil proceeding.
    D. all of the above.

_____ 6. The routine review of prehospital care reports for conformity to current medical and organizational standards is a process called:
    A. initial feedback.   **C.** stress debriefing.
    B. quality improvement.   **D.** system research.

_____ 7. Each individual box on a prehospital care report is called a(n):
    A. narrative.   **C.** key punch.
    B. data element.   **D.** assessment.

_____ 8. According to the U.S. Department of Transportation, in addition to other data elements, the minimum data set on a prehospital care report should include all of the following <u>except</u>:
    A. respiratory rate and effort and skin color and temperature.
    B. times of incident, dispatch, and arrival at the patient.
    C. patient's Social Security number.
    D. capillary refill for patients less than 6 years old.

_____ 9. The minimum data set includes all of the following <u>except</u>:
    A. vital signs.   **C.** chief complaint.
    B. vehicle mileage.   **D.** times of the call.

_____ 10. The time of dispatch is an example of _____ data on the prehospital care report (PCR).
    A. assessment   **C.** patient
    B. run   **D.** narrative

_____ 11. Examples of patient data on a prehospital care report would be:
   A. date of birth and age.
   B. time of arrival at the hospital.
   C. ambulance identification number.
   D. the hospital transported to.

_____ 12. Experienced EMTs consider a good prehospital care report as one that:
   A. protects them against a QA review.
   B. is vague enough to prevent lawsuits.
   C. paints a picture of the patient.
   D. identifies symptoms overlooked by the patient.

_____ 13. A statement such as "The patient has a swollen, deformed extremity" on the narrative portion of the prehospital care report is an example of:
   A. subjective information.
   B. objective information.
   C. pertinent negative information.
   D. nonstandard abbreviations.

_____ 14. All the following are examples of information that should be put in quotation marks on the prehospital care report except:
   A. bystander statements.
   B. chief complaint.
   C. objective information.
   D. police officer's statements.

_____ 15. In the narrative section of a prehospital care report, the EMT should:
   A. list his or her conclusions about the situation.
   B. include pertinent negatives.
   C. use the radio codes for each treatment.
   D. list the vital signs and times obtained.

_____ 16. Medical abbreviations should be used on a prehospital care report (PCR):
   A. to save space in the narrative section.
   B. to replace all words you cannot spell.
   C. only if they are standardized.
   D. to ensure correct interpretation by physicians.

_____ 17. The prehospital care report form itself and the information on it should be considered:
   A. the property of the ambulance service.
   B. confidential information.
   C. privileged information.
   D. the patient's property.

_____ 18. When a patient refuses transport, before the EMT leaves the scene, he or she should:
   A. document assessment findings and care given.
   B. try again to persuade the patient to go to a hospital.
   C. ensure the patient is able to make a rational, informed decision.
   D. do all of the above.

_____ 19. When completing a prehospital care report on a patient refusal, the EMT should document all of the following except:
   A. that he or she was willing to return if the patient changed his or her mind.
   B. the complete patient assessment.
   C. that alternative methods of care were offered.
   D. the patient's diagnosis.

©2009 Pearson Education, Inc.
Emergency Care, 11th Ed.

_____ **20.** If the EMT forgot to administer a treatment that is required by a state protocol, he or she should:
   A. document on the PCR only treatment actually given.
   B. be sure to document an excuse for why the treatment was skipped.
   C. record that the patient was given the forgotten treatment.
   D. do none of the above.

_____ **21.** Falsification of information on a prehospital care report may lead to:
   A. suspension or revocation of your license or certification.
   B. better EMT education.
   C. longer response times.
   D. none of the above.

_____ **22.** To correct an error discovered while writing the prehospital care report, the EMT should:
   A. scribble out the error so it cannot be seen.
   B. draw a line through the error, initial it, and write the correct information.
   C. place his or her initials over the error.
   D. erase the error completely, and then write the correction.

_____ **23.** If information was omitted on a prehospital care report, the EMT should:
   A. prepare another report and substitute that for the earlier one.
   B. notify the service Medical Director immediately.
   C. add a note with the correct information, the date, and initial it.
   D. do nothing, as information should never be added after the call.

_____ **24.** An example of an instance in which it would <u>not</u> be unusual for the EMT to obtain only a limited amount of information is:
   A. during a multiple-casualty incident.
   B. during an interhospital transfer.
   C. while performing a nonemergency run.
   D. when encountering a child abuse case.

_____ **25.** Special situation reports:
   A. document events that should be reported to local regulatory authorities.
   B. can be submitted at any time after the call.
   C. need not be accurate and/or objective.
   D. are required on each call.

_____ **26.** Ambulance services are required by the _____ to take steps to safeguard patient confidentiality.
   A. OSHA law   **C.** NHTSA
   B. HIPAA   **D.** U.S. DOT

_____ **27.** An example of a method that an ambulance service would use to safeguard patient confidentiality would include:
   A. requiring employees to place completed PCRs in a locked box.
   B. only using patient last names during radio transmissions.
   C. only allowing PCRs with patient names to be distributed during QA meetings.
   D. none of the above is an acceptable procedure.

_____ **28.** The policy an ambulance service develops concerning patient rights and confidentially must take into consideration:
   A. state regulations.
   B. local regulations.
   C. HIPAA.
   D. all of the above.

©2009 Pearson Education, Inc.
Emergency Care, 11th Ed.

COMPLETE THE FOLLOWING

1. List ten examples of patient data on a prehospital care report (PCR).

A. _____

B. _____

C. _____

D. _____

E. _____

F. _____

G. _____

H. _____

I. _____

J. _____

2. List five guidelines to help the EMT prepare the narrative portion of the PCR.

A. _____

B. _____

C. _____

D. _____

E. _____

STREET SCENES DISCUSSION

Review the Street Scene on p. 351 of the textbook. Then answer the questions below.

1. What legal problem might have been created if you had forgotten to record the patient's distal pulses, motor function, and sensation (PMS) before and after immobilization?

2. What might it mean if the documentation had been sloppy and difficult to read?

3. Imagine that the patient had told you that he was drunk. Should you document that information? If so, how?

4. What will the emergency department staff do with your prehospital care report?

ON THE WEB

To help you review and practice basic skills, visit the *Emergency Care 11th Ed. Companion Website* at www.prenhall.com/limmer. For Online Test Preparation, visit www.prenhall.com/emtachieve.

EMT SKILLS PERFORMANCE CHECKLIST

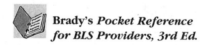 Brady's *Pocket Reference for BLS Providers, 3rd Ed.*

▶ **PATIENT REFUSAL PROCEDURE (PP. 342–345)**

❑ Spend time effectively communicating with patient (includes reasoning, persistence, and strategies to convince patient to go to hospital).

❑ Clearly inform patient of consequences of not going to hospital.

❑ Consult with medical direction.

❑ Contact family to help convince patient.

❑ Call law enforcement, who may be able to order or "arrest" serious patient in order to force patient to go to hospital.

❑ Try to determine why patient is refusing care.

❑ Complete thorough documentation of refusal, have patient sign refusal release, and have witness sign the release (e.g., bystander, police, family).

NOTE: Procedure may differ by state and jurisdiction. Always follow your Medical Director's advice.

CHAPTER 15

General Pharmacology

MATCH TERMINOLOGY/ DEFINITIONS

A. Specific signs or circumstances under which it is appropriate to administer a drug to a patient

B. Spray device with a mouthpiece that contains an aerosol form of a medication that a patient can spray directly into his or her airway

C. Semisolid paste form of a drug

D. Medication given by mouth to treat a conscious patient (one who is able to swallow) with an altered mental status and a history of diabetes

E. Brand name of a medication

F. Drug that helps to constrict the blood vessels and relax airway passages; it may be used to counter a severe allergic reaction

G. Solid form of a drug; compressed powder

H. Powder, usually premixed with water, that will adsorb some poisons and help prevent them from being absorbed by the body

I. This gas, in its pure form, is used as a drug to treat any patient whose medical or traumatic condition causes them to be hypoxic, or low in oxygen

J. Liquid form of a drug in which a powder is mixed with a slurry or water

K. Any action of a drug other than the desired action

L. Specific signs or circumstances under which it is not appropriate and may be harmful to administer a drug to a patient

_____ **1.** Activated charcoal

_____ **2.** Epinephrine

_____ **3.** Gel

_____ **4.** Indications

_____ **5.** Inhaler

_____ **6.** Oral glucose

_____ **7.** Oxygen

_____ **8.** Suspension

_____ **9.** Tablet

_____ **10.** Trade name

_____ **11.** Contraindications

_____ **12.** Side effect

MULTIPLE-CHOICE REVIEW

_____ **1.** The study of drugs, their sources, and their effects is called:
   A. anatomy.   **C.** medicinology.
   B. physiology.   **D.** pharmacology.

_____ **2.** Medications that are routinely carried on the EMS unit are:
   A. activated charcoal, oral glucose, and oxygen.
   B. oxygen and nitroglycerin.
   C. epinephrine and prescribed inhalers.
   D. all of the above.

_____ **3.** Activated charcoal is an example of a:
   A. powder, usually premixed with water.
   B. prescribed inhaler.
   C. liquid for injection.
   D. fine powder for inhalation.

_____ **4.** Activated charcoal is given to a patient because it:
   A. displaces poisons by surface tension.
   B. will bind some poisons to its surface.
   C. prevents the patient from vomiting.
   D. can be used in a patient without a gag reflex.

_____ **5.** Poorly managed diabetes can cause:
   A. hypoxia, or low oxygen.   **C.** dilation of the coronary arteries.
   B. altered mental status.   **D.** absorption of poisons.

_____ **6.** Oral glucose is given between the patient's cheek and gum because:
   A. this area contains blood vessels that allow easy absorption into the bloodstream.
   B. it will not be aspirated if the patient suddenly becomes unconscious.
   C. this area will cause the patient to regurgitate the stomach's contents.
   D. it will assist in dilating the coronary vessels as much as possible.

_____ **7.** Examples of medications a patient may have in his or her possession that the EMT may assist the patient in taking under the appropriate circumstances are:
   A. activated charcoal, glucose injections, and anticonvulsants.
   B. home oxygen, antihypertensives, and anti-inflammatories.
   C. epinephrine auto-injector, a prescribed inhaler, and nitroglycerin.
   D. insulin, antihypertensives, and anticonvulsants.

_____ **8.** Patients who have a medical history of asthma, emphysema, and chronic bronchitis may carry:
   A. nitroglycerin.   **C.** a bronchodilator.
   B. an epinephrine auto-injector. **D.** a bronchoconstrictor.

_____ **9.** The drug nitroglycerin is used to _____ vessels.
   A. dilate the peripheral   **C.** dilate the coronary
   B. constrict the peripheral   **D.** constrict the coronary

_____ **10.** The government publication listing all drugs in the United States is called the:
   A. _Physician's Desk Reference._   **C.** _U.S. Pharmacopoeia._
   B. _Hazmat Guidebook._   **D.** _National Medicine Guidebook._

_____ **11.** The name that the manufacturer uses in marketing a drug is called the _____ name.
   A. generic   **C.** official
   B. trade   **D.** original

_____ **12.** A circumstance in which a drug should not be used because it may cause harm to the patient or offer no effect in improving the patient's condition or illness is called a(n):
  A. indication.
  B. side effect.
  C. adverse reaction.
  D. contraindication.

_____ **13.** An action of a drug that is other than the desired action is called a(n):
  A. side effect.
  B. overdose.
  C. contraindication.
  D. systemic effect.

_____ **14.** Prior to administering a medication to a patient, you must know all the following except:
  A. the route of administration.
  B. the proper dose to administer.
  C. the actions the medication will take.
  D. both the generic and chemical names.

_____ **15.** Drugs prescribed for pain relief are called:
  A. antidysrhythmics.
  B. analgesics.
  C. anticonvulsants.
  D. antihypertensives.

_____ **16.** Drugs prescribed to reduce high blood pressure are called:
  A. antidysrhythmics.
  B. analgesics.
  C. anticonvulsants.
  D. antihypertensives.

_____ **17.** Drugs prescribed for heart rhythm disorders are called:
  A. antidiabetics.
  B. bronchodilators.
  C. antidysrhythmics.
  D. anticonvulsants.

_____ **18.** Drugs prescribed to relax the smooth muscles of the bronchial tubes are called:
  A. bronchospasms.
  B. bronchodilators.
  C. anticonvulsants.
  D. bronchoconstrictors.

_____ **19.** Drugs prescribed for prevention and control of seizures are called:
  A. antidiabetics.
  B. antihypertensives.
  C. anticonvulsants.
  D. antidepressants.

_____ **20.** Drugs prescribed to help regulate the emotional activity of patients to minimize the psychological and emotional peaks and valleys are called:
  A. antidepressants.
  B. analgesics.
  C. antidysrhythmics.
  D. anticonvulsants.

COMPLETE THE FOLLOWING

1. List six medications an EMT can administer or assist a patient in taking.

A. _____

B. _____

C. _____

D. _____

E. _____

F. _____

©2009 Pearson Education, Inc.
Emergency Care, 11th Ed.

2. List the four "rights" to adhere to when administering a medication.

A. _____

B. _____

C. _____

D. _____

STREET SCENES DISCUSSION

Review the Street Scene on pp. 365–366 of the textbook. Then answer the questions below.

1. Suppose the patient's wife had administered the nitroglycerin tablets before your arrival. What side effect should you be alert for?

2. What effect does a patient with chest pain expect from the nitroglycerin tablet? How does this effect occur?

3. Are there any "pertinent negatives" in the Sample Documentation? If so, what are they?

ON THE WEB

To help you review and practice basic skills, visit the *Emergency Care 11th Ed. Companion Website* at www.prenhall.com/limmer. For Online Test Preparation, visit www.prenhall.com/emtachieve.

16

Respiratory Emergencies

MATCH TERMINOLOGY/ DEFINITIONS

A. Active process in which the intercostal muscles and the diaphragm contract, expanding the size of the chest cavity and causing air to flow into the lungs; also called inhalation

B. Sporadic, irregular breaths that are usually seen just before respiratory arrest

C. Blockage of the bronchi that lead from the trachea to the lungs

D. Pulling in of the accessory muscles to breathe

E. Passive process in which the intercostal muscles and the diaphragm relax, causing the chest cavity to decrease in size and forcing air from the lungs; also called exhalation

F. Another term for inspiration

_____ **1.** Agonal respirations

_____ **2.** Bronchoconstriction

_____ **3.** Expiration

_____ **4.** Inspiration

_____ **5.** Retractions

_____ **6.** Inhalation

MULTIPLE-CHOICE REVIEW

_____ **1.** The structure that divides the chest cavity from the abdominal cavity is called the _____ muscle:
  A. intercostal
  B. sternocleidomastoid
  C. diaphragm
  D. inguinal

_____ **2.** Expiration is a(n):
  A. active process that involves the relaxation of the intercostal muscles and the diaphragm.
  B. passive process that involves the relaxation of the intercostal muscles and the diaphragm.
  C. active process that involves the contraction of the intercostal muscles and the diaphragm.
  D. passive process that involves the contraction of the intercostal muscles and the diaphragm.

_____ 3. To determine the <u>quality</u> of breathing, check for all of the following <u>except</u>:
   A. presence of breath sounds.
   B. chest expansion.
   C. breathing rhythm.
   D. depth of respirations.

_____ 4. An unresponsive patient with shallow, gasping breaths with only a few breaths per minute requires:
   A. oxygen given via nasal cannula.
   B. immediate transport to a medical facility.
   C. immediate artificial ventilation with supplemental oxygen.
   D. oxygen given via nonrebreather mask.

_____ 5. The muscles in the neck and abdomen that sometimes assist in breathing are called _____ muscles.
   A. extra   C. subdiaphragmatic
   B. accessory   D. smooth

_____ 6. Since oxygenation of the body's tissue is reduced in a patient with inadequate breathing, the skin may be _____ in color and feel _____.
   A. pale; dry and cool   C. yellow; dry and warm
   B. red; clammy and hot   D. blue; clammy and cool

_____ 7. If an unresponsive adult patient makes _____ sounds, she may have a serious airway problem requiring immediate intervention.
   A. snoring or gurgling   C. sniffling
   B. slight wheezing   D. whistling or grunting

_____ 8. Statistically, a leading killer of infants and children is:
   A. motor vehicle collisions.   C. respiratory conditions.
   B. heart attacks.   D. infection.

_____ 9. The structure of an infant's or child's airway is different from an adult's in each of the following ways <u>except</u>:
   A. all airway structures are smaller and more easily obstructed.
   B. their tongues are proportionately larger than an adult's.
   C. the trachea is softer and more flexible.
   D. the cricoid cartilage is more rigid.

_____ 10. Because the chest wall is softer in infants and children, they:
   A. must inhale twice the amount of air to breathe.
   B. depend more heavily on the diaphragm for breathing.
   C. grunt and gurgle whenever they breathe.
   D. expend less energy than adults do when breathing.

_____ 11. The signs of inadequate breathing in infants and children include all of the following <u>except</u>:
   A. nasal flaring.   C. "seesaw breathing."
   B. grunting.   D. quivering jaw.

_____ 12. Which one of the following would be <u>most</u> important to observe related to a patient's breathing?
   A. presence of breathing and pulse rate
   B. breathing pattern and adequacy of breathing
   C. presence of breathing and adequacy of breathing
   D. patient position and adequacy of breathing

_____ 13. The best method for providing artificial ventilation is the:
   A. pocket face mask with supplemental oxygen.
   B. two-person bag-valve mask with supplemental oxygen.
   C. flow-restricted, oxygen-powered ventilation device.
   D. one-person bag-valve mask with supplemental oxygen.

_____ **14.** If you are unsure whether a patient requires artificial ventilation, you should:
  A. contact medical direction immediately.
  B. move to the ambulance and transport rapidly.
  C. increase the liter flow rate to the nonrebreather mask.
  D. provide artificial ventilation.

_____ **15.** The adequate rate of artificial ventilations for a nonbreathing adult patient is _____ breaths per minute.
  A. 8   **C.** 16
  B. 12   **D.** 20

_____ **16.** The adequate rate of artificial ventilations for a nonbreathing infant or child patient is _____ breaths per minute.
  A. 10   **C.** 20
  B. 15   **D.** 25

_____ **17.** If an infant or a child has _____ in the setting of a respiratory emergency, this usually indicates trouble.
  A. a fever   **C.** a low pulse
  B. cold skin   **D.** a rapid pulse

_____ **18.** You are artificially ventilating an adult patient in respiratory arrest. The chest does not rise and fall with each ventilation. The <u>first</u> action to take is to:
  A. increase the oxygen flow rate.
  B. increase the force of ventilations.
  C. change the ventilatory device.
  D. recheck the airway.

_____ **19.** Why is it important to try to distinguish between a lower airway and an upper airway problem in an infant and a child?
  A. Suctioning can cause spasms with some lower respiratory diseases.
  B. You will need to give this information to the emergency department.
  C. Finger sweeps will not help to clear an upper airway obstruction.
  D. The lower airway may wheeze when treated with oxygen.

_____ **20.** The sign(s) of a lower airway problem include all of the following <u>except</u>:
  A. wheezing.
  B. increased breathing effort upon exhalation.
  C. rapid breathing without stridor.
  D. yellow skin color.

_____ **21.** If your patient is able to speak only in short choppy sentences, this may mean she:
  A. may have a language problem.
  B. is unable to hear you clearly.
  C. is experiencing breathing difficulty.
  D. is afraid of you.

_____ **22.** When an EMT states that the patient was in the tripod position due to respiratory distress, this means the patient was:
  A. holding self up by two legs and one arm.
  B. leaning forward with hands resting on knees.
  C. in the recovery position.
  D. supine with knees flexed against the chest.

_____ **23.** Which pair of signs/symptoms is <u>not</u> commonly associated with breathing difficulty?
  A. crowing/restlessness
  B. retractions/shortness of breath
  C. increased pulse/tightness in chest
  D. vomiting/headache

©2009 Pearson Education, Inc.
Emergency Care, 11th Ed.

_____ **24.** If a patient is suffering from breathing difficulty and is breathing adequately, administer oxygen via:
  A. nasal cannula.
  B. nonrebreather mask.
  C. pocket face mask.
  D. bag-valve mask with supplemental oxygen.

_____ **25.** If a patient is experiencing breathing difficulty and is breathing adequately, it is usually best to place him in the _____ position.
  A. tripod   **C.** sitting-up
  B. supine   **D.** none of the above

_____ **26.** A patient with respiratory problems that cause bronchoconstriction may carry a(n):
  A. bronchoconstrictor.   **C.** inhaler or puffer.
  B. metered dose aspirator. **D.** antihypertensive medication.

_____ **27.** Once you receive permission from medical direction to assist a patient with an inhaler, make sure you have all of the following <u>except</u>:
  A. the right dose.
  B. an inhaler that is not expired.
  C. a large enough syringe.
  D. a patient who is alert enough to cooperate.

_____ **28.** Prior to coaching the patient in the use of an inhaler, the EMT should:
  A. shake the inhaler vigorously.
  B. test the unit by spraying into the air.
  C. ensure that the patient is no longer alert.
  D. call the patient's personal physician.

_____ **29.** To ensure that the most medication is absorbed when using an inhaler, you should try to encourage the patient to:
  A. take short, shallow breaths.
  B. hold the breath as long as possible.
  C. take a short nap.
  D. hyperventilate.

_____ **30.** The best way to document that a patient has a respiratory complaint is to:
  A. describe your opinion of the patient's problem in detail.
  B. see if the patient can answer all the SAMPLE and OPQRST questions.
  C. ask the patient to describe the difficulty in his own words.
  D. carefully count the patient's breathing rate for at least two minutes.

_____ **31.** A physician realizes that his patient may become anxious and use his inhaler improperly. To help improve the volume of the medication that the patient is able to self-administer when in distress, the physician may prescribe a:
  A. tranquilizer.   **C.** spacer device.
  B. decongestant.   **D.** heat treatment.

_____ **32.** Of the prescribed inhalers listed below, which is <u>not</u> considered a medication that would be used in an emergency to reverse airway constriction, as its use is aimed at prevention of attacks by reducing inflammation?
  A. Ventolin   **C.** Proventil
  B. Advair   **D.** Albuterol

_____ **33.** When assessing the lungs of a patient in respiratory distress, you hear a fine bubbling sound upon inspiration. This sound is caused by fluid in the alveoli and is called:
  A. wheezes.   **C.** rhonchi.
  B. stridor.   **D.** crackles.

_____ **34.** A device commonly used in the hospital setting that is now frequently used by COPD patients in their homes for respiratory treatments is called a(n):

A. nonrebreather mask. **C.** small-volume nebulizer.

B. endotracheal tube. **D.** Combitube.

COMPLETE THE FOLLOWING

1. List nine conditions of inadequate breathing.

A. _____

B. _____

C. _____

D. _____

E. _____

F. _____

G. _____

H. _____

I. _____

2. List four signs of inadequate breathing in infants and children.

A. _____

B. _____

C. _____

D. _____

3. List eight signs of breathing difficulty.

A. _____

B. _____

C. _____

D. _____

E. _____

F. _____

G. _____

H. _____

©2009 Pearson Education, Inc.
Emergency Care, 11th Ed.

4. PULSE OXIMETER READINGS

Oxygen should be administered to all patients with respiratory distress regardless of their oxygen saturation readings. The oximeter reading in a normal, healthy person is typically (A) _____ . An oximeter reading below (B) _____ indicates hypoxia. A reading of (C) _____ indicates mild hypoxia, (D) _____ indicates moderate hypoxia, and (E) _____ indicates severe hypoxia.

LABEL THE DIAGRAMS

Fill in each phase of respiration on the line provided.

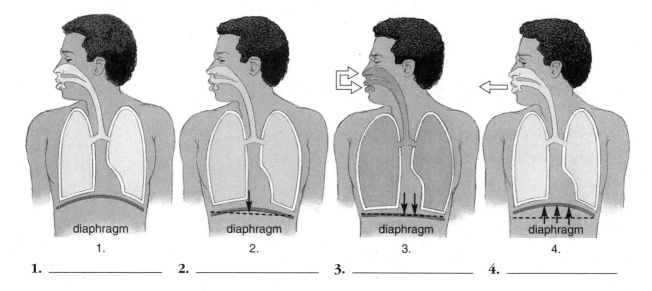

diaphragm 1. diaphragm 2. diaphragm 3. diaphragm 4.

1. _____ 2. _____ 3. _____ 4. _____

STREET SCENES DISCUSSION

Review the Street Scene on pp. 387–388 of the textbook. Then answer the questions below.

1. You have already reported that the patient has emphysema. Imagine that you were also told the patient was coughing earlier in the day. Would it be worth documenting the cough on your PCR? Why or why not?

2. If advanced life support (ALS) had been available, would it have been appropriate to request its assistance?

3. Is it possible to assist the ventilations of a patient who is in a semi-sitting position?

ON THE WEB

To help you review and practice basic skills, visit the *Emergency Care 11th Ed. Companion Website* at www.prenhall.com/limmer. For Online Test Preparation, visit www.prenhall.com/emtachieve.

EMT SKILLS
PERFORMANCE CHECKLIST

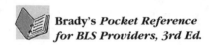 **Brady's *Pocket Reference for BLS Providers, 3rd Ed.***

▶ **PRESCRIBED INHALER (PP. 382–383)**

❑ Conduct a scene size-up.

❑ Take Standard Precautions.

❑ Perform initial assessment.

❑ Perform focused history and physical exam.

❑ Confirm indications for inhaler use.

❑ Obtain medical direction for prescribed patient-assisted inhaler. (generics: albuterol, isoetharine, metaproterenol, etc.)

❑ Check contraindications for inhaler use.

❑ Assure right patient, right medication, right dose, right route, and patient is alert enough to use inhaler.

❑ Check expiration date of inhaler.

❑ Check if patient has already taken any doses.

❑ Assure inhaler is at room temperature or warmer.

❑ Shake inhaler vigorously several times.

❑ Have patient exhale deeply.

❑ Have patient put lips around the opening of inhaler.

❑ Have patient depress the handheld inhaler as he begins to inhale deeply.

❑ Instruct patient to hold breath for as long as comfortable so medication can be absorbed.

❑ Put oxygen back on patient.

❑ Allow patient to breathe a few times, and repeat dose if so ordered by medical direction.

❑ If patient has a spacer device for inhaler, it should be used.

CHAPTER 17

Cardiac Emergencies

MATCH TERMINOLOGY/ DEFINITIONS

▶ **PART A**

A. Buildup of fatty deposits on the inner walls of arteries

B. Dilation, or ballooning, of a weakened section in the wall of an artery

C. Condition of excessive fluid buildup in the lungs and/or other organs and body parts because of the inadequate pumping of the heart

D. Condition in which artery walls become hard and stiff due to calcium deposits

E. When the heart has ceased generating electrical impulses

F. Blanket term for any kind of heart problem

G. Irregular, or absent, heart rhythm

H. Diseases that affect the arteries of the heart

I. Condition in which a portion of the myocardium dies as a result of oxygen starvation; often called a heart attack by laypersons

J. Pain in the chest that occurs when the blood supply to the heart is reduced and a portion of the heart muscle is not receiving enough oxygen

_____ **1.** Acute myocardial infarction

_____ **2.** Aneurysm

_____ **3.** Angina pectoris

_____ **4.** Arrhythmia

_____ **5.** Arteriosclerosis

_____ **6.** Asystole

_____ **7.** Atherosclerosis

_____ **8.** Cardiac compromise

_____ **9.** Congestive heart failure

_____ **10.** Coronary artery disease

A. Condition in which the heart's electrical impulses are disorganized, preventing the heart muscle from contracting normally

B. Blockage

C. Accumulation of fluid in the feet or ankles

D. Cardiac arrest that occurs within 2 hours of the onset of symptoms

E. Accumulation of fluid in the lungs

F. Condition in which the heartbeat is quite rapid; if rapid enough, it will not allow the heart's chambers to fill with enough blood between beats to produce blood flow sufficient to meet the body's needs

G. Clot of blood and plaque that has broken loose from the wall of an artery and then moves to smaller arteries and blocks blood flow

H. Clot formed of blood and plaque attached to the inner wall of an artery

I. Condition in which the heart's electrical rhythm remains relatively normal, yet the mechanical pumping activity fails to follow the electrical activity, causing cardiac arrest

J. Swelling resulting from a buildup of fluid in tissues

_____ **1.** Edema

_____ **2.** Embolism

_____ **3.** Occlusion

_____ **4.** Pedal edema

_____ **5.** Pulmonary edema

_____ **6.** Pulseless electrical activity (PEA)

_____ **7.** Sudden death

_____ **8.** Thrombus

_____ **9.** Ventricular fibrillation

_____ **10.** Ventricular tachycardia

MULTIPLE-CHOICE REVIEW

_____ **1.** Cardiac compromise is a blanket term that refers to:
 A. a heart attack.
 B. sudden death.
 C. any kind of problem with the heart.
 D. a period of time when the heart stops.

_____ **2.** Chest pain from the heart is typically described by the patient as any of the following except:
 A. dull.   **C.** tearing.
 B. squeezing.   **D.** crushing.

_____ **3.** The pain or discomfort from a heart problem commonly radiates to the:
 A. arms and jaw.
 B. feet and head.
 C. stomach and lower abdomen.
 D. right arm and lower abdomen.

_____ **4.** In addition to chest pain or discomfort, the patient with cardiac compromise will also complain of:
 A. diarrhea.   **C.** dyspnea.
 B. shivering.   **D.** headache.

_____ **5.** Patients with heart problems may complain of any of the following except:
 A. pain in the center of the chest.
 B. mild chest discomfort.
 C. sudden onset of sharp abdominal pain.
 D. difficulty breathing.

6. If the heart is beating too fast or too slow, the patient with cardiac compromise may also:
  A. have stomach pain.
  B. lose consciousness.
  C. have a seizure or convulsion.
  D. have right-side weakness.

7. The signs and symptoms of cardiac compromise include all of the following except:
  A. difficulty breathing and abnormal pulse rate.
  B. sudden onset of sweating with nausea or vomiting.
  C. sharp lower abdominal pain and a fever.
  D. pain in the chest or upper abdomen.

8. The emergency medical care of the patient with cardiac compromise should include all of the following except:
  A. placing the patient in the position of comfort.
  B. administering high concentration oxygen by nonrebreather mask.
  C. administering high flow oxygen by a nasal cannula.
  D. assisting the patient with nitroglycerin administration if medical direction authorizes.

9. What is the typical "position of comfort" for a conscious patient who is having chest pain and difficulty breathing?
  A. Fowler's   **C.** prone
  B. supine   **D.** lying down with knees bent

10. All the following cardiac compromise patients are candidates for immediate transport except a patient with:
  A. no history of cardiac problems.
  B. a history of cardiac problems, who does not have nitroglycerin.
  C. prescribed nitroglycerin.
  D. a systolic blood pressure of less than 100.

11. You should consider using nitroglycerin when the patient:
  A. is hypertensive and has a headache.
  B. has his own nitroglycerin and has crushing chest pain.
  C. loses consciousness after feeling dizzy.
  D. has chest pain for over 5 minutes and is hypotensive.

12. Which of the following is the best description of the role of medical direction in the treatment of a cardiac compromise patient?
  A. authorizing the EMT to administer oxygen via nonrebreather mask
  B. prescribing nitroglycerin that the EMT can then assist the patient in taking
  C. authorizing the EMT to assist the patient in taking his prescribed nitroglycerin
  D. contacting the patient's physician to ensure the patient's nitroglycerin prescription is not out-of-date

13. A patient is complaining of chest pain. In order for the EMT to administer nitroglycerin, all the following conditions must be met except:
  A. medical direction should authorize its administration.
  B. the patient's physician should have prescribed the medication.
  C. the patient's blood pressure is lower than 100 systolic.
  D. the patient's blood pressure is greater than 100 systolic.

14. The maximum number of doses of nitroglycerin routinely given in the field is:
  A. one.   **C.** three.
  B. two.   **D.** four.

_____ **15.** After administering three doses of nitroglycerin, if the patient's blood pressure falls below 100 systolic, you should:
   A. administer another dose of nitroglycerin.
   B. reassess the patient's vital signs.
   C. treat for shock and transport promptly.
   D. do all of the above.

_____ **16.** Nitroglycerin is contraindicated for the patient who has:
   A. a head injury.
   B. a systolic blood pressure of 110.
   C. not yet taken the maximum dose.
   D. been complaining of the pain for at least 20 minutes.

_____ **17.** Which of the following is <u>not</u> a common side effect of nitroglycerin?
   A. hypotension
   B. headache
   C. pulse rate changes
   D. palpitations

_____ **18.** After administering nitroglycerin, it is important to:
   A. immediately administer the next dose.
   B. discontinue the oxygen therapy.
   C. reassess the vital signs.
   D. lay the patient down.

_____ **19.** Most cardiovascular emergencies are caused, directly or indirectly, by all of the following <u>except</u>:
   A. changes in the inner walls of arteries.
   B. problems with the heart's electrical function.
   C. problems with the heart's mechanical function.
   D. complications resulting from cardiovascular surgery.

_____ **20.** When the body is subjected to exertion or stress, the heart rate will normally:
   A. increase.
   B. decrease.
   C. become irregular.
   D. stop temporarily.

_____ **21.** Two conditions commonly cause narrowing or blocking of the arteries. One condition is atherosclerosis, and the other is:
   A. aneurysm.
   B. dysrhythmia.
   C. arteriosclerosis.
   D. congestive heart failure.

_____ **22.** Factor(s) that put a person at risk for developing coronary artery disease and acute coronary syndromes include:
   A. lack of exercise.
   B. cigarette smoking.
   C. obesity.
   D. all of the above.

_____ **23.** Which of the following risk factors can be modified to reduce the risk of coronary artery disease?
   A. age
   B. heredity
   C. hypertension
   D. none of the above

_____ **24.** The reason an emergency occurs in most cardiac-related medical emergencies is due to:
   A. reduced blood flow to the myocardium.
   B. cardiac arrest.
   C. loss of consciousness.
   D. breathing difficulty.

_____ **25.** Angina pectoris means, literally:
   A. a small heart attack.
   B. a pain in the chest.
   C. paralyzed chest muscles.
   D. breathing difficulty.

_____ **26.** Why is nitroglycerin administered to the patient with chest pain?
   A. It increases blood flow to the brain.
   B. It dilates the blood vessels and decreases the work of the heart.
   C. It constricts the blood vessels and raises the blood pressure.
   D. It is easy to administer in unconscious patients.

_____ **27.** A condition in which a portion of the myocardium dies as a result of oxygen starvation is known as:
   A. coronary occlusion.
   B. acute myocardial infarction.
   C. myocardial starvation.
   D. acute angina attack.

_____ **28.** When a cardiac arrest occurs within 2 hours of the onset of cardiac symptoms, this is referred to as:
   A. prehospital death.
   B. prehospital arrest.
   C. sudden death.
   D. ventricular tachycardia.

_____ **29.** Unfortunately, nearly _____ of the patients who experience a cardiac arrest within 2 hours of the onset of symptoms have no previous history of cardiac problems.
   A. 10%   **C.** 60%
   B. 25%   **D.** 80%

_____ **30.** Changes in the field care of acute coronary syndromes have made _____ and _____ two of the most important treatment methods.
   A. oxygen, PASG   **C.** fibrinolytics, defibrillation
   B. rapid transport, surgery   **D.** none of the above

_____ **31.** Congestive heart failure is a(n):
   A. clotting of the coronary artery.
   B. condition in which excessive fluids build up in the lungs and/or other organs.
   C. infection in the heart that makes it difficult to oxygenate the blood.
   D. chronic lung condition that requires a low concentration of oxygen administration.

_____ **32.** When there is damage to the left ventricle and blood backs up into the lungs, this usually presents in the form of:
   A. pedal edema.   **C.** thrombolytics (fibrinolyitics).
   B. pulmonary edema.   **D.** diaphoresis.

_____ **33.** The elements of the chain of survival include early access to all of the following except:
   A. CPR.   **C.** advanced care.
   B. defibrillation.   **D.** diagnosis.

_____ **34.** Ways to decrease the EMS access time include:
   A. installing a 911 system.
   B. placing 911 stickers on telephones.
   C. providing public information workshops.
   D. all of the above.

_____ **35.** Which of the following steps is not necessary to ensure that CPR can be delivered earlier to cardiac arrest victims?
   A. Send CPR-trained professionals to patients faster.
   B. Ensure that heart specialists are involved in CPR training.
   C. Train laypeople in CPR.
   D. Have EMDs instruct callers in how to perform CPR.

_____ **36.** Who is the typical cardiac arrest victim?
  A. a male in his sixties
  B. a female in her forties
  C. a male in his seventies
  D. There is no pattern to cardiac arrests.

_____ **37.** The most common witness to a cardiac arrest is a:
  A. male in his forties.   **C.** man in his sixties.
  B. female in her forties.   **D.** female in her sixties.

_____ **38.** The single most important factor in determining survival from cardiac arrest is:
  A. nitroglycerin administration.
  B. training middle-aged and older people in CPR.
  C. early CPR.
  D. early defibrillation.

_____ **39.** If the response time from the moment a call is received to arrival of the defibrillator is longer than _____ minutes, virtually no one survives a cardiac arrest.
  A. 6   **C.** 10
  B. 8   **D.** 12

_____ **40.** When treating a cardiac arrest patient and there is no ACLS unit in the community, the EMT should:
  A. discontinue resuscitative efforts and pronounce the patient dead.
  B. package quickly and transport to the closest medical facility.
  C. call for ACLS from another town and wait for its arrival.
  D. continue to provide CPR at the scene until the patient regains a pulse.

_____ **41.** In order to manage a patient in cardiac arrest, the EMT should be able to do all of the following except:
  A. use a bag-valve-mask device with oxygen.
  B. use an automated external defibrillator.
  C. request advanced life support backup (when available).
  D. administer epinephrine via IV.

_____ **42.** Which of the following steps is *not* necessary for the EMT to take when using a fully automated defibrillator?
  A. Assess the patient.
  B. Turn on the power.
  C. Put the pads on the patient's chest.
  D. Press the button to deliver the shock.

_____ **43.** The primary electrical disturbance resulting in cardiac arrest is:
  A. asystole.   **C.** ventricular tachycardia.
  B. ventricular fibrillation.   **D.** pulseless electrical activity.

_____ **44.** The shockable rhythms include all of the following except:
  A. asystole and PEA.   **C.** pulseless ventricular tachycardia.
  B. ventricular fibrillation.   **D.** ventricular tachycardia.

_____ **45.** A nonshockable rhythm that can be the result of a terminally sick heart or severe blood loss is called:
  A. pulseless electrical activity.
  B. ventricular tachycardia.
  C. pulseless ventricular tachycardia.
  D. ventricular fibrillation.

_____ **46.** A nonshockable rhythm that is commonly called "flatline" is named:
  A. pulseless electrical activity. **C.** asystole.
  B. ventricular tachycardia.   **D.** ventricular fibrillation.

©2009 Pearson Education, Inc.
Emergency Care, 11th Ed.

_____ **47.** When the AED is analyzing the patient's heart rhythm, the EMT must:
- **A.** continue the CPR compressions.
- **B.** avoid touching the patient.
- **C.** hyperventilate the patient.
- **D.** reassess for a carotid pulse.

_____ **48.** The AED should routinely be used on:
- **A.** trauma victims.
- **B.** patients under 55 pounds.
- **C.** all patients under 8 years of age.
- **D.** adults and children with shockable rhythms.

_____ **49.** The AED pads are first attached to the cables. Then the pad attached to the _____ cable goes on the _____ lower ribs.
- **A.** white, left
- **B.** white, right
- **C.** red, left
- **D.** red, right

_____ **50.** After the first shock, the patient has a strong carotid pulse. The patient is also breathing adequately. You should then _____ and transport.
- **A.** give high-concentration oxygen via bag-valve mask
- **B.** provide artificial ventilations with high-concentration oxygen
- **C.** give high-concentration oxygen via nonrebreather mask
- **D.** administer two more shocks

_____ **51.** After three shocks, the EMT should _____ unless local protocol says otherwise.
- **A.** give two more in a row
- **B.** transport the patient
- **C.** terminate the arrest
- **D.** increase the rate of ventilation

_____ **52.** Which of the following is <u>not</u> a general principle of AED use?
- **A.** Hook up oxygen before beginning defibrillation.
- **B.** Avoid contact with patient during rhythm analysis.
- **C.** Be sure everyone is "clear" before delivering each shock.
- **D.** Avoid defibrillation in a moving ambulance.

_____ **53.** Of the cardiac arrest patients listed below, which one can be defibrillated immediately?
- **A.** soaking wet patient lying in the rain
- **B.** trauma patient with severe blood loss
- **C.** patient on a metal deck being cradled by another person
- **D.** patient with an implanted defibrillator

_____ **54.** If it is necessary to remove a nitroglycerin patch to defibrillate a patient, you should:
- **A.** wear gloves.
- **B.** wear goggles.
- **C.** ensure you have a replacement patch.
- **D.** cleanse the patient's skin with alcohol.

_____ **55.** If a patient has a cardiac pacemaker and needs to be defibrillated, the EMT should:
- **A.** perform the procedure as he or she would for other cardiac patients.
- **B.** remove the pacemaker before defibrillation.
- **C.** place the pad several inches away from the pacemaker battery.
- **D.** double the power setting on the AED.

COMPLETE THE FOLLOWING

1. List the four elements of the chain of survival.

A. _____

B. _____

C. _____

D. _____

LABEL THE DIAGRAM

Fill in the name of each component of the cardiovascular system on the line provided.

1. _____

2. _____

3. _____

4. _____

5. _____

6. _____

7. _____

8. _____

9. _____

10. _____

11. _____

12. _____

13. _____

©2009 Pearson Education, Inc.
Emergency Care, 11th Ed.

STREET SCENES DISCUSSION

Review the Street Scene on pp. 428–429 of the textbook. Then answer the questions below.

1. It was decided very quickly that ALS should be dispatched. This was an appropriate decision. Why is ALS needed in this type of call?

2. If the patient had prescribed nitroglycerin, would it have been appropriate to assist her in the administration of it? (Assume that you have a standing order to assist with nitroglycerin.)

3. If you had applied the AED and it did not shock the patient, what would that have meant?

4. How often should vital signs be taken on this patient? What is her priority?

ON THE WEB

To help you review and practice basic skills, visit the *Emergency Care 11th Ed. Companion Website* at www.prenhall.com/limmer. For Online Test Preparation, visit www.prenhall.com/emtachieve.

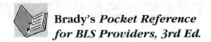
▶ NITROGLYCERIN ASSIST (P. 398)

❑ Take Standard Precautions.

❑ Perform focused assessment for cardiac patient.

❑ Take BP (systolic pressure must be above 90 mmHg).

❑ Contact medical direction for authorization to administer.

❑ Assure patient is alert.

❑ Assure right patient, right medication, right dose, and right route.

❑ Check expiration date.

❑ Assist patient with nitroglycerin administration.

❑ Reassess vital signs and chest pain after each dose. Document findings.

NOTE: If the blood pressure falls below 90 systolic, treat the patient for shock (hypoperfusion). Transport promptly.

▶ CARDIAC ARREST MANAGEMENT AND THE AED (PP. 412–415)

❑ Take Standard Precautions.

❑ Assess patient for breathing and a pulse (maximum 10 seconds).

❑ If no pulse is present, direct CPR while attaching AED to patient.

❑ Direct rescuer to stop CPR.

❑ Verify absence of spontaneous pulse.

❑ Turn on defibrillator power.

❑ Ensure all individuals are standing clear of patient.

❑ Initiate analysis of rhythm.

❑ Deliver shock.

❑ Verify presence or absence of spontaneous pulse. If absent:

- Direct resumption of CPR.
- Gather additional information on arrest event.
- Confirm effectiveness of CPR (ventilation and compressions).
- Direct insertion of an airway adjunct (oropharyngeal/nasopharyngeal).
- Direct ventilation of patient with high-concentration oxygen.
- Assure CPR continues without unnecessary/prolonged interruption.

❑ After 2 minutes of CPR, reevaluate patient.

❑ Repeat defibrillator sequence.

❑ Check carotid pulse.

❑ If there is a spontaneous pulse, check patient's breathing.

❑ If breathing is adequate, provide high-concentration oxygen by nonrebreather mask. If breathing is inadequate, ventilate patient with high-concentration oxygen.

❑ Transport patient without delay.

©2009 Pearson Education, Inc.
Emergency Care, 11th Ed.

▶ CHECKING THE AED (P. 424)

❑ Check the AED for the following:

- Unit, cables, connectors for cleanliness and condition.
- Supplies carried with AED.
- Power supply and its operation.
- Indicators on ECG display.
- ECG recorder operation.
- Charge display cycle with a simulator.
- Pacemaker feature, if applicable.

❑ File a written report on status of AED.

NOTE: This list is derived from FDA Automated Defibrillator: Operator's Shift Checklist.

▶ USING THE THUMPER (P. 426)

❑ Take Standard Precautions.

❑ Assure CPR is in progress and effective.

❑ Attach Thumper® base plate to long backboard.

❑ Stop CPR to slide long backboard under patient.*

❑ Restart CPR and attach shoulder straps to patient.

❑ Slide Thumper® piston plate into position on base plate (away from chest).

❑ Stop CPR and quickly pivot piston arm into place, measuring anterior/posterior and middle sternum placement.*

❑ Slowly adjust depth of compression to appropriate diagram.

❑ Adjust ventilations.

❑ Turn off compressions temporarily for pulse checks and defibrillation.*

❑ Upon termination of arrest or return of spontaneous circulation, power down unit.

*NOTE: Always limit interruptions in chest compressions to 10 seconds or less.

▶ USING THE AUTO-PULSE® (P. 426)

❑ Take Standard Precautions.

❑ Assure CPR is in progress and effective.

❑ Align the patient on the Auto-Pulse® platform.*

❑ Close the Lifeband chest band over the patient's chest.

❑ Press the start (Auto-Pulse® is designed to do the compressions automatically).

❑ Provide bag mask ventilation at a rate of 2 ventilations for every 30 compressions. Each ventilation should be given over 1 second to provide visible chest rise.

❑ If an advanced airway is in place (ETT, LMA, or Combitube) there are no longer cycles of compressions to ventilations. The compression rate is a continuous 100/min. and ventilation rate is 8–10/min.

❑ After 2 minutes of CPR reassess for pulse and/or shockable rhythm.*

*NOTE: Always limit interruptions in chest compressions to 10 seconds or less.

18

Acute Abdominal Emergencies

MATCH TERMINOLOGY/ DEFINITIONS

A. A localized pain that arises from the parietal peritoneum, the lining of the abdominal cavity

B. The membrane that lines the abdominal cavity and covers the organs within it

C. Pain that is felt in a location other than where the pain originates

D. Sharp pain that feels as if body tissues are being torn apart

E. A poorly localized, dull, or diffuse pain that arises from the abdominal organs or viscera

_____ **1.** Tearing pain

_____ **2.** Peritoneum

_____ **3.** Visceral pain

_____ **4.** Parietal pain

_____ **5.** Referred pain

MULTIPLE-CHOICE REVIEW

_____ **1.** The membrane that covers the abdominal organs is called the _____ peritoneum.
    A. pleural
    B. visceral
    C. parietal
    D. serius

_____ **2.** The organs outside the peritoneum that are found between the abdomen and the back are in the:
    A. posterior pelvic spine.
    B. subxiphoid space.
    C. retroperitoneal space.
    D. dorsal back space.

_____ **3.** Pain originating from an organ in the abdomen is called:
    A. somatic.
    B. parital.
    C. referred.
    D. visceral.

_____ **4.** Pain from an organ is often described as:
    A. dull.
    B. achy.
    C. diffuse.
    D. any of the above.

©2009 Pearson Education, Inc.
Emergency Care, 11th Ed.

_____ **5.** When a patient has colicky pain, this is often _____ pain from a _____ organ in the abdomen.
  A. tearing, hollow
  B. referred, solid
  C. visceral, hollow
  D. parietal, solid

_____ **6.** Why is it common for the patient who has a gallbladder attack to complain of pain in his right shoulder blade?
  A. Because the gallbladder is located under the right shoulder blade in most adult patients.
  B. Nerve pathways from the gallbladder return to the spinal cord by way of shared pathways with the shoulder.
  C. Because the muscle that holds the gallbladder in position is attached to the right scapula.
  D. It is not common for this to happen at all.

_____ **7.** Why would last oral intake be important to ask if the patient has a chief complaint of abdominal discomfort?
  A. The food may have been spoiled.
  B. Food can lead to altered mental state in many instances.
  C. Visceral pain is more severe on an empty stomach.
  D. Referred pain is more severe on a full stomach.

_____ **8.** Why would an EMT ask a young, adult female patient, who is complaining of abdominal discomfort, where she is in her menstrual cycle?
  A. to file a complete PCR
  B. to begin to focus on the possibility of an ectopic pregnancy
  C. to definitively rule out an ectopic pregnancy
  D. to rule out the possibility that the patient could be pregnant

_____ **9.** When it is necessary to palpate the abdomen, palpate the area with the _____ pain.
  A. last
  B. first
  C. second
  D. third

_____ **10.** When managing a patient who has a complaint of abdominal pain and has no difficulty breathing, yet has vital signs consistent with shock or hypoperfusion, the EMT should:
  A. transport in the semi-Fowler's position.
  B. administer 10–15 lpm oxygen by nonrebreather mask.
  C. apply a cervical collar and long spine board.
  D. contact medical direction for permission to assist the patient with a nitro.

COMPLETE THE FOLLOWING

1. List four solid organs found in the abdomen.

  A. _____   **C.** _____

  B. _____   **D.** _____

2. List six hollow organs found in the abdomen.

  A. _____   **D.** _____

  B. _____   **E.** _____

  C. _____   **F.** _____

Major Body Organs

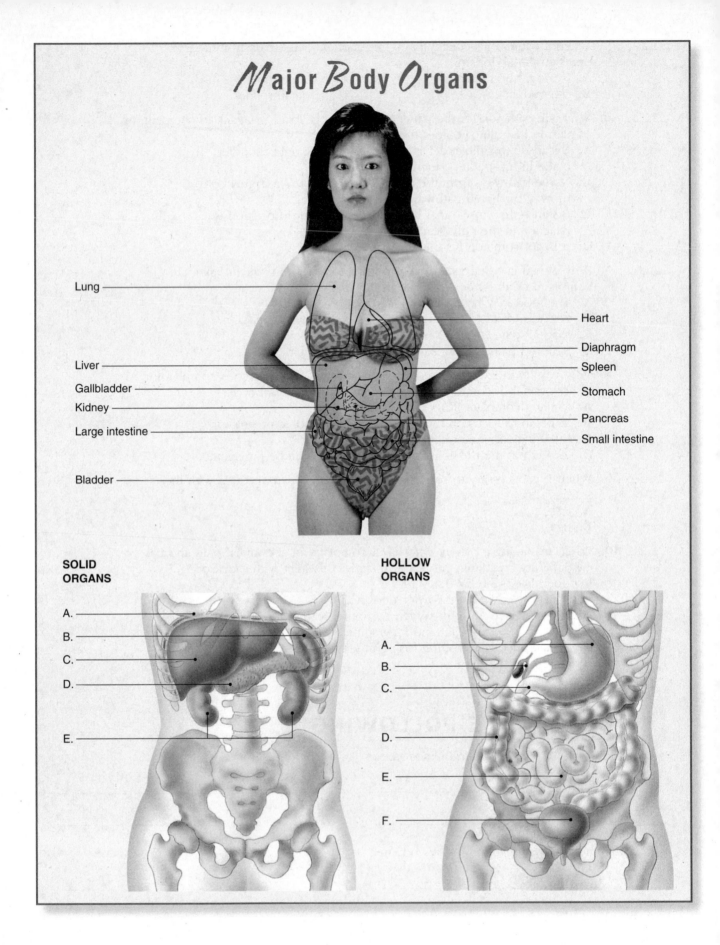

Lung

Heart

Diaphragm

Liver

Spleen

Gallbladder

Stomach

Kidney

Pancreas

Large intestine

Small intestine

Bladder

SOLID ORGANS

A.

B.

C.

D.

E.

HOLLOW ORGANS

A.

B.

C.

D.

E.

F.

©2009 Pearson Education, Inc.
Emergency Care, 11th Ed.

LABEL THE DIAGRAMS

Fill in the name of each structure on the line provided.

SOLID ORGANS

A. _____

B. _____

C. _____

D. _____

E. _____

HOLLOW ORGANS

A. _____

B. _____

C. _____

D. _____

E. _____

F. _____

STREET SCENES DISCUSSION

Review the Street Scene on pp. 445–446 of the textbook. Then answer the questions below.

1. Suppose this patient was 25 years old. Would you have more potential causes of her illness to consider, and if so, what would be the most serious ones?

2. If when examining her abdomen you noticed that she has a mass that seems to have a pulse and she has a tearing sensation in her abdomen radiating into her back, what could this be and is it a priority?

3. If the patient suddenly begins to complain of pain in the epigastric area and breaks out in a cold sweat, what should you consider?

ON THE WEB

To help you review and practice basic skills, visit the *Emergency Care 11th Ed. Companion Website* at www.prenhall.com/limmer. For Online Test Preparation, visit www.prenhall.com/emtachieve.

Diabetic Emergencies and Altered Mental Status

MATCH TERMINOLOGY/ DEFINITIONS

A. Form of sugar that provides the body's basic source of energy

B. Condition brought about by decreased insulin production; also called "sugar diabetes" or simply "diabetes"

C. Hormone produced by the pancreas or taken as a medication by many diabetics that helps cells use glucose

D. Uncontrolled muscular movements

E. Prolonged seizure, or when a person suffers two or more convulsive seizures without regaining full consciousness

F. Low blood sugar

G. Medical condition that sometimes causes seizures

H. High blood sugar

I. Sudden change in sensation, behavior, or movement that can, in its most severe form, produce convulsions

J. Blockage or bursting of a major blood vessel supplying the brain

_____ **1.** Convulsions

_____ **2.** Diabetes mellitus

_____ **3.** Epilepsy

_____ **4.** Glucose

_____ **5.** Hyperglycemia

_____ **6.** Hypoglycemia

_____ **7.** Insulin

_____ **8.** Seizure

_____ **9.** Status epilepticus

_____ **10.** Stroke

©2009 Pearson Education, Inc.
Emergency Care, 11th Ed.

145

MULTIPLE-CHOICE REVIEW

_____ **1.** The relationship of glucose to insulin is often described as:
  A. oppositional.
  B. synergistic.
  C. a lock-and-key mechanism.
  D. antagonistic.

_____ **2.** The condition brought about by decreased insulin production is known as:
  A. diabetes mellitus.
  B. hypotension.
  C. hypoglycemia.
  D. stroke.

_____ **3.** The most common medical emergency for the diabetic patient is called:
  A. diabetes mellitus.
  B. hypotension.
  C. hypoglycemia.
  D. stroke.

_____ **4.** When a diabetic overexercises or overexerts, a medical condition called _____ can develop.
  A. hypoglycemia
  B. hyperglycemia
  C. diabetes mellitus
  D. acute pulmonary edema

_____ **5.** Which of the following is <u>not</u> a cause of hypoglycemia?
  A. The patient may have taken too much insulin by mistake.
  B. The patient ate a box of candy too fast.
  C. The patient has been vomiting.
  D. The patient has been fasting.

_____ **6.** If sugar is not replenished quickly for the hypoglycemic patient, the:
  A. patient may have permanent brain damage.
  B. patient may go into pulmonary edema.
  C. patient will have chest pain.
  D. body can live off its internal sugar supply for up to 2 weeks.

_____ **7.** The clues that a patient is a diabetic include all of the following <u>except</u>:
  A. a medical identification bracelet.
  B. the presence of insulin in the refrigerator.
  C. low-fat food in the freezer.
  D. information provided by family members.

_____ **8.** Which one of the following is <u>not</u> a common oral medication used to treat diabetes?
  A. Humulin
  B. Sugunoil
  C. Glucotrol
  D. Micronase

_____ **9.** An intoxicated appearance and uncharacteristic behavior are typical of:
  A. shock.
  B. dehydration.
  C. cardiac arrest.
  D. diabetic emergency.

_____ **10.** Diabetics often present the EMT with all of the following signs and symptoms <u>except</u>:
  A. cold, clammy skin.
  B. decreased heart rate.
  C. anxiety.
  D. combativeness.

_____ **11.** In order for the EMT to consider administering oral glucose, the patient must have an altered mental status, a:
  A. history of diabetes, and be awake enough to swallow.
  B. prescribed medication, and an absent gag reflex.
  C. history of seizures, and be awake.
  D. Medic Alert® tag that says "diabetic," and a head injury.

©2009 Pearson Education, Inc.
Emergency Care, 11th Ed.

_____ **12.** When reassessing a patient to whom you have administered oral glucose, you note the patient's condition has not improved. What action should you take?
  A. Call the patient's personal physician.
  B. Give glucose in orange juice.
  C. Consult medical direction about whether to administer more glucose.
  D. Administer oxygen by nasal cannula.

_____ **13.** Which position is most appropriate for transport of the diabetic patient who is not awake enough to swallow and does not need ventilation?
  A. supine   **C.** recovery
  B. prone   **D.** Fowler's

_____ **14.** Which statement is most correct related to children with diabetes?
  A. Children are more likely than adults to eat correctly.
  B. Children are less likely than adults to exhaust blood sugar levels.
  C. Children are more at risk than adults for developing hypoglycemia.
  D. Children have a greater risk for medical emergencies than adults.

_____ **15.** Which of the following would <u>most</u> likely indicate an alteration in the patient's blood sugar level?
  A. right lower abdominal pain   **C.** change in mental status
  B. nausea and vomiting   **D.** rigid abdomen on palpation

_____ **16.** Before and after administering oral glucose, make sure you:
  A. check for distal pulses in both arms.
  B. document the mental status of the patient.
  C. increase the oxygen flow rate by 5 liters per minute.
  D. have the patient drink a glass of water.

_____ **17.** A trade name for oral glucose is:
  A. D_5W.   **C.** Insulin.
  B. Lactose.   **D.** Insta-glucose.

_____ **18.** A patient is very confused and disoriented. Before deciding the patient has a behavioral problem, the EMT should consider all of the following <u>except</u>:
  A. a potential head injury.   **C.** hypoxia.
  B. a brain tumor.   **D.** glucose allergy.

_____ **19.** People with diabetes routinely test the level of sugar in their blood using a(n):
  A. capnograph.   **C.** urinal.
  B. glucose meter.   **D.** oximeter.

_____ **20.** Complications of diabetes include:
  A. kidney failure.   **C.** blindness.
  B. heart disease.   **D.** any of the above.

_____ **21.** The reading on the device described in question number 19 is reported in:
  A. grams of sugar per liter of blood.
  B. centimeters of blood per decimeter of sugar.
  C. milligrams of glucose per deciliter of blood.
  D. none of the above.

_____ **22.** If the diabetic is symptomatic and has a sugar level below _____, he is considered hypoglycemic.
  A. 140   **C.** 100
  B. 120   **D.** 80

_____ **23.** If the diabetic is symptomatic and has a sugar level above _____, he is considered hyperglycemic.
  A. 120   **C.** 80
  B. 100   **D.** 60

_____ **24.** The <u>most</u> common cause of seizures in adults is:
   A. taking a double dose of antiseizure medication.
   B. taking a small dose of antiseizure medication.
   C. not taking antiseizure medication.
   D. use of illicit street drugs.

_____ **25.** Seizures are commonly caused by all the following <u>except</u>:
   A. cold exposure.
   B. a high fever.
   C. a brain tumor.
   D. an infection.

_____ **26.** Which of the following is <u>not</u> a characteristic of an idiopathic seizure?
   A. lasts longer than 10 minutes
   B. occurs spontaneously
   C. has an unknown cause
   D. often starts in childhood

_____ **27.** Convulsive seizures may be seen with:
   A. epilepsy or hypoglycemia.
   B. hyperventilation or AMI.
   C. anaphylaxis or pulmonary embolism.
   D. hyperglycemia or asthma.

_____ **28.** The best-known condition that results in seizures is:
   A. a stroke.
   B. epilepsy.
   C. measles.
   D. eclampsia.

_____ **29.** Most people associate a _____ seizure with epilepsy.
   A. generalized tonic-clonic
   B. complex partial
   C. simple partial
   D. idiopathic

_____ **30.** When obtaining the medical history of a seizure patient, find out from bystanders all of the following <u>except</u>:
   A. how long the seizure lasted.
   B. what the patient did after the seizure.
   C. what the patient was doing prior to the seizure.
   D. what the family's reaction was to the seizure.

_____ **31.** A seizure patient becomes cyanotic. After convulsions have ended, what action should you take?
   A. Wait for the patient's color to return to normal.
   B. Place a nonrebreather mask with oxygen on the patient.
   C. Provide artificial ventilations with supplemental oxygen.
   D. Monitor the pulse closely for 2 minutes.

_____ **32.** You notice that a bystander has placed a tongue blade in the corner of a seizure patient's mouth. What should you do?
   A. Begin oxygen therapy with a nonrebreather mask.
   B. Carefully remove the object from the patient's mouth.
   C. Immobilize the patient on a long spine board.
   D. Immediately transport to the hospital.

_____ **33.** A seizure will normally last about _____ minutes.
   A. 1 to 3
   B. 4 to 6
   C. 7 to 10
   D. 30

_____ **34.** A patient has two or more back-to-back seizures without regaining full consciousness. This is called:
   A. repeating seizure.
   B. status epilepticus.
   C. status asthmaticus.
   D. convulsions.

_____ **35.** If you suspect a conscious patient has had a stroke, you should transport her in the _____ position.
   A. recovery
   B. supine
   C. prone
   D. semi-sitting

_____ **36.** A stroke patient has difficulty saying what he is thinking even though he clearly understands you. This is called:
  A. receptive aphasia.
  B. expressive aphasia.
  C. miscommunication.
  D. confusion.

_____ **37.** The patient can speak clearly but cannot understand what you are saying. This is called:
  A. expressive aphasia.
  B. hyperactivity.
  C. receptive aphasia.
  D. petit mal seizure.

_____ **38.** A common sign of a stroke is:
  A. tingling in both legs.
  B. diminished urine flow.
  C. low blood pressure.
  D. headache.

_____ **39.** Signs and symptoms of a stroke include:
  A. vomiting.
  B. seizures.
  C. loss of bladder control.
  D. all of the above.

_____ **40.** When a patient has many of the signs and symptoms of a stroke, which completely resolve in less than 24 hours, this is called a(n):
  A. altered mental status (AMS).
  B. transient ischemic attack (TIA).
  C. acute myocardial infarction (AMI).
  D. hypoglycemic incident.

_____ **41.** When a patient faints, the medical term to describe this is usually a(n):
  A. hypoglycemic incident.
  B. stroke.
  C. syncopal episode.
  D. hyperglycemic incident.

_____ **42.** Lightheadedness or dizziness is often due to:
  A. too much blood being circulated to the brain.
  B. poor perfusion to the brain.
  C. too much fluid intake in too short a period of time.
  D. standing erect for too long a period of time.

COMPLETE THE FOLLOWING

1. List six signs and symptoms associated with a diabetic emergency.

A. _____

B. _____

C. _____

D. _____

E. _____

F. _____

2. Give four reasons a diabetic may develop <u>hyperglycemia</u>.

A. _____

B. _____

C. _____

D. _____

STREET SCENES DISCUSSION

Review the Street Scene on pp. 471–472 of the textbook. Then answer the questions below.

1. What advice should be given to this patient and his friend before they walk away?

2. Aside from not eating all day, what are other possible causes of hypoglycemia?

3. If you did not have oral glucose with you, what else could you have used to help bring up this patient's sugar level?

ON THE WEB

To help you review and practice basic skills, visit the *Emergency Care 11th Ed. Companion Website* at www.prenhall.com/limmer. For Online Test Preparation, visit www.prenhall.com/emtachieve.

EMT SKILLS PERFORMANCE CHECKLIST

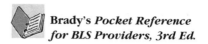

▶ **ORAL GLUCOSE ADMINISTRATION (P. 456)**

❏ Conduct a scene size-up.

❏ Take Standard Precautions.

❏ Perform initial assessment.

❏ Perform focused history and physical exam and take vital signs. Record mental status before glucose administration.

❏ Consult medical direction.

❏ Assure signs and symptoms of altered mental status with a history of diabetes.

❏ Assure patient is awake with a gag reflex.

❏ Place glucose on tongue depressor between cheek and gum.

❏ Perform ongoing assessment. Record mental status after glucose administration.

▶ **USING A BLOOD GLUCOSE METER (EMT SKILL WITH MEDICAL DIRECTION AUTHORIZATION) (P. 453)**

❏ Take Standard Precautions.

❏ Prepare the blood glucose meter and supplies (i.e., lancet, test strip, band-aid, sharps container, alcohol prep).

❏ Cleanse the skin with an alcohol prep. Allow the alcohol to dry before performing the stick.

❏ Use the lancet to perform a stick. Wipe away the first drop of blood that appears. Squeeze the puncture wound to get a second drop of blood.

❏ Apply the blood to the test strip. This may be done by holding strip to the finger to draw the blood into the strip.

❏ Dispose of the lancet in a sharps container.

❏ Read the blood glucose level displayed on the glucose meter. It may take from 15 to 60 seconds for the device to provide a reading. (Newer devices take 5 seconds and less blood).

❏ Assess the puncture site and apply direct pressure or a band-aid to control the bleeding.

The reading is in mg/dl (milligrams of glucose per deciliter of blood). Normal "fasting" blood sugar values are 70–110 mg/dl. If the patient has a value less than 60–80 mg/dl and is symptomatic, treatment should be provided following local medical control.

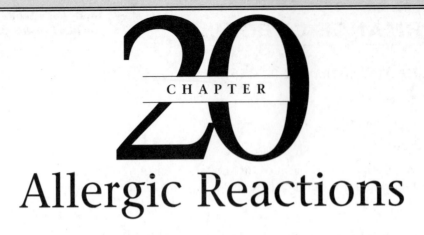

CHAPTER 20

Allergic Reactions

MATCH TERMINOLOGY/ DEFINITIONS

A. Red, itchy, possibly raised blotches on the skin that often result from an allergic reaction

B. Severe or life-threatening allergic reaction in which the blood vessels dilate, causing a drop in blood pressure, and the tissues lining the respiratory system swell, interfering with the airway

C. Something that causes an allergic reaction

D. Hormone produced by the body; as a medication, it constricts blood vessels and dilates respiratory passages and is used to relieve severe allergic reactions

E. Syringe, preloaded with medication, that has a spring-loaded device that pushes the needle through the skin when the tip of the device is pressed firmly against the body

_____ **1.** Allergen

_____ **2.** Anaphylaxis

_____ **3.** Auto-injector

_____ **4.** Epinephrine

_____ **5.** Hives

MULTIPLE-CHOICE REVIEW

_____ **1.** An exaggerated response of the body's immune system to any substance is called a(n) _____ reaction.
   A. vasoconstricting
   B. immune
   C. allergic
   D. syncopal

_____ **2.** Why are allergic reactions sometimes treated as a high priority?
   A. The patient can vomit.
   B. The patient can become covered with hives.
   C. They can speed up the heart rate.
   D. They can cause airway obstruction.

©2009 Pearson Education, Inc.
Emergency Care, 11th Ed.

_____ **3.** The first time a person is exposed to an allergen, the person's immune system:
   A. reacts violently.
   B. shuts down.
   C. forms antibodies.
   D. ignores the allergen.

_____ **4.** The second time a person is exposed to an allergen, the body reactions may include all of the following except:
   A. destruction of antibodies.
   B. difficulty breathing.
   C. massive swelling.
   D. dilation of the blood vessels.

_____ **5.** Common causes of allergic reactions include all of the following except:
   A. hornet stings.
   B. eggs and milk.
   C. poison ivy and penicillin.
   D. red fruits and vegetables.

_____ **6.** Why is it important to find out if a patient is allergic to latex?
   A. so you do not wear gloves that could cause an allergic reaction
   B. because the patient will also be allergic to milk
   C. because latex allergy can produce antitoxins
   D. because a latex allergy causes immediate cardiac arrest

_____ **7.** The respiratory signs and symptoms of anaphylactic shock include all of the following except:
   A. rapid breathing.
   B. hives.
   C. cough.
   D. stridor.

_____ **8.** The effects on the cardiac system of an allergic reaction could include _____ heart rate and _____ blood pressure.
   A. decreased, decreased
   B. increased, increased
   C. decreased, increased
   D. increased, decreased

_____ **9.** To be considered a severe allergic reaction, a patient must have signs and symptoms of shock or:
   A. a history of allergies.
   B. massive swelling.
   C. respiratory distress.
   D. increased blood pressure.

_____ **10.** After administering epinephrine, the EMT should:
   A. prepare another dose.
   B. reassess the patient after 2 minutes.
   C. decrease the oxygen being administered.
   D. allow the patient to remain at home.

_____ **11.** If you see a patient who has no history of allergies and is having her first allergic reaction, you should:
   A. consult with medical direction.
   B. treat for shock and transport immediately.
   C. administer epinephrine via auto-injector.
   D. attempt to determine the cause immediately.

_____ **12.** If a patient has an epinephrine auto-injector, besides helping him take the medication, you should always:
   A. ask if the patient has any spare auto-injectors for the trip to the hospital.
   B. call the patient's physician and request another dosage of the medication.
   C. determine if other family members have a history of allergic reactions.
   D. take the insect or substance that caused the reaction to the hospital.

_____ **13.** The recommended location for injection with the auto-injector is the:
  A. center of the back.
  B. lateral mid-thigh.
  C. buttocks.
  D. biceps.

_____ **14.** Epinephrine auto-injectors come in two different sizes. The child size contains:
  A. 0.05 mg.   **C.** 0.5 mg.
  B. 0.15 mg.   **D.** 1.0 mg.

_____ **15.** Which statement is true related to anaphylactic reactions in infants and children?
  A. Infants frequently experience anaphylactic reactions.
  B. Children "outgrow" allergies as they mature.
  C. Anaphylactic reactions are common in younger children.
  D. Parents seldom can provide useful information about the child's medical history.

COMPLETE THE FOLLOWING

1. List ten signs and symptoms of allergic reaction or anaphylactic shock.

  A. _____

  B. _____

  C. _____

  D. _____

  E. _____

  F. _____

  G. _____

  H. _____

  I. _____

  J. _____

2. For a patient to be considered in anaphylaxis, list two signs, either of which must be evident.

  A. _____

  B. _____

©2009 Pearson Education, Inc.
Emergency Care, 11th Ed.

LABEL THE DIAGRAMS

Fill in the name of each substance that may cause an allergic reaction on the line provided.

1. _____

2. _____

3. _____

4. _____

1.

2.

3.

4.

STREET SCENES DISCUSSION

Review the Street Scene on pp. 487–488 of the textbook. Then answer the questions below.

1. If the patient had an epinephrine auto-injector, would it be appropriate to use it in this situation? If so, where would you inject it?

2. Would it be appropriate to call for an estimated time of arrival (ETA) on the ALS unit? Why or why not?

3. If the patient went into cardiac arrest, what would be your patient-care priorities?

ON THE WEB

To help you review and practice basic skills, visit the *Emergency Care 11th Ed. Companion Website* at www.prenhall.com/limmer. For Online Test Preparation, visit www.prenhall.com/emtachieve.

EMT SKILLS PERFORMANCE CHECKLIST

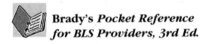 Brady's *Pocket Reference for BLS Providers, 3rd Ed.*

▶ **EPINEPHRINE AUTO-INJECTOR ASSIST* (PP. 482–485)**

❑ Take Standard Precautions.

❑ Perform an initial assessment. Provide high-concentration oxygen by nonrebreather mask.

❑ Obtain SAMPLE history.

❑ Take patient's vital signs.**

❑ Contact medical direction for authorization (or follow written standing order).

❑ Obtain patient's prescribed auto-injector.

❑ Check medication for expiration date.

❑ Check medication for cloudiness or discoloration.

❑ Remove safety cap from the injector.

❑ Assure injector is prescribed for patient.

❑ Remove cap from auto-injector. Place tip of auto-injector against patient's thigh (lateral portion, midway between waist and knee).

❑ Push injector firmly against thigh until injector activates.

❑ Hold injector in place until medication is injected (at least 10 seconds).

❑ Properly discard auto-injector in biohazard container.

❑ Document patient's response to medication and time.

❑ Perform ongoing assessment, paying special attention to the patient's ABCs and vital signs, while transporting.

*NOTE: These patients change very quickly so move quickly!

**NOTE: Initial reassessment 2 minutes post-epi administration.

©2009 Pearson Education, Inc.
Emergency Care, 11th Ed.

CASE STUDY

▶ **THE LAKEFRONT EMERGENCY**

You respond to a camp on the lake for a call from a woman having difficulty breathing. Upon your arrival, after ensuring the scene is safe, you find a woman in her forties who is clutching her chest and is having obvious breathing difficulty.

1. Is there a need for another ambulance?

2. Should you call for an ALS unit to respond?

After taking Standard Precautions, you begin your initial assessment. There is no reason to suspect trauma, and the patient has an open airway. She is responsive, although she talks in short, choppy sentences. She knows her name, where she is, and the day of the week.

3. Why is she talking in short, choppy sentences?

4. What would be your assessment of her level of responsiveness?

A high-pitched musical tone is heard as she breathes. She shows other signs of respiratory distress.

5. What is the name of her breathing sound, and what are some of the potential causes of this sound?

6. What are some additional signs of breathing difficulty that you may observe in this patient?

You decide that beginning oxygen administration is an appropriate thing to do at this time.

7. How would you deliver the oxygen, and how many liters per minute would you administer?

You note the patient has a weak and rapid radial pulse. There is no reason to suspect any life-threatening external bleeding in this instance. The patient is very pale and is sweating profusely. She also complains of chest tightness and dizziness, which she denies she has ever had before.

8. Would you prioritize this patient as a low or high priority? Why?

9. What would be the best position in which to transport the patient and why?

As you begin to prepare the patient for transport, you start the focused history and physical exam. The patient has chest tightness and breathing difficulty, which came on suddenly. The pain is across the upper chest, doesn't radiate, and is constant. Nothing the patient does makes the pain go away; she states it is a 7 on a scale of 1 to 10 with 10 being the worst pain she ever had. The pain has been present for approximately 15 minutes. You assign a crew member to obtain a complete set of vital signs as you quickly listen to her lungs. She has a weak and rapid pulse at 110, respirations are labored at 26 per minute, and her blood pressure is 88/50 mmHg.

©2009 Pearson Education, Inc.
Emergency Care, 11th Ed.

10. As you load the patient into the ambulance, what additional history should you obtain?

Your patient states she was cleaning out the gutter and may have been stung by a bee. She previously reacted severely to a bee sting and carries a "bee-sting kit."

11. A) What medicine is usually in these kits? **B)** Should you help her take the medicine?

12. A) Is it necessary to call a doctor? **B)** What must be checked prior to administering the medicine?

As you leave the scene, the driver arranges for an ALS intercept on the way to the hospital. Other than reassessing the patient after administering the medication, you continue to monitor the patient. About 5 minutes en route, your driver pulls the ambulance to the side of the road momentarily as the ALS paramedic jumps in with his equipment. Then you proceed to the hospital.

13. What would be your quick report to the paramedic on **A)** the patient's chief complaint, **B)** your assessment of the situation, and **C)** the treatment you have given?

14. What care would you expect to see the paramedic give en route to the hospital?

MATCH TERMINOLOGY/ DEFINITIONS

A. Any substance that can harm the body by altering cell structure or functions

B. Stimulants, such as amphetamines, that affect the central nervous system to excite the user

C. State in which a patient's body reacts severely when deprived of an abused substance

D. Poisons that are taken into the body through unbroken skin

E. Depressants, such as barbiturates, that depress the central nervous system

F. Poisons that are swallowed

G. Class of drugs that affect the nervous system and change many normal body activities; their legal use is for relief of pain

H. Substance that adsorbs many poisons and prevents them from being absorbed by the body

I. Thinning down or weakening by mixing with something else

J. Severe reaction that can be part of alcohol withdrawal, characterized by sweating, trembling, anxiety, and hallucinations

K. Poisons that are breathed in

L. Mind-affecting or mind-altering drugs that act on the central nervous system to produce excitement and distortion of perceptions

_____ **1.** Absorbed poisons

_____ **2.** Activated charcoal

_____ **3.** Antidote

_____ **4.** Delirium tremens

_____ **5.** Dilution

_____ **6.** Downers

_____ **7.** Hallucinogens

_____ **8.** Ingested poisons

_____ **9.** Inhaled poisons

_____ **10.** Narcotics

_____ **11.** Poison

_____ **12.** Toxin

_____ **13.** Uppers

_____ **14.** Volatile chemicals

_____ **15.** Withdrawal

©2009 Pearson Education, Inc.
Emergency Care, 11th Ed.

M. Poisonous substance secreted by bacteria, plants, or animals

N. Vaporizing compounds, such as cleaning fluid, that are breathed in by an abuser to produce a "high"

O. Substance that will neutralize a poison or its effects

MULTIPLE-CHOICE REVIEW

_____ **1.** Which of the following is an environmental clue at the scene that can be used to help you determine that your patient may have been poisoned?
   A. The patient appears to have been vomiting.
   B. There is an empty pill bottle on the night table.
   C. The patient has an altered mental status.
   D. The patient states that he or she has a headache.

_____ **2.** Which of the following is the most accurate definition of a poison?
   A poison is any:
   A. substance that can harm the body, sometimes seriously enough to create a medical emergency.
   B. foreign substance swallowed by the patient.
   C. substance that could kill the patient if it is injected into the body.
   D. substance labeled with a hazardous material placard or label.

_____ **3.** Most of the over one million poisonings in the United States yearly are due to:
   A. suicide attempts by adults.
   B. attempts to murder someone.
   C. accidents involving young children.
   D. teenagers on illicit drugs.

_____ **4.** A substance secreted by plants, animals, or bacteria that is poisonous to humans is called a:
   A. chemical.   **C.** narcotic.
   B. toxin.   **D.** drug.

_____ **5.** Due to the poisons they produce, plants such as _____ can be dangerous to humans or pets.
   A. mistletoe   **C.** rubber plants
   B. mushrooms   **D.** all of the above

_____ **6.** Bacteria may produce toxins that cause deadly diseases such as:
   A. HIV.   **C.** penicillin.
   B. botulism.   **D.** steroids.

_____ **7.** For most poisonous substances, the reaction is more serious in:
   A. the evening hours.
   B. the elderly and the ill.
   C. smaller concentrations.
   D. summer.

_____ **8.** Which one of the following is <u>not</u> a way that poisons damage the body?
   A. destroying skin and other tissues
   B. enhancing normal biochemical processes
   C. overstimulating the central nervous system
   D. displacing oxygen on the hemoglobin

_____ **9.** Poisons may enter the body through any of the following routes <u>except</u>:
   A. inhalation.   **C.** injection.
   B. ingestion.   **D.** excretion.

_____ 10. Carbon monoxide, chlorine, and sulfur are examples of _____ poisons:
   A. ingested
   B. injected
   C. inhaled
   D. swallowed

_____ 11. Examples of absorbed poisons include:
   A. insecticides and agricultural chemicals.
   B. carbon monoxide and chlorine.
   C. insect stings and snake bites.
   D. aspirin and LSD.

_____ 12. The venom of a snake bite is an example of an _____ poison.
   A. ingested
   B. injected
   C. inhaled
   D. absorbed

_____ 13. Why is it important to determine when the ingestion of a poison occurred?
   A. Different poisons act on the body at different rates.
   B. Those who ingest poison in the evening tend to vomit more.
   C. Dilution of the poison is not effective after 10 minutes.
   D. The antidote will work more effectively once the poison is in the intestines.

_____ 14. If you suspect poisoning by ingestion, after assuring a child has a patent airway, ask the parent for the child's:
   A. name.
   B. weight.
   C. last visit to a physician.
   D. favorite drink.

_____ 15. The most common results of poison ingestion are:
   A. altered mental status and diarrhea.
   B. nausea and vomiting.
   C. abdominal pain and diarrhea.
   D. chemical burns around the mouth and stomach pain.

_____ 16. Activated charcoal is used to:
   A. act as an antidote.
   B. dilute the poisonous substance.
   C. reduce the amount of poison absorbed by the body.
   D. speed up the digestion of most chemicals in the body.

_____ 17. The difference between activated charcoal and regular charcoal is that:
   A. activated charcoal is manufactured to have many cracks and crevices.
   B. regular charcoal is too large to swallow.
   C. activated charcoal is mixed with a substance to cause vomiting.
   D. regular charcoal is not diluted when used.

_____ 18. The decision on when to use activated charcoal is best made:
   A. en route to the hospital.
   B. upon arrival at the emergency department.
   C. with medical direction or poison-control center consultation.
   D. in consultation with the patient's family physician.

_____ 19. Activated charcoal is <u>not</u> routinely used with ingestion of:
   A. caustic substances.
   B. strong acids.
   C. strong alkalis.
   D. all of the above.

_____ 20. Examples of caustic substances include all of the following <u>except</u>:
   A. lye.
   B. venom.
   C. toilet bowl cleaner.
   D. oven cleaner.

_____ 21. A patient who continues to cough violently after a gasoline ingestion should:
   A. not be given activated charcoal.
   B. not be given oxygen.
   C. be transported immediately.
   D. be treated like a patient with an airway obstruction.

_____ 22. When a physician orders dilution of an ingested substance, you can use either water or:
  A. a cola drink.
  B. coffee.
  C. milk.
  D. apple juice.

_____ 23. The most common inhaled poison is:
  A. carbon dioxide.
  B. nitrogen.
  C. carbon monoxide.
  D. phosgene.

_____ 24. As you approach a patient who has passed out while cleaning a large tank, you smell an unusual odor. What should you do?
  A. Stand back and attempt to learn more about the chemical involved.
  B. Rapidly remove the patient from the area using a drag maneuver.
  C. Ignore the smell; it is probably a normal odor around industrial sites.
  D. Ask his coworkers to bring the patient to your ambulance.

_____ 25. The principal prehospital treatment of a patient who has inhaled poison is:
  A. administering activated charcoal to the patient.
  B. administering high-concentration oxygen.
  C. providing full spinal immobilization.
  D. administering an antidote.

_____ 26. Besides motor vehicle exhaust, where else might you find carbon monoxide?
  A. in the patient compartment of your ambulance
  B. wherever you can smell its odor
  C. around an improperly vented wood-burning stove
  D. around the foundation of a house

_____ 27. How does carbon monoxide affect the body?
  A. It causes severe respiratory burns.
  B. It prevents the normal carrying of oxygen by the red blood cells.
  C. It causes the tissues in the airway to swell, making breathing difficult.
  D. It stimulates the central nervous system to decrease oxygen consumption.

_____ 28. A conscious patient who you suspect has carbon monoxide poisoning may exhibit any of the following except:
  A. cyanosis.
  B. altered mental status.
  C. dizziness.
  D. cherry red lips.

_____ 29. If a patient has been contaminated by a poisonous powder, how should she be treated?
  A. Brush off as much powder as possible, then irrigate.
  B. Immediately start irrigation with very cold water.
  C. Leave the powder in place and transport immediately.
  D. Irrigate with water for 20 minutes.

_____ 30. If you smell alcohol on the breath or clothes of a patient, you should:
  A. call for police immediately.
  B. not let this sidetrack you from doing a complete assessment.
  C. ask the patient how much he has had to drink today.
  D. assume that the patient will not give you the entire truth about his condition.

_____ 31. Of the following signs and symptoms, which one is not seen with alcohol abuse but is seen with a diabetic emergency?
  A. acetone breath
  B. hallucinations
  C. slurred speech
  D. swaying and unsteadiness of movement

_____ 32. The sweating, trembling, anxiety, and hallucinations found in the alcohol withdrawal patient are called:
  A. withdrawal signs.
  B. seizures.
  C. delirium tremens.
  D. Parkinson's tremors.

_____ **33.** A patient who has mixed alcohol and drugs will exhibit:
   A. uncontrolled shivering.
   B. depressed vital signs.
   C. extreme calmness.
   D. all of the above.

_____ **34.** When interviewing an intoxicated patient, do not begin by asking if he has taken any drugs. The reason for this statement is that:
   A. the presence of drugs will negate the presence of the alcohol.
   B. the patient may feel you are accusing him of a crime.
   C. alcoholics generally do not take drugs.
   D. the patient would probably not tell the truth.

_____ **35.** Drugs that stimulate the nervous system to excite the user are called:
   A. uppers.   **C.** narcotics.
   B. downers.   **D.** antihypertensives.

_____ **36.** Tranquilizers or sleeping pills are examples of:
   A. uppers.   **C.** narcotics.
   B. downers.   **D.** hallucinogens.

_____ **37.** Drugs that have a depressant effect on the central nervous system are called:
   A. uppers.   **C.** narcotics.
   B. downers.   **D.** hallucinogens.

_____ **38.** Drugs capable of producing stupor or sleep that are often used to relieve pain are called:
   A. uppers.   **C.** narcotics.
   B. downers.   **D.** hallucinogens.

_____ **39.** Mind-altering drugs that act on the nervous system to produce an intense state of excitement or distortion of the user's perceptions are called:
   A. uppers.   **C.** narcotics.
   B. downers.   **D.** hallucinogens.

_____ **40.** A class of drugs that have few legal uses and are dissolved in the mouth are called:
   A. narcotics.   **C.** hallucinogens.
   B. uppers.   **D.** downers.

_____ **41.** Cleaning fluid, glue, and model cement are examples of:
   A. hallucinogens.   **C.** diuretics.
   B. volatile chemicals.   **D.** narcotics.

_____ **42.** A patient who has overdosed on an upper may have signs and symptoms such as:
   A. excitement, increased pulse and breathing rates, dilated pupils, and rapid speech.
   B. sluggishness, sleepiness, and lack of coordination of body and speech.
   C. fast pulse rate, dilated pupils, flushed face, and "see" or "hear" things.
   D. reduced pulse rate and rate and depth of breathing, constricted pupils, and sweating.

_____ **43.** A patient who has overdosed on a downer may have signs and symptoms such as:
   A. excitement, increased pulse and breathing rates, dilated pupils, and rapid speech.
   B. sluggishness, sleepiness, and lack of coordination of body and speech.
   C. fast pulse rate, dilated pupils, flushed face, and "see" or "hear" things.
   D. reduced pulse rate and rate and depth of breathing, constricted pupils, and sweating.

©2009 Pearson Education, Inc.
Emergency Care, 11th Ed.

_____ **44.** A patient who has overdosed on a hallucinogen may have signs and symptoms such as:
  A. excitement, increased pulse and breathing rates, dilated pupils, and rapid speech.
  B. sluggishness, sleepiness, and lack of coordination of body and speech.
  C. fast pulse rate, dilated pupils, flushed face, and "see" or "hear" things.
  D. reduced pulse rate and rate and depth of breathing, constricted pupils, and sweating.

_____ **45.** A patient who has overdosed on a narcotic may have signs and symptoms such as:
  A. excitement, increased pulse and breathing rates, dilated pupils, and rapid speech.
  B. sluggishness, sleepiness, and lack of coordination of body and speech.
  C. fast pulse rate, dilated pupils, flushed face, and "see" or "hear" things.
  D. reduced pulse rate and rate and depth of breathing, constricted pupils, and sweating.

COMPLETE THE FOLLOWING

1. What information should the EMT document for medical direction when treating a patient he or she suspects was poisoned?

A. _____

B. _____

C. _____

D. _____

E. _____

F. _____

G. _____

H. _____

2. List at least six signs and symptoms of alcohol abuse.

A. _____

B. _____

C. _____

D. _____

E. _____

F. _____

LABEL THE DIAGRAMS

Fill in the way that each type of poison enters the body.

1. _____

2. _____

3. _____

4. _____

1.

Cleaning fluid

Sprays

2.

Drugs

3.

Lye

Rat poison

Drain cleaners

4.

Household cleaners

Insecticides

COMPLETE THE CHART

Fill in the type of commonly abused drug on the line provided. Indicate on the chart whether each drug is an upper, downer, narcotic, mind-altering, or volatile chemical.

AMPHETAMINE   1. _____

CODEINE   2. _____

LSD   3. _____

PSILOCYBIN   4. _____

GASOLINE   5. _____

SECOBARBITAL   6. _____

METHAQUALONE   7. _____

COCAINE   8. _____

DEXTROAMPHETAMINE   9. _____

CHLORAL HYDRATE   10. _____

MESCALINE   11. _____

MORNING GLORY SEEDS	12. _____
STP	13. _____
HEROIN	14. _____
BUTYL NITRATE	15. _____
PCP	16. _____
PRELUDIN	17. _____
METHADONE	18. _____
BARBITURATES	19. _____
DEMEROL	20. _____
PHENOBARBITAL	21. _____
MARIJUANA	22. _____
OPIUM	23. _____
AMYL NITRATE	24. _____
CARBON TETRACHLORIDE	25. _____

STREET SCENES DISCUSSION

Review the Street Scene on pp. 514–515 of the textbook. Then answer the questions below.

1. Imagine you were confronted with an infant who had an altered mental status, as well as evidence of ingested poison. Would you quickly administer activated charcoal to the patient? Why or why not?

2. If the infant continues to vomit, what emergency care should be your highest priority?

3. Why is it necessary to take the oil to the hospital?

ON THE WEB

To help you review and practice basic skills, visit the *Emergency Care 11th Ed.*
Companion Website at www.prenhall.com/limmer. For Online Test Preparation,
visit www.prenhall.com/emtachieve.

EMT SKILL
PERFORMANCE CHECKLISTS

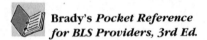

Brady's *Pocket Reference*
for BLS Providers, 3rd Ed.

▶ **MANAGEMENT OF INGESTED POISONS (P. 495)**

❑ Take Standard Precautions.

❑ Conduct an initial assessment.

❑ Maintain an open airway.

❑ Perform a focused history and physical exam, including SAMPLE history
and vital signs.

❑ Quickly gather information about the substance.

❑ Call medical direction on the scene or en route.

❑ If directed, administer activated charcoal.

❑ Position patient for vomiting and save all vomitus. Have suction ready.

❑ Perform an ongoing assessment.

❑ Transport as soon as possible.

▶ **MANAGEMENT OF INHALED POISONS (P. 500)**

❑ Size-up the situation, and take the necessary precautions to prevent injury
to yourself and your crew.*

❑ Take Standard Precautions. Remove patient from the source. Avoid
contaminating yourself with poison.

❑ Maintain open airway. Stay alert for vomiting. Properly position the patient
and have suction equipment ready.

❑ Conduct an initial assessment.

❑ Administer high-concentration oxygen by nonrebreather mask.

❑ Perform a focused history and physical exam, including SAMPLE history.

❑ Remove contaminated clothing and other articles (e.g., shoes, jewelry).

❑ Assess baseline vital signs.

❑ Quickly gather information about the product (containers, bottles, and labels).

❑ Call medical direction on the scene or en route.

❑ Transport as soon as possible.

❑ Perform ongoing assessment en route.

*SAFETY NOTE: In the presence of hazardous fumes or gases, wear protective clothing and
self-contained breathing apparatus or wait for those who are properly trained and equipped
to enter the scene and bring the patient out to a safe area.

▶ MANAGEMENT OF ABSORBED POISONS (P. 502)

- ❑ Size-up the situation, and take the necessary precautions to prevent injury to yourself and your crew.

- ❑ Take Standard Precautions.

- ❑ Remove the patient from the source. Avoid contaminating yourself with the poison.

- ❑ Conduct an initial assessment.

- ❑ Maintain an open airway.

- ❑ Administer high-concentration oxygen.

- ❑ Perform a focused history and physical exam, including SAMPLE history and vital signs.

- ❑ Brush powders from the patient. Be careful not to abrade the patient's skin.

- ❑ Remove contaminated clothing and other articles such as shoes and jewelry.

- ❑ Quickly gather information about the product.

- ❑ If appropriate, irrigate with a large amount of clear water for at least 20 minutes. Call medical direction.

- ❑ Perform an ongoing assessment.

- ❑ Be alert for shock, and transport as soon as possible.

CHAPTER 22

Environmental Emergencies

MATCH TERMINOLOGY/ DEFINITIONS

▶ **PART A**

A. Change from liquid to gas; as perspiration on the skin vaporizes, the body experiences a cooling effect

B. Abbreviation that stands for arterial gas embolism

C. Application of an external heat source to rewarm the body of a hypothermic patient

D. Carrying away of heat by currents of air or water or other gases or liquids

E. Death caused by changes in the lungs resulting from immersion in water

F. Direct transfer of heat from one material to another through direct contact

G. Condition resulting from nitrogen trapped in the body's tissues caused by coming up too quickly from a deep, prolonged dive

H. Application of heat to the lateral chest, neck, armpits, and groin of a hypothermic patient

I. Increase in body temperature above normal; life-threatening in its extreme

J. Gas bubble in the bloodstream; more accurately called an arterial gas embolism

_____ **1.** Active rewarming

_____ **2.** AGE

_____ **3.** Air embolism

_____ **4.** Central rewarming

_____ **5.** Conduction

_____ **6.** Convection

_____ **7.** Decompression sickness

_____ **8.** Drowning

_____ **9.** Evaporation

_____ **10.** Hyperthermia

PART B

A. The process of experiencing respiratory impairment from submersion or immersion in liquid; the person may live or die

B. Covering a hypothermic patient and taking other steps to prevent further heat loss and help the body rewarm itself

C. Sending out energy, such as heat, in waves into space

D. Breathing; during this process, the body loses heat as warm air is exhaled from the body

E. Cooling or freezing of particular parts of the body

F. Generalized cooling that reduces body temperature below normal; life-threatening in its extreme

G. Substances produced by animals or plants that are poisonous to humans

H. Chilling caused by conduction of heat from the body when the body or clothing is wet

I. Toxin produced by certain animals such as snakes, spiders, and some marine life-forms

J. Chilling caused by convection of heat from the body in the presence of air currents

_____ 1. Hypothermia

_____ 2. Local cooling

_____ 3. Drowning

_____ 4. Passive rewarming

_____ 5. Radiation

_____ 6. Respiration

_____ 7. Toxins

_____ 8. Venom

_____ 9. Water chill

_____ 10. Wind chill

MULTIPLE-CHOICE REVIEW

_____ 1. Water conducts heat away from the body _____ than still air.
   A. 25 times faster
   B. 25 times slower
   C. 50 times faster
   D. 50 times slower

_____ 2. The body loses heat from respiration, radiation, conduction, convection, and:
   A. excretion.
   B. induction.
   C. evaporation.
   D. condensation.

_____ 3. When there is _____ wind, there is _____ heat loss.
   A. more, less
   B. less, greater
   C. more, greater
   D. no, maximum

_____ 4. Most radiant heat loss occurs from a person's:
   A. arms and legs.
   B. chest and back.
   C. head and neck.
   D. feet and hands.

_____ 5. Predisposing factors to hypothermia include all of the following except:
   A. burns.
   B. diabetes.
   C. spinal-cord injuries.
   D. headache.

_____ 6. Which one of the following is not a reason infants and children are more prone to hypothermia?
   A. They have small muscle mass.
   B. They have large skin surface in relation to their total body mass.
   C. They are unable to shiver effectively.
   D. They have more body fat than adults do.

_____ 7. You are treating an elderly patient with a possible leg fracture who was found lying on his cold garage floor where he had been all night. You should also consider:
A. stroke.
B. hypothermia.
C. pulmonary edema.
D. hyperperfusion.

_____ 8. When a patient's core body temperature drops below 90°F, the patient:
A. may be shivering uncontrollably.
B. may no longer be shivering.
C. will be pulseless.
D. will suddenly become alert.

_____ 9. All of the following are signs and symptoms of hypothermia <u>except</u>:
A. high blood pressure and low pulse.
B. stiff or rigid posture.
C. cool abdominal skin temperature.
D. loss of motor coordination.

_____ 10. Passive rewarming involves:
A. applying heat packs to the patient.
B. covering the patient.
C. administering heated oxygen to the patient.
D. massaging the patient's limbs.

_____ 11. The treatment of the hypothermic patient who is alert and responding may include all of the following <u>except</u>:
A. removal of all of the patient's wet clothing.
B. actively rewarming the patient during transport.
C. rapidly giving the patient plenty of hot liquids.
D. providing care for shock and providing oxygen.

_____ 12. When actively rewarming a patient:
A. apply heat to the chest, neck, armpits, and groin.
B. quickly rewarm the patient.
C. give the patient stimulants to drink.
D. immerse the arms and feet in hot water.

_____ 13. The reason why you should rewarm the body's core first is to:
A. prevent blood from collecting in the extremities due to vasodilation.
B. quickly circulate cold blood throughout the body.
C. speed up the blood flow to the extremities.
D. increase blood flow to the brain to prevent unconsciousness.

_____ 14. When transporting an alert patient with mild hypothermia, it is recommended that you:
A. transport in Fowler's position.
B. massage the legs so the patient can walk.
C. keep the patient at rest.
D. leave the wet clothes in place.

_____ 15. In a heat emergency, EMT care of a patient with moist, pale, normal-to-cool skin includes all of the following <u>except</u>:
A. place the patient in an air-conditioned ambulance.
B. fan the patient so he begins to shiver.
C. elevate the patient's legs.
D. administer oxygen.

_____ 16. In a heat emergency, if a patient with moist, pale, normal-to-cool skin is responsive and not nauseated, the EMT should:
A. skip the oxygen.
B. place cold packs in the patient's armpits.
C. have the patient drink water.
D. do all of the above.

©2009 Pearson Education, Inc.
Emergency Care, 11th Ed.

_____ **17.** When treating the unresponsive patient with severe hypothermia:
   A. keep the patient's head raised above the feet for the transport to the hospital.
   B. place the patient in a warm bathtub for at least 20 minutes.
   C. provide high-concentration oxygen that has been passed through a warm humidifier.
   D. massage the extremities for 35–45 seconds.

_____ **18.** Because patients with extreme hypothermia may not reach biological death for over 30 minutes, the medical philosophy is:
   A. if there is a pulse, start CPR.
   B. they are not dead until they're warm and dead.
   C. resuscitate for no longer than 30 minutes.
   D. always resuscitate very aggressively.

_____ **19.** A cold injury usually occurring to exposed areas of the body that is brought about by direct contact with a cold object or exposure to cold air is called:
   A. an early local cold injury.   **C.** frostbite.
   B. a superficial late cold injury.   **D.** a deep local cold injury.

_____ **20.** The skin color of a patient with a superficial local cold injury will change from _____ to _____ .
   A. red, white   **C.** red, blue
   B. white, red   **D.** white, blue

_____ **21.** If a superficial local cold injury is on an extremity, the EMT should:
   A. splint and leave uncovered.
   B. rub the extremity briskly.
   C. not re-expose the injury to cold.
   D. immerse the extremity in hot water.

_____ **22.** When muscles, bones, deep blood vessels, and organ membranes become frozen, this type of injury is called:
   A. a superficial local cold injury.   **C.** a deep local cold injury.
   B. frostnip.   **D.** local cooling.

_____ **23.** In frostbite, the affected area first appears:
   A. black and stiff.   **C.** red and blotchy.
   B. white and waxy.   **D.** blue and abraded.

_____ **24.** Do not allow the frostbite patient to smoke or drink alcohol because:
   A. the patient may suffer altered mental status or fall asleep.
   B. these would stimulate the patient to move, which could cause further injury.
   C. constriction of blood vessels and decreased circulation to the injured tissues may result.
   D. either could contaminate the frostbitten area.

_____ **25.** Active rewarming of a frozen part:
   A. is seldom recommended in the field.
   B. includes using very hot water.
   C. is performed without removing the patient's clothing.
   D. includes covering the patient's face.

_____ **26.** When assessing a patient you suspect is in extreme hypothermia, check the carotid pulse for _____ seconds.
   A. 5–10   **C.** 30–45
   B. 15–25   **D.** 50–60

_____ **27.** The environment associated with hyperthermia includes heat and:
   A. high winds.   **C.** high humidity.
   B. light rain.   **D.** low humidity.

_____ 28. The higher the humidity is, the:
   A. less you perspire.
   B. less your perspiration evaporates.
   C. less you radiate heat.
   D. more you lose heat from your body.

_____ 29. The medical problems resulting from dry heat are often worse than those from moist heat because:
   A. dry heat is more common.
   B. moist heat tires people quickly.
   C. dry heat causes more sunburn.
   D. dry heat affects the respiratory system more quickly.

_____ 30. When salts are lost by the body through sweating, the patient may have all of the following except:
   A. muscle cramps.
   B. weakness or exhaustion.
   C. dizziness or periods of faintness.
   D. fluid buildup in the lungs.

_____ 31. A patient with heat exhaustion will present with:
   A. dry, hot skin.   C. a lack of sweating.
   B. moist, pale, normal-to-cool skin.   D. rapid strong pulse.

_____ 32. The signs and symptoms of a heat emergency in patients who have hot, dry or moist skin include:
   A. slow and shallow breathing.   C. constricted pupils.
   B. seizures.   D. muscle cramps.

_____ 33. The signs and symptoms of a heat emergency in patients who have hot, dry or moist skin include all the following except:
   A. generalized weakness.
   B. loss of consciousness or altered mental status.
   C. profuse perspiration.
   D. full and rapid pulse.

_____ 34. Which of the following is a large contributor to adolescent and adult drownings?
   A. inexperience with equipment   C. stomach cramps
   B. substance abuse   D. car crash immersions

_____ 35. During a drowning submersion incident, water flowing past the epiglottis causes:
   A. a reflex to close the mouth.
   B. the victim to gasp for more air.
   C. a reflex spasm of the larynx.
   D. the victim to begin hyperventilating.

_____ 36. About 10% of drowning submersion victims die from:
   A. too much fluid in their lungs.   C. cervical spine injuries.
   B. lack of air.   D. crushing chest injury.

_____ 37. If you are not an experienced swimmer, you should:
   A. never attempt to go into the water to do a rescue.
   B. don a floatation device prior to going into the water.
   C. use a boat as your first approach to conduct the rescue.
   D. coach the patient in floating techniques.

_____ 38. If you suspect that a patient still in the pool has a possible spine injury:
   A. spineboard the patient as you pull him from the water.
   B. immobilize and spineboard the patient while still in the water.
   C. quickly remove the patient from the water to prevent hypothermia.
   D. encourage the patient to swim to the side of the pool.

©2009 Pearson Education, Inc.
Emergency Care, 11th Ed.

_____ 39. Two special medical problems seen in scuba-diving accidents are decompression sickness and:
   A. carbon monoxide poisoning.   C. air embolism.
   B. oxygen toxicity.   D. arthritis.

_____ 40. The risk of decompression sickness is increased by:
   A. air travel within 12 hours of a dive.
   B. breathing 100% oxygen immediately after the dive.
   C. drinking fluids before and after the dive.
   D. none of the above.

_____ 41. A toxin produced by some animals that is harmful to humans is called:
   A. poison.   C. venom.
   B. lymph.   D. allergen.

_____ 42. Typical sources of injected poisons include _____ bites or stings.
   A. spider   C. snake
   B. scorpion   D. all of the above

_____ 43. While cleaning out the crawl space below the house, you experience blotchy skin, redness in your arm, weakness, and nausea. It is possible that you:
   A. are developing heat stroke.
   B. were bitten by a poisonous spider.
   C. are having a diabetic reaction.
   D. are allergic to something in the air.

_____ 44. Signs and symptoms of injected poisoning include all of the following except:
   A. lack of sensation in one side of the body.
   B. puncture marks.
   C. muscle cramps, chest tightening, and joint pains.
   D. excessive saliva formation and profuse sweating.

_____ 45. If you suspect that your patient has been bitten by a snake, you should do all of the following except:
   A. call for medical direction.
   B. clean the injection site with soap and water.
   C. remove rings, bracelets, or other constricting items on the bitten limb.
   D. capture the live snake and bring it in the ambulance to the emergency department.

COMPLETE THE FOLLOWING

1. List six signs and symptoms of heat exhaustion.

A. _____

B. _____

C. _____

D. _____

E. _____

F. _____

2. List six signs and symptoms of heat stroke.

A. _____

B. _____

C. _____

D. _____

E. _____

F. _____

3. List ten signs and symptoms of an insect, spider, or scorpion bite or sting.

A. _____

B. _____

C. _____

D. _____

E. _____

F. _____

G. _____

H. _____

I. _____

J. _____

4. List five signs and/or symptoms of a snake bite.

A. _____

B. _____

C. _____

D. _____

E. _____

STREET SCENES DISCUSSION

Review the Street Scene on pp. 545–546 of the textbook. Then answer the questions below.

1. If the condition of the patient requires that you actively rewarm him, what should you do?

2. At the scene, if the patient goes into cardiac arrest, should CPR be performed?

3. Usually patients in hypothermia have a slow pulse. In this case, the vital signs showed tachycardia. What might this indicate in a patient?

ON THE WEB

To help you review and practice basic skills, visit the *Emergency Care 11th Ed. Companion Website* at www.prenhall.com/limmer. For Online Test Preparation, visit www.prenhall.com/emtachieve.

EMT SKILL PERFORMANCE CHECKLISTS

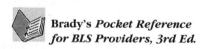 **Brady's *Pocket Reference for BLS Providers*, 3rd Ed.**

▶ **ACTIVE RAPID REWARMING OF FROZEN PARTS (PP. 525–526)**

❑ Take Standard Precautions.

❑ Conduct an initial assessment.

❑ Conduct focused history and physical exam, including baseline vital signs.

❑ Consider administering oxygen by nonrebreather mask.

❑ Heat water to a temperature between 100°F and 105°F.

❑ Fill a container with the heated water and prepare the injured part by removing clothing, jewelry, bands, or straps.

(continued next page)

- Fully immerse the injured part. Do not allow the injured area to touch the sides or bottom of the container. Do not place any pressure on the affected part. Continuously stir the water. When the water cools below 100°F, remove the affected part and add more warm water. The patient may complain of moderate pain as the affected area rewarms or may experience some period of intense pain.

- If you complete rewarming of the part, gently dry the affected area and apply a dry sterile dressing.

- Place dry sterile dressings between fingers and toes before dressing hands and feet.

- Cover the site with blankets or whatever is available to keep the affected area warm. Do not allow these coverings to come in contact with the injured area or to put pressure on the site.

- Keep the patient at rest. Do not allow the patient to walk if a lower extremity has been frostbitten or frozen.

- Keep the entire patient warm.

- Continue to monitor the patient.

- Assist circulation according to local protocol. (Some systems recommend rhythmically and carefully raising and lowering the affected limb.)

- Do not allow the limb to refreeze.

- Transport patient as soon as possible with the affected limb slightly elevated.

▶ WATER RESCUE—POSSIBLE SPINAL INJURY (PP. 532–533)

- Take Standard Precautions.

- Conduct an initial assessment.

- Splint patient's head and neck with arms.*

- Roll patient over into supine position.

- Ensure airway and breathing. (Note: If patient is not breathing, remove him from the water on a backboard as soon as possible.)

- Provide manual stabilization of the head and neck.

- Assess pulses, motor function, and sensation (PMS) in all four extremities.

- Slide backboard under patient.

- Apply properly sized rigid extrication collar.

- Tie down torso, then the head and neck with straps.

- Float board to the edge of the water.

- Remove patient from water with as much assistance as needed.

- Obtain baseline vital signs.

- Conduct focused history and physical exam.

- Reassess pulses, motor function, and sensation (PMS) in all four extremities.

- Administer oxygen, and prepare to transport patient.

*SAFETY NOTE: Unless you are a very good swimmer and trained in water rescue, do not go into the water to save someone.

©2009 Pearson Education, Inc.
Emergency Care, 11th Ed.

CASE STUDY

▶ TOO COLD FOR COMFORT

You respond to a call for a child with an altered mental status in the backyard of a private residence. It is late in the afternoon on a windy day, so you grab your uniform jacket as you jump into the ambulance. On arrival, you are met by three children, ages approximately 9 to 12, who state that their little sister has been acting "funny." Their parent is at the store, and they called her on the cell phone. She was the one who called 911 and should be home momentarily.

Apparently the children have been practicing diving in the pool for the past 4 hours. The youngest child, Robin—a very thin, small 7-year-old—is sitting by the edge of the pool shivering.

1. What are your initial assessment concerns with the patient?

2. Is it necessary for you to wait until the parent arrives to question the children?

3. Besides obtaining a set of baseline vital signs, what additional history may be helpful to obtain?

Upon questioning, you find that Robin has not been playing as a part of the group for at least the last hour. When you ask the children if they were cold, they say they did not notice the temperature, just the wind, until a few minutes ago when the sun went down. They also are able to confirm that Robin has no medical history, takes no meds, has no allergies, and has not eaten since lunchtime. When you question Robin, it is clear that she is confused and shivering, cool to the touch, and breathing rapidly.

4. After ruling out trauma, you place the child on your stretcher. What would be the best position?

5. When the mother arrives, you advise her of your findings. She is in agreement that the child should be checked in the hospital. What do you suspect may be wrong with this child?

6. Would it be appropriate to administer oxygen to Robin?

7. If you took her temperature, what do you suspect you would find?

8. Why might this child be prone to hypothermia?

The parent tells you that the children are all very good swimmers and they are practicing for a diving competition. She only ran out for a half hour to go to the store. The children are quick to call her on the cell phone whenever there is a problem. She also says that she told them to get out of the pool before she left for the store.

9. When she asks you how a similar incident could be prevented in the future, what should you say?

©2009 Pearson Education, Inc.
Emergency Care, 11th Ed.

Behavioral Emergencies

MATCH TERMINOLOGY/ DEFINITIONS

A. Humane device made of leather used to hold a patient still to prevent the patient from injuring himself or others

B. Display of emotions, such as fear, grief, or anger, in response to an accident, serious illness, or death

C. Death of a person due to a body position that restricts breathing for a prolonged time

D. When a patient's behavior is not typical for the situation; when the patient's behavior is unacceptable or intolerable to the patient, his family, or the community; or when the patient may harm himself or others

E. Manner in which a person acts

_____ **1.** Behavior

_____ **2.** Behavioral emergency

_____ **3.** Positional asphyxia

_____ **4.** Soft restraint

_____ **5.** Stress reaction

MULTIPLE-CHOICE REVIEW

_____ **1.** Physical causes of altered behavior include all of the following <u>except</u>:
   A. inadequate blood flow to the brain.
   B. mind-altering substances.
   C. excessive heat or cold.
   D. differing lifestyles.

_____ **2.** Altered behavior ranging from irritability to altered mental status can be due to any of the following <u>except</u>:
   A. lack of oxygen.   **C.** hypoactivity.
   B. head trauma.   **D.** hypoglycemia.

_____ **3.** To calm a patient who is experiencing a stress reaction, you should:
   A. complete your assessment as quickly as possible.
   B. allow the patient to control the situation.
   C. explain things to the patient honestly.
   D. restrain the patient quickly.

_____ **4.** Which one of the following is <u>not</u> usually a common presentation of a patient experiencing a behavioral emergency?
   A. panic or anxiety
   B. neat appearance
   C. repetitive motions
   D. pressured-sounding speech

_____ **5.** When you are called to care for a patient who has attempted suicide or is about to attempt suicide, your first concern should be:
   A. how you will restrain the patient.
   B. your personal safety.
   C. determining the patient's method for suicide.
   D. the patient's and family's safety.

_____ **6.** High suicide rates occur at ages:
   A. 15–25.
   B. 25–30.
   C. 30–35.
   D. 35–40.

_____ **7.** Which one of the following is <u>not</u> an example of a self-destructive activity?
   A. a defined lethal plan of action that has been verbalized
   B. giving away personal possessions
   C. denial of suicidal thoughts
   D. previous suicide threats

_____ **8.** When a suicidal patient exhibits sudden improvement from depression, the EMT should consider that the patient is:
   A. no longer suicidal.
   B. now ready to accept care.
   C. still at risk for suicide.
   D. none of the above.

_____ **9.** When assessing an aggressive patient for a possible threat to you or your crew, take all of the following actions <u>except</u>:
   A. try to determine the patient's history of aggressive behavior.
   B. pay attention to the patient's vocal activity.
   C. take note of the patient's posturing.
   D. assess the patient in the kitchen.

_____ **10.** If a patient stands in a corner of the room with fists clenched and screaming obscenities, you should:
   A. request police backup and keep the doorway in sight.
   B. raise your voice to a higher level than the patient's.
   C. challenge the patient in an attempt to calm him.
   D. explain that you would respond in the same way.

_____ **11.** Use of reasonable force to restrain a patient should involve an evaluation of all of the following <u>except</u> the:
   A. patient's size and strength.
   B. family's ability to pay for your services.
   C. patient's mental status.
   D. available methods of restraint.

_____ **12.** The use of force by an EMT is allowed:
   A. to defend against an attack by an emotionally disturbed patient.
   B. only when the police are present.
   C. whenever a patient refuses any of your treatments.
   D. whenever you suspect the patient has been drinking.

_____ **13.** Once the decision has been made to restrain a patient, which one of the following steps should be avoided?
   A. Use multiple straps to restrain the patient.
   B. Reassure the patient throughout the procedure.
   C. Reassess the patient's distal circulation frequently.
   D. Use two rescuers to secure the patient.

_____ **14.** A restrained patient who is spitting on rescuers can best be managed by:
  A. placement in a prone position on the stretcher.
  B. wrapping the patient's mouth with roller gauze.
  C. placing 3-inch tape across the patient's mouth.
  D. placing a surgical mask on the patient's face.

_____ **15.** When a patient is a danger to himself or others and needs to be transported against his will, the EMT should:
  A. restrain the patient immediately.
  B. transport the patient with the family's assistance.
  C. contact the police for assistance.
  D. contact the patient's physician.

COMPLETE THE FOLLOWING

1. List nine potential risk factors for suicide.

  A. _____

  B. _____

  C. _____

  D. _____

  E. _____

  F. _____

  G. _____

  H. _____

  I. _____

2. List four precautions for your safety and that of your crew when you feel your patient may hurt himself or others.

  A. _____

  B. _____

  C. _____

  D. _____

STREET SCENES DISCUSSION

Review the Street Scene on pp. 560–561 of the textbook. Then answer the questions below.

1. Suppose that the patient had suddenly become violent, flailing his arms and screaming obscenities. Should you help the police hold him down?

2. Once the patient is down, how should he be restrained?

3. Since the patient is having a behavioral emergency, is it acceptable to skip taking vital signs?

EMT SKILLS PERFORMANCE CHECKLIST

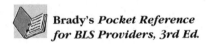

Brady's *Pocket Reference for BLS Providers*, 3rd Ed.

▶ **RESTRAINING A PATIENT* (P. 557)**

❏ Plan your approach to the patient in advance and remain outside of reach of arms and legs until you are ready to act.

❏ Assign one EMT to each limb and approach the patient at the same time.

❏ Place the patient on the stretcher as his condition and local protocols indicate. Do not let go until he is properly secured.

❏ Use multiple straps or other soft restraints to secure the patient to the stretcher.

❏ When the patient is secure, assess his distal circulation and monitor his airway and breathing continually.

*Never perform skill when the patient is prone.

ON THE WEB

To help you review and practice basic skills, visit the *Emergency Care 11th Ed. Companion Website* at www.prenhall.com/limmer. For Online Test Preparation, visit www.prenhall.com/emtachieve.

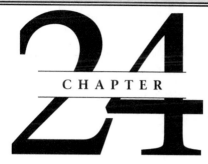

CHAPTER 24

Obstetrics and Gynecological Emergencies

MATCH TERMINOLOGY/ DEFINITIONS

▶ **PART A**

A. Normal head-first birth

B. Neck of the uterus at the entrance to the birth canal

C. Implantation of the fertilized egg in an oviduct, the cervix of the uterus, or in the abdominopelvic cavity

D. Placenta, membranes of the amniotic sac, part of the umbilical cord, and some tissues from the lining of the uterus that are delivered after the birth of the baby

E. Baby developing in the womb

F. Condition in which the placenta separates from the uterine wall; a cause of prebirth bleeding

G. Deliberate actions taken to stop a pregnancy

H. When more than one baby is born during a single delivery

I. Spontaneous (miscarriage) or induced termination of pregnancy

J. Three stages of the delivery of a baby that begin with the contractions of the uterus and end with the expulsion of the placenta

K. Thin, membranous "bag of waters" that surrounds the developing fetus

L. Amniotic fluid that is greenish or brownish-yellow rather than clear; an indication of possible maternal or fetal distress during labor

_____ **1.** Abortion

_____ **2.** Abruptio placentae

_____ **3.** Afterbirth

_____ **4.** Amniotic sac

_____ **5.** Breech presentation

_____ **6.** Cephalic presentation

_____ **7.** Cervix

_____ **8.** Crowning

_____ **9.** Ectopic pregnancy

_____ **10.** Fetus

_____ **11.** Induced abortion

_____ **12.** Labor

_____ **13.** Meconium staining

_____ **14.** Multiple birth

_____ **15.** Perineum

_____ **16.** APGAR

M. When the buttocks or both legs of a baby deliver first during birth

N. The surface area between the vagina and the anus

O. When the presenting part of the baby first appears through the vaginal opening

P. A way to assign a number to a newborn's condition and is the total of five values, ranging from 0 to 10

▶ **PART B**

A. When the umbilical cord presents first and is squeezed between the vaginal wall and the baby's head

B. Dizziness and a drop in blood pressure caused when the mother is in a supine position and the weight of the uterus, infant, placenta, and amniotic fluid compresses the inferior vena cava, reducing return of blood to the heart and cardiac output

C. When the fetus and placenta deliver before the 28th week of pregnancy, commonly called a miscarriage

D. Muscular abdominal organ where the fetus develops; also called the womb

E. Born dead

F. Any newborn weighing less than 5½ pounds or one that is born before the 37th week of pregnancy

G. Fetal structure containing the blood vessels that carry blood to and from the placenta

H. Organ of pregnancy where exchange of oxygen, foods, and wastes occurs between a mother and fetus

I. Condition in which the placenta is formed in an abnormal location (usually low in the uterus and close to or over the cervical opening) that will not allow for a normal delivery of the fetus

J. Birth canal

_____ **1.** Placenta

_____ **2.** Placenta previa

_____ **3.** Premature infant

_____ **4.** Prolapsed umbilical cord

_____ **5.** Spontaneous abortion

_____ **6.** Stillborn

_____ **7.** Supine hypotensive syndrome

_____ **8.** Umbilical cord

_____ **9.** Uterus

_____ **10.** Vagina

MULTIPLE-CHOICE REVIEW

_____ **1.** The 9 months of pregnancy are divided into 3-month trimesters. During the second trimester, the:
  A. fetus is being formed and there is little uterine growth during this period.
  B. uterus grows very rapidly while the woman's blood volume, cardiac output, and heart rate increase.
  C. uterus is often seen reaching up to the epigastrium by this time.
  D. uterus develops to full size.

_____ **2.** The normal birth position is _____ and is called a _____ birth.
  A. head first, breech
  B. head first, cephalic
  C. feet first, breech
  D. feet first, cephalic

_____ **3.** The first stage of labor starts:
   A. with conception.
   B. at the 9-month point.
   C. with regular contractions of the uterus.
   D. when the cervix is dilated.

_____ **4.** The second stage of labor starts with:
   A. the birth of the baby.
   B. regular contractions of the uterus.
   C. the delivery of the afterbirth.
   D. the entry of the baby into the birth canal.

_____ **5.** The third stage of labor begins with:
   A. the birth of the baby.   **C.** dilation of the cervix.
   B. delivery of the afterbirth.   **D.** full growth of the uterus.

_____ **6.** The third stage of labor is complete when:
   A. the baby is born.
   B. the afterbirth is expelled.
   C. 20 minutes have passed since the delivery.
   D. the uterus is firm again.

_____ **7.** The process by which the cervix gradually widens and thins out is called:
   A. delivery.   **C.** staining.
   B. dilation.   **D.** contraction.

_____ **8.** As the fetus moves downward and the cervix dilates, normally the amniotic sac breaks and fluid leaks out. If this fluid is greenish or brownish-yellow in color, this may indicate:
   A. fetal or maternal distress.
   B. the fetus is dead.
   C. the mother is pushing too hard.
   D. the amniotic sac broke too early.

_____ **9.** The greenish or brownish-yellow fluid expelled from the amniotic sac is called:
   A. a bloody show.
   B. vena cava syndrome.
   C. meconium staining.
   D. amniotic bile.

_____ **10.** When a mother in labor states she feels the need to move her bowels, this means the:
   A. birth will be delayed.   **C.** birth moment is nearing.
   B. uterus is almost dilated.   **D.** baby is in distress.

_____ **11.** The contraction duration is timed from the:
   A. start of the pain until the delivery of the infant.
   B. beginning of the contraction to when the uterus relaxes.
   C. end of a contraction to the beginning of the next one.
   D. peak of the contraction to the end of the contraction.

_____ **12.** The contraction interval, or frequency, is timed from the:
   A. start of one contraction to the start of the next.
   B. beginning of the contraction to when the uterus relaxes.
   C. peak of the contraction to the end of the contraction.
   D. start of the pain until the delivery of the infant.

_____ **13.** Delivery is imminent when the contractions last _____ seconds and are _____ minutes apart.
   A. 15; 5 to 8   **C.** 45; 8 to 10
   B. 30; 2 to 3   **D.** 90; 5 to 8

_____ 14. The EMT's primary roles at a normal childbirth scene are to determine whether the delivery will occur at the scene and, if so, to:
   A. determine if the delivery can be delayed.
   B. assist the mother as she delivers the infant.
   C. carefully deliver the infant.
   D. immobilize the patient.

_____ 15. The sterile obstetrical kit does <u>not</u> contain:
   A. a rubber bulb syringe for suctioning.
   B. several individually wrapped sanitary napkins.
   C. heavy flat twine to tie the cord.
   D. cord clamps or hemostats.

_____ 16. When evaluating the mother for a possible home delivery, the EMT should ask:
   A. if pregnancy problems run in the family.
   B. the frequency and duration of contractions.
   C. if the mother feels she needs to urinate.
   D. the father's blood type and medical history.

_____ 17. It is important to ask the mother if you can examine for crowning if the mother:
   A. is straining during contractions.
   B. is in her ninth month of pregnancy.
   C. is pregnant for the first time.
   D. It is not important to ask permission to examine the mother.

_____ 18. You are treating a 25-year-old female who is 8 months pregnant. She states she has contractions every 15 minutes or so, which last for about 20 seconds. She is not exactly sure what labor pain is like because this is her first pregnancy. Her vitals are pulse of 96, blood pressure of 130/70, and respirations of 22. What should you do next?
   A. Administer oxygen and transport immediately.
   B. Prepare for a home delivery immediately.
   C. Ask if her water broke and prepare for a quiet ride to the hospital.
   D. Tell her to call you back when the contractions are more frequent.

_____ 19. If you determine that the delivery is imminent based on the presence of crowning and other signs, you should:
   A. contact medical direction.
   B. transport as quickly as possible.
   C. ask the mother to go the bathroom first.
   D. ask the mother to hold her legs closed.

_____ 20. When a full-term pregnant woman in a supine position complains of dizziness and you note a drop in blood pressure, this could be due to a condition called _____ syndrome.
   A. diabetes mellitus
   B. supine hypotension
   C. Cushing's reflex
   D. fluid retention

_____ 21. To counteract the pressure of the uterus on the inferior vena cava, you should:
   A. raise the patient's legs.
   B. transport the patient on her left side.
   C. raise the patient's head.
   D. apply the PASG.

_____ 22. During a delivery, the EMT will need all the following infection control gear <u>except</u>:
   A. surgical gloves.
   B. a mask.
   C. eye protection.
   D. a Tyvek suit.

©2009 Pearson Education, Inc.
Emergency Care, 11th Ed.

_____ 23. During delivery, encourage the mother to:
    A. breathe rapidly and deeply.
    B. hold her breath every 2 minutes.
    C. close her mouth and breathe through her nose.
    D. breathe deeply through her mouth.

_____ 24. When supporting the baby's head during a delivery, the EMT should do all of the following <u>except</u>:
    A. pull on the baby's shoulders when they appear.
    B. apply gentle pressure to control the delivery.
    C. place one hand below the baby's head.
    D. spread fingers evenly around the baby's head.

_____ 25. If the amniotic sac has not broken by the time the baby's head is delivered, you should:
    A. stop the delivery and transport immediately.
    B. use your finger to puncture the membrane.
    C. contact medical direction immediately.
    D. delay the delivery until it breaks.

_____ 26. If you cannot loosen or unwrap the umbilical cord from around the infant's neck, you should:
    A. stop the delivery and transport immediately.
    B. tell the mother to push more forcefully.
    C. clamp the cord in two places and cut between the clamps.
    D. contact medical direction for advice.

_____ 27. Most babies are born:
    A. face down and then rotate to either side.
    B. face up and then rotate to either side.
    C. feet and buttocks first and do not rotate.
    D. face up and do not rotate.

_____ 28. When suctioning a newborn:
    A. compress the bulb syringe when inside the baby's mouth.
    B. compress the bulb syringe before placing it in the baby's mouth.
    C. suction the nose and then the mouth.
    D. insert the syringe about 22 inches into the baby's mouth.

_____ 29. Once the baby's feet are delivered:
    A. pick the baby up by the feet using a firm grasp.
    B. lay the baby on her side with head slightly lower than her torso.
    C. lay the baby on her side and massage her back.
    D. pick the baby up by the feet and massage her back.

_____ 30. To assess the newborn, the EMT should do all of the following <u>except</u>:
    A. note ease of breathing.
    B. check movement in the extremities.
    C. note skin coloration.
    D. check the response to a sternal rub.

_____ 31. Why is it necessary to suction the baby's mouth before the nose?
    A. so the baby can gasp and begin breathing
    B. so the baby is stimulated to cry
    C. to prevent aspiration of materials from her mouth
    D. because this will open the nasopharynx passageway

_____ 32. If assessment of the infant's breathing reveals shallow, slow, or absent respirations, the EMT should:
    A. provide oxygen by nonrebreather mask.
    B. use a gentle but vigorous rubbing of the infant's back.
    C. provide artificial ventilations at 40 to 60 per minute.
    D. provide artificial ventilations at 20 to 30 per minute.

_____ **33.** In a normal birth, the infant must be breathing on her own:
  A. before you clamp and cut the cord.
  B. prior to transportation to the hospital.
  C. prior to considering ventilation.
  D. in order to use an oral airway.

_____ **34.** The first umbilical cord clamp should be placed about _____ inches from the baby.
  A. 4   **C.** 8
  B. 6   **D.** 10

_____ **35.** The second umbilical cord clamp should be placed about _____ inches from the baby.
  A. 3   **C.** 7
  B. 5   **D.** 9

_____ **36.** If the placenta does not deliver within _____ minutes of the baby's birth, transport the mother and baby to a medical facility without delay.
  A. 5   **C.** 15
  B. 10   **D.** 20

_____ **37.** It is not uncommon for the mother to tear part of the perineum during a delivery. If this occurs:
  A. massage the uterus for at least 15 minutes.
  B. apply a sanitary napkin and gentle pressure.
  C. transport the patient on her left side immediately.
  D. contact medical direction immediately.

_____ **38.** Which of the following is an appropriate action to take for a breech presentation?
  A. Place the mother on her left side.
  B. Provide low-concentration oxygen.
  C. Pull on the baby's legs to deliver.
  D. Initiate rapid transport upon recognition.

_____ **39.** If you see the umbilical cord presenting first:
  A. gently push up on the baby's head or buttocks to take pressure off of the cord.
  B. use two gloved fingers to check the cord for a pulse and keep the cord cool.
  C. raise the mother's head and lower buttocks to lessen pressure on the birth canal.
  D. attempt to push the cord back if it is not wrapped around the baby's neck.

_____ **40.** When a baby's limb presents first, the EMT should:
  A. push gently on the extremity to prevent it from advancing.
  B. pull gently on the limb to encourage delivery.
  C. administer low-concentration oxygen to the mother.
  D. begin rapid transport of the patient immediately.

_____ **41.** When assisting with the delivery of twins:
  A. the afterbirth will be delivered after each individual infant.
  B. clamp the cord of the first baby before the second baby is born.
  C. labor contractions will stop after the first delivery.
  D. transport the mother immediately.

_____ **42.** Premature infants are at high risk for hypothermia because:
  A. they are smaller than most babies.
  B. their brains are less developed than those of full-term babies.
  C. they lack fat deposits that would normally keep them warm.
  D. their temperature-regulating structures are not fully developed.

_____ **43.** When oxygen is administered to an infant, it should be given by:
   A. a nonrebreather mask.
   B. flowing it past the baby's face.
   C. a pediatric nasal cannula.
   D. a transport ventilator.

_____ **44.** If you suspect meconium staining when the infant is born:
   A. contact medical direction for advice.
   B. avoid stimulating the infant before suctioning the oropharynx.
   C. suction the nose, then the mouth.
   D. provide oxygen to the mother.

_____ **45.** A condition in which the placenta is formed low in the uterus and close to the cervical opening, preventing the normal delivery of the fetus, is called:
   A. abruptio placentae.
   B. stillborn birth.
   C. placenta toxemia.
   D. placenta previa.

_____ **46.** Which one of the following is true of seizures in pregnancy?
   A. They are usually associated with low blood pressure.
   B. They tend to occur early in pregnancy.
   C. They pose a threat to the mother but not the unborn baby.
   D. They are usually associated with extreme swelling of the extremities.

_____ **47.** The greatest danger associated with blunt trauma to the pregnant woman's abdomen and pelvis is:
   A. cramping abdominal pains.
   B. spontaneous abortion.
   C. massive bleeding and shock.
   D. elevated blood pressure.

_____ **48.** Which one of the following is true about the physiology of a pregnant woman?
   A. Vital signs may be interpreted as suggestive of shock when they are actually normal.
   B. The pregnant woman has a pulse rate that is 10–15 beats per minute slower than the nonpregnant female.
   C. A woman in later pregnancy may have a blood volume that is up to 48% lower than her nonpregnant state.
   D. Assessing for shock is easier in the pregnant patient than for a nonpregnant patient.

_____ **49.** Unless a back or neck injury is suspected, all pregnant women who have suffered blunt trauma injury should be transported in the _____ position.
   A. supine
   B. left lateral recumbent
   C. Trendelenburg
   D. Fowler's

_____ **50.** Which of the following is true of the treatment necessary for a woman with vaginal bleeding associated with abdominal pain?
   A. Massage the abdomen vigorously.
   B. Assume the woman is pregnant and transport.
   C. Treat as if she has a potentially life-threatening condition.
   D. Determine the cause before treatment is begun.

COMPLETE THE FOLLOWING

1. List seven things you should do when evaluating the expectant mother.

   A. _____

   B. _____

   C. _____

   D. _____

   E. _____

   F. _____

   G. _____

2. List eight steps you should take when providing care for the premature infant.

   A. _____

   B. _____

   C. _____

   D. _____

   E. _____

   F. _____

   G. _____

   H. _____

3. Complete the following:

APGAR SCORE

	0	1	2
Appearance	Blue (or pale) all over	**(A)**	Pink all over
Pulse	0	<100	**(B)**
Grimace (reaction to suctioning or flicking of the feet)	**(C)**	Facial grimace	Sneeze, cough, or cry
Activity	No movement	**(D)**	Moving around normally
Respiratory effort	None	Slow or irregular breathing, weak cry	**(E)**

LABEL THE DIAGRAMS

Fill in the name of each structure of pregnancy on the line provided.

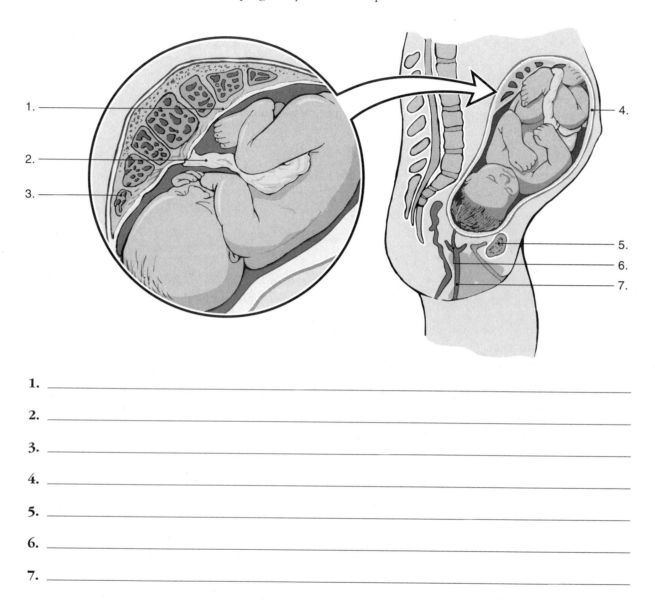

1. _____

2. _____

3. _____

4. _____

5. _____

6. _____

7. _____

STREET SCENES DISCUSSION

Review the Street Scene on pp. 598–599 of the textbook. Then answer the questions below.

1. Imagine that when you observe crowning, you also observe that the amniotic sac is intact. What should you do?

2. When the amniotic fluid is expelled from the bag, you notice that it is dark green. What is this called? What does it indicate? What should you do about it?

3. Suppose that after delivery of the placenta, you observe that the mother is continuing to bleed excessively. Is there anything you can do to help her?

ON THE WEB

To help you review and practice basic skills, visit the *Emergency Care 11th Ed. Companion Website* at www.prenhall.com/limmer. For Online Test Preparation, visit www.prenhall.com/emtachieve.

EMT SKILLS
PERFORMANCE CHECKLIST

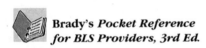 Brady's *Pocket Reference for BLS Providers, 3rd Ed.*

▶ **EVALUATING THE MOTHER FOR IMMINENT DELIVERY (PP. 571–574)**

❑ Take Standard Precautions.

❑ Conduct an initial assessment.

❑ Obtain mother's history to determine active labor. History includes:
  - Length of pregnancy.
  - Number of previous pregnancies and births.
  - If the "bag of waters" has broken.
  - Frequency and duration of uterine contractions.
  - Recent vaginal discharge or hemorrhage.
  - If she is straining or feels the urge to move her bowels.

❑ With mother's permission, examine her for crowning.

❑ Feel for uterine contractions when she says she is having a contraction.

❑ Take another set of vitals and make the decision to prepare for a delivery or to begin transport.

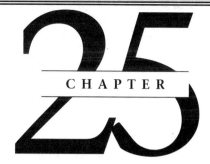

Putting It All Together for the Medical Patient

MATCH TERMINOLOGY/ DEFINITIONS

A. Passageway by which air enters or leaves the body

B. Respiration, or process by which a person inhales and exhales air

C. Movement of blood throughout the body

D. Form of sugar, the body's basic source of energy

E. Action taken to correct a patient's problem

F. Pain in the chest, occurring when blood supply to the heart is reduced and a portion of the heart muscle is not receiving enough oxygen

G. Orders from the on-duty physician given directly to an EMT in the field by radio or telephone

H. Decision on the seriousness of the patient's condition

_____ **1.** Intervention

_____ **2.** Circulation

_____ **3.** Airway

_____ **4.** Priority determination

_____ **5.** On-line medical direction

_____ **6.** Breathing

_____ **7.** Angina pectoris

_____ **8.** Glucose

MULTIPLE-CHOICE REVIEW

_____ 1. The limited number of interventions an EMT can provide include all of the following except:
A. administration of intravenous fluids.
B. application of an AED.
C. application of oxygen.
D. insertion of oral or nasal airways.

_____ 2. When a patient presents with more than one condition, or a familiar condition but under unusual circumstances, the EMT should:
A. call medical direction right away.
B. call for an ALS unit right away.
C. assess the patient as usual.
D. assign a higher priority to the patient.

_____ 3. When a patient tells you he has a disease with which you are not familiar, it is best to respond by saying:
A. I'm not familiar with that disease. Could you tell me about it?
B. That doesn't concern me. My job is to treat emergencies.
C. Interesting disease. I studied it during EMS training.
D. I'm not a physician. Just tell me what's wrong today.

_____ 4. When a patient has two or more medical conditions that are presenting symptoms at the same time, it is good to:
A. treat them all at once.
B. treat them one at a time.
C. consult with medical direction for advice.
D. just manage the ABCs and forget the rest.

_____ 5. The patient with slurred speech may have had:
A. a stroke.   C. a seizure.
B. an overdose.   D. any combination of the above.

_____ 6. The patient with chest pain may have any of the following conditions except:
A. angina.   C. seizure.
B. acute myocardial infarction. D. rib fracture.

_____ 7. A patient who is vomiting coffee-ground-like material probably has:
A. internal bleeding.
B. a seizure history.
C. gall bladder problems.
D. ingested a strong acid.

_____ 8. A wheeze is a common breathing sound found in a patient having:
A. an asthma attack.
B. an allergic reaction.
C. bronchospasm.
D. any one of the above.

_____ 9. There is no specific EMT intervention for the patient with:
A. chest pain.   C. a fractured leg.
B. abdominal pain.   D. a serious laceration.

_____ 10. Each one of the following is an example of patient problems that have no specific EMT intervention except:
A. headache.
B. sickle-cell crisis.
C. hyperthermia.
D. post-surgical complications.

©2009 Pearson Education, Inc.
Emergency Care, 11th Ed.

COMPLETE THE FOLLOWING

1. List six examples of EMT interventions for medical patients.

   A. _____

   B. _____

   C. _____

   D. _____

   E. _____

   F. _____

STREET SCENES DISCUSSION

Review the Street Scene on pp. 610–611 of the textbook. Then answer the questions below.

1. Imagine that in addition to his fever, the patient had vomiting and a rash. What Standard Precautions should you take?

2. If the patient also complains of dizziness when he stands up, how might it change your emergency care?

3. Suppose this patient had a history of diabetes and also has cool, clammy skin. Would this change your management of the patient?

ON THE WEB

To help you review and practice basic skills, visit the *Emergency Care 11th Ed. Companion Website* at www.prenhall.com/limmer. For Online Test Preparation, visit www.prenhall.com/emtachieve.

Interim Exam 2

Use the answer sheet on pages 207–208 to complete this exam. It is perforated so it can be easily removed from this workbook.

1. During the initial assessment, all of the following are assessed <u>except</u>:
   A. airway.
   B. mental status.
   C. circulation.
   D. blood pressure.

2. Which is <u>not</u> a component of the initial assessment?
   A. determining patient priority
   B. evaluating extremity mobility
   C. forming a general impression
   D. assessing breathing

3. When forming your general impression of a child's condition, the environment can provide clues. An example would be a child:
   A. complaining of nausea or vomiting.
   B. holding pieces of a toy in his or her hand.
   C. with a blood pressure of 120/80.
   D. with a rapid heart beat.

4. When forming a general impression, the EMT takes into consideration all of the following <u>except</u> the patient's:
   A. position.   C. blood pressure.
   B. age and sex.   D. sounds.

5. After forming a general impression, the next step of the initial assessment is:
   A. assessing breathing.
   B. assessing mental status.
   C. determining the priority of the patient.
   D. assessing airway.

6. The "V" in "AVPU" stands for:
   A. virtual.   C. verbal.
   B. visible.   D. vertex.

7. The "P" in "AVPU" stands for:
   A. pulse.   C. paralysis.
   B. painful.   D. paresthesia.

8. The lowest and the most serious mental status is:
   A. A.   C. P.
   B. V.   D. U.

9. If a patient's level of responsiveness is lower than Alert, you should:
   A. apply a cervical collar.
   B. administer high-concentration oxygen.
   C. place him in a recovery position.
   D. bandage all bleeding wounds.

10. If a patient is talking or crying, assume the patient:
    A. is in little pain.
    B. has no life-threatening bleeding.
    C. has an open airway.
    D. has an "A" mental status.

11. If the patient is not alert and her breathing rate is slower than 8 breaths per minute, the EMT should:
    A. insert an oral airway.
    B. place the patient in a prone position.
    C. assist ventilations with a bag-valve mask.
    D. apply the PASG.

12. If the skin is pale and clammy, this indicates:
    A. nervous system damage.
    B. poor circulation.
    C. extremely high temperature.
    D. an airway problem.

13. A patient who gives a poor general impression should be considered a _____ priority.
    A. high
    B. low
    C. delayed
    D. stable

14. Which one of the following is <u>not</u> an example of a high-priority condition?
    A. difficulty breathing
    B. nausea and vomiting
    C. a severed artery
    D. a mental status of "U"

15. The initial assessment takes different forms, which depend on the age of the patient and whether or not he:
    A. has a medical problem or a trauma problem.
    B. is alert or conscious.
    C. has a history of diabetes.
    D. has a history of head injury.

16. When evaluating circulation in infants, the EMT should use the:
    A. femoral pulse.
    B. distal pulse check.
    C. capillary refill test.
    D. radial pulse.

17. The mental status of an unconscious infant is typically checked by:
    A. splashing cold water on him.
    B. shouting and flicking his feet.
    C. performing a pin prick on the feet.
    D. applying a sternal rub.

18. Which is not a high-priority condition?
    A. shock
    B. a fever with a rash
    C. a complicated childbirth
    D. severe pain anywhere

19. The difference between the general impression steps for a medical patient and those for a trauma patient is:
    A. manual stabilization of the head for a trauma patient.
    B. no SAMPLE is taken for a trauma patient.
    C. the medical patient is treated faster.
    D. the AVPU is not used for a medical patient.

20. When the EMT documents that the chest pain patient denies shortness of breath, this is most appropriately termed:
    A. an informative objective.
    B. advisory information.
    C. a pertinent negative.
    D. run data information.

21. When writing the narrative section of a pre-hospital care report, the EMT should do all of the following except:
    A. use medical terminology correctly.
    B. avoid nonstandard abbreviations.
    C. write legibly and use correct spelling.
    D. state one's personal opinion of the patient's condition.

22. Which statement best describes an important concept of documentation?
    A. Always fill out a continuation sheet.
    B. If it's not written down, you didn't do it.
    C. It should include plenty of medical terms.
    D. Document everything you see.

23. If the patient does not wish to go to the hospital, the EMT should:
    A. document with a refusal-of-care form.
    B. take the patient to the hospital anyway.
    C. end the assessment immediately.
    D. call for another crew to subdue him.

24. When an important part of the assessment or care was not performed, this is called:
    A. submission.   C. inhibition.
    B. omission.   D. commission.

25. When an EMT makes up a set of vitals for inclusion on the prehospital care report, this is called:
    A. assault.   C. falsification.
    B. libel.   D. battery.

26. An objective statement is:
    A. one that is made from a particular point of view.
    B. one that is made by the patient or a family member.
    C. one that describes observable or measurable information.
    D. one's own assessment of what is wrong with the patient.

27. When the EMT writes "The patient is alert and oriented" on the prehospital care report, this is an example of:
    A. objective information.
    B. a statement beyond his or her training.
    C. subjective information.
    D. nonfactual information.

28. When you are documenting exactly what a patient told you on the prehospital care report, you should:
    A. paraphrase for brevity.
    B. summarize the key points.
    C. use medical terminology.
    D. use quotes around the statement.

29. Writing a statement such as "The patient's daughter was rude to us" on a prehospital care report is:
    A. not relevant.
    B. objective information.
    C. run data information.
    D. an example of what should be included in quotes.

30. The next step in the initial assessment after establishing unresponsiveness is to:
    A. ensure an open airway.
    B. check for adequate breathing.
    C. check for circulation.
    D. look for profuse bleeding.

31. The term "sixth sense" is used to describe:
    A. an EMT's clinical judgment.
    B. the six steps in an initial assessment.
    C. a patient's sensory functions.
    D. the ability to hear.

32. Which one of the following is a true vital sign?
    A. nausea
    B. skin temperature
    C. level of responsiveness
    D. age

33. The normal pulse rate for an adult at rest is between _____ beats per minute.
   A. 50 and 70   **C.** 65 and 95
   B. 60 and 100   **D.** 80 and 100

34. During the determination of vital signs, the initial pulse rate for patients 1 year and older is normally taken at the _____ pulse.
   A. carotid   **C.** pedal
   B. femoral   **D.** radial

35. When the force of the pulse is weak and thin, it is described as:
   A. shallow.   **C.** partial.
   B. full.   **D.** thready.

36. Normal at-rest respiration rates for adults vary from _____ breaths per minute.
   A. 5 to 10   **C.** 15 to 30
   B. 12 to 20   **D.** 20 to 32

37. A noisy, harsh sound heard during inhalation that indicates a partial airway obstruction is:
   A. gurgling.
   B. snorting.
   C. stertorous respirations.
   D. crowing.

38. Systolic blood pressure indicates the arterial pressure created as the:
   A. artery contracts.
   B. artery relaxes.
   C. heart contracts.
   D. heart relaxes.

39. Diastolic blood pressure indicates the arterial pressure created as the:
   A. heart contracts.   **C.** artery contracts.
   B. heart refills.   **D.** artery relaxes.

40. The technique of measuring blood pressure with a sphygmomanometer and a stethoscope is called:
   A. palpation.   **C.** oscillation.
   B. auscultation. **D.** priapism.

41. Determining blood pressure by palpation is:
   A. not as accurate as the auscultation method.
   B. used when there is no noise around a patient.
   C. is documented as the "palp/diastolic."
   D. used whenever the patient is hypertensive.

42. Information that you can see, hear, feel, and smell is called:
   A. signs.   **C.** symptoms.
   B. sensations.   **D.** assessments.

43. When the EMT asks the patient "Have you recently had any surgery or injuries?" he is inquiring about the:
   A. patient's medications.
   B. patient's pertinent past history.
   C. events leading up to the illness.
   D. allergies that the patient may have.

44. When the EMT asks the patient "Are you on birth control pills?" she is inquiring about the:
   A. patient's medications.
   B. patient's pertinent past history.
   C. events leading up to the illness.
   D. allergies that the patient may have.

45. An acronym used to remember what questions to ask about the patient's present problem and past history is:
   A. AVPU.   **C.** SAMPLE.
   B. DCAP-BTLS.   **D.** PEARL.

46. When conducting a patient interview on an adult patient, the EMT should do all of the following except:
   A. position oneself close to the patient.
   B. identify oneself and reassure the patient.
   C. gently touch the patient's shoulder or rest a hand over the patient's hand.
   D. avoid asking the patient's age.

47. Normal diastolic pressures range from _____ mmHg.
   A. 50 to 80   **C.** 60 to 80
   B. 50 to 90   **D.** 60 to 90

48. Using the formula presented in the text, a 36-year-old man would have an estimated systolic blood pressure of _____ mmHg.
   A. 116   **C.** 136
   B. 126   **D.** 146

49. Using the formula presented in the text, a 26-year-old woman would have an estimated systolic blood pressure of _____ mmHg.
   A. 106   **C.** 126
   B. 116   **D.** 136

50. Why should the stethoscope not be placed under the cuff and then inflated when evaluating the blood pressure?
   A. It may give a false reading.
   B. It can dent the stethoscope.
   C. The patient will not like the feeling.
   D. It will prevent pumping the cuff to the proper pressure.

51. When taking a patient's blood pressure, the stethoscope is placed over the _____ artery.
   A. carotid   **C.** brachial
   B. radial   **D.** femoral

©2009 Pearson Education, Inc.
Emergency Care, 11th Ed.

52. The best indication of potential injury is the:
    A. type of accident.
    B. type of injury.
    C. mechanism of injury.
    D. position of the patient.

53. When there are no apparent hazards at the scene of a collision, the danger zone should extend _____ feet in all directions from the wreckage.
    A. 25   C. 75
    B. 50   D. 100

54. In the up-and-over injury pattern, the patient is most likely to sustain _____ injuries.
    A. knee   C. head
    B. hip   D. leg

55. A keen awareness that there may be injuries based on the mechanism of injury is called a(n):
    A. sixth sense.
    B. general impression.
    C. index of suspicion.
    D. kinesthetic sense.

56. The purpose of the initial assessment is to:
    A. take the patient's vital signs.
    B. gather information about the collision.
    C. discover and treat life-threatening conditions.
    D. obtain the patient's history.

57. The first step in the focused history and physical exam for <u>any</u> trauma patient is to:
    A. make a status decision.
    B. check for an open airway.
    C. reconsider the mechanism of injury.
    D. treat life-threatening conditions.

58. The "A" in DCAP-BTLS stands for:
    A. allergies.   C. abrasions.
    B. alert.   D. arrhythmia.

59. All of the following are clues that help an EMT determine the need for cervical immobilization <u>except</u>:
    A. mechanism of injury.
    B. level of responsiveness.
    C. location of injuries.
    D. breathing rate.

60. Which of the following is true of the rapid trauma assessment?
    A. It begins with examination of the posterior body and ends with examination of the head.
    B. It evaluates areas of the body where the greatest threats to the patient may be.
    C. It is performed on a trauma patient who has no significant mechanism of injury.
    D. It includes careful examination of the face, eyes, ears, nose, and mouth.

61. On which type of patient is the detailed physical exam most often performed?
    A. trauma patient with a significant mechanism of injury
    B. trauma patient with no significant mechanism of injury
    C. responsive medical patient
    D. unresponsive medical patient

62. To obtain a history of a patient's present illness:
    A. ask the OPQRST questions.
    B. conduct the subjective interview.
    C. ask the SAMPLE questions.
    D. use the look, listen, feel, and smell method.

63. The "P" in OPQRST stands for:
    A. punctures.
    B. penetrations.
    C. provokes.
    D. pulses.

64. The steps in the focused history and physical exam of the unresponsive medical patient include the following:
    1. Obtain baseline vital signs.
    2. Gather the history of the present illness from bystanders and family.
    3. Conduct a rapid physical exam.
    4. Gather a SAMPLE history from bystanders and family.

    Which is the correct order in which the above steps should be performed?
    A. 3, 1, 2, 4
    B. 2, 3, 4, 1
    C. 3, 2, 4, 1
    D. 1, 2, 3, 4

65. For a stable patient, the EMT should perform the ongoing assessment every _____ minutes.
    A. 5   C. 15
    B. 10   D. 20

66. During the ongoing assessment, whenever you believe there may have been a change in the patient's condition, you should immediately:
    A. repeat the initial assessment.
    B. transport the patient immediately.
    C. document trends in vital signs.
    D. repeat the rapid trauma assessment.

67. Cool, clammy skin most likely indicates:
    A. high fever.
    B. exposure to cold.
    C. mild fever.
    D. hypoperfusion (shock).

68. As an EMT, your overriding concern at all times is:
   A. the patient's safety.
   B. the safety of patients and bystanders.
   C. the patient's life.
   D. your own safety.

69. During the detailed physical exam of the head of a trauma patient, inspect the:
   A. ears and nose for blood or clear fluids.
   B. inner surface of the eyelids.
   C. skin color of the cheeks.
   D. mouth for blood and clear fluids.

70. Infants and young children under the age of _____ are abdominal breathers.
   A. 2
   B. 4
   C. 8
   D. 16

71. Repeaters are:
   A. phones that transmit radio signals over air waves instead of wires.
   B. devices used to transmit radio signals over long distances.
   C. patients who consistently call 911.
   D. a type of cellular phone used in EMS.

72. Which one of the following is an appropriate interpersonal communication technique?
   A. standing above a patient
   B. avoiding eye contact
   C. directly facing a patient
   D. standing, arms crossed

73. What is the first item given to the hospital in your medical radio report to the receiving facility?
   A. the patient's age and sex
   B. unit identification/level of provider
   C. estimated time of arrival
   D. emergency medical care given

74. Which of the following is not considered an essential component of the verbal report to the receiving facility?
   A. patient's chief complaint
   B. additional treatment given en route
   C. additional vital signs taken en route
   D. patient's attitude.

75. Which of the following is true of the medical radio report? You:
   A. use codes to communicate patient information.
   B. ensure that you give the hospital your patient diagnosis.
   C. paint a picture of the patient's problem in words.
   D. speak rapidly to limit transmission time.

76. To avoid misunderstanding and miscommunication when speaking with medical direction, you should do all of the following except:
   A. give information clearly and accurately.
   B. repeat back the order you are given word for word.
   C. ask the physician to repeat the order if it is unclear.
   D. avoid questioning the physician about the order.

77. Medications that are carried on the ambulance and that EMTs can administer include activated charcoal, oxygen, and
   A. oral glucose.
   B. nitroglycerin.
   C. epinephrine.
   D. all of the above.

78. Any action of a drug other than the desired action is called a/an:
   A. contraindication.
   B. indication.
   C. reflex.
   D. side effect.

79. When a drug is administered subcutaneously, this means the drug is:
   A. dissolved under the tongue.
   B. injected into a vein.
   C. rubbed into a muscle.
   D. injected under the skin.

80. Which of the following is true of the structure of infants' and children's airways?
   A. The trachea is more rigid and less flexible than an adult's.
   B. The tongue is proportionately smaller than an adult's.
   C. The cricoid cartilage is more rigid than an adult's.
   D. They depend more on the diaphragm for respiration than adults do.

81. The means of providing artificial ventilation are:
   1. Pocket face mask with supplemental oxygen.
   2. Two-person bag-valve mask with supplemental oxygen.
   3. Flow-restricted, oxygen-powered ventilator.
   4. One-person bag-valve mask with supplemental oxygen.

   What is the best method to use?
   A. 1
   B. 2
   C. 3
   D. 4

82. The adequate rate of artificial ventilations for a nonbreathing adult patient is _____ breaths per minute.
   A. 6–8
   B. 10–12
   C. 14–16
   D. 18–20

©2009 Pearson Education, Inc.
Emergency Care, 11th Ed.

83. The adequate rate of artificial ventilations for a nonbreathing infant or child patient is _____ breaths per minute.
   A. 8–10
   B. 6–8
   C. 12–20
   D. 22–25

84. Which of the following respiratory sounds made by an unresponsive adult most likely indicates a serious airway problem requiring immediate intervention?
   A. snoring or gurgling
   B. slight wheezing
   C. sniffling
   D. whistling or grunting

85. The skin of a patient with inadequate breathing will most likely be:
   A. pale, cool, and dry
   B. red, hot, and clammy
   C. yellow, warm, and dry
   D. blue, cool, and clammy

86. If a patient is experiencing breathing difficulty, but is breathing adequately, it is usually best to place him in the _____ position.
   A. tripod
   B. supine
   C. sitting-up
   D. recovery

87. Which one of the following is a cause of adult chest pain due to a decreased blood supply to the heart muscle?
   A. stroke
   B. arrhythmia
   C. congestive heart failure
   D. angina pectoris

88. Most heart attacks are caused by the narrowing or occlusion of a _____ artery.
   A. cephalic
   B. brachial
   C. coronary
   D. carotid

89. Which of the following is the condition in which a portion of the myocardium dies because of oxygen starvation?
   A. angina pectoris
   B. mechanical pump failure
   C. cardiogenic shock
   D. acute myocardial infarction

90. An irregular heart rhythm is called:
   A. mechanical pump failure.
   B. arrhythmia.
   C. cardiogenic shock.
   D. congestive heart failure.

91. Which term applies to a pulse slower than 60 beats per minute?
   A. bradycardia
   B. ventricular fibrillation
   C. tachycardia
   D. atrial fibrillation

92. An at-rest heart beating faster than 100 beats per minute is referred to as:
   A. bradycardia.
   B. ventricular fibrillation.
   C. tachycardia.
   D. atrial fibrillation.

93. Which of the following is the condition caused by excessive fluid buildup in the lungs because of the inadequate pumping of the heart?
   A. congestive heart failure
   B. acute heart failure
   C. acute myocardial infarction
   D. chronic myocardial infarction

94. The conscious patient with a possible heart attack is best transported in the:
   A. recovery position.
   B. medical coma position.
   C. traumatic coma position.
   D. position of comfort.

95. A diabetic found with a weak, rapid pulse and cold, clammy skin who complains of hunger pangs suffers from:
   A. hypoglycemia.
   B. cardiogenic shock.
   C. hyperglycemia.
   D. ulcers.

96. Which of the following conditions frequently results in an acetone smell on the patient's breath?
   A. stroke
   B. hyperglycemia
   C. ulcers
   D. hypoglycemia

97. A conscious hypoglycemic patient who is able to swallow is frequently administered
   A. oral glucose.
   B. insulin.
   C. nitroglycerin.
   D. epinephrine.

98. If you cannot administer glucose to the diabetic patient because she is not alert enough to swallow, you should:
   A. wait until her mental status improves.
   B. contact medical direction immediately.
   C. treat her like any other patient with altered mental status.
   D. place her in a position of comfort.

99. The first time a person is exposed to an allergen, the immune system:
   A. reacts violently.
   B. shuts down.
   C. forms antibodies.
   D. ignores the allergen.

100. To be considered a severe allergic reaction, a patient must have signs and symptoms of shock and/or:
  A. a history of allergies.
  B. massive swelling.
  C. respiratory distress.
  D. increased blood pressure.

101. A patient has no history of allergies and is having his first allergic reaction. What action should you take?
  A. Consult with medical direction.
  B. Treat for shock and transport immediately.
  C. Administer epinephrine via auto-injector.
  D. Attempt to determine the cause immediately.

102. Carbon monoxide, chlorine, and ammonia are examples of _____ poisons.
  A. ingested   C. inhaled
  B. injected   D. absorbed

103. It is important for the EMT to determine when the ingestion of a poison occurred because:
  A. different poisons act on the body at different rates.
  B. those who ingest poison in the evening tend to vomit frequently.
  C. dilution of the poison is never effective after 10 minutes.
  D. the antidote is more effective once the poison reaches the stomach.

104. The principal prehospital treatment of a patient who has inhaled poisonous gas is:
  A. administering activated charcoal.
  B. administering high-concentration oxygen.
  C. rapidly administering an antidote.
  D. irrigating the respiratory tract with water.

105. Drinking alcohol along with taking other drugs frequently results in:
  A. uncontrolled shivering.
  B. depressed vital signs.
  C. extreme agitation.
  D. all of the above.

106. Activated charcoal is contraindicated for patients who have ingested:
  A. alkalis.   C. acids.
  B. gasoline.   D. all of the above.

107. Most cases of poisoning:
  A. are intentional in nature.
  B. involve elderly patients.
  C. involve young children.
  D. lead to disability or death.

108. Poisons that are swallowed are _____ poisons.
  A. absorbed   C. ingested
  B. inhaled   D. injected

109. For a heat emergency, the patient with _____, dry skin requires rapid cooling and immediate transport.
  A. pale   C. cool
  B. hot   D. warm

110. As frostbite progresses and exposure continues, the skin will turn from white and waxy to:
  A. blotchy and grayish yellow.
  B. pale and pinkish red.
  C. deep blue at the nose and cheeks.
  D. cherry red, except for the extremities.

111. To treat a patient with deep frostbite:
  A. immerse the limb in 105°F water and transport the patient.
  B. rub snow on the frozen area or apply cold packs if available.
  C. cover the frostbitten area, handle it as gently as possible, and transport patient.
  D. protect the frostbitten area by keeping it cold and transport the patient.

112. With frostbite, the:
  A. underlying tissues feel frozen to the touch.
  B. skin is commonly mottled and grayish blue.
  C. skin blisters and swells.
  D. affected area feels frozen, but only on the surface.

113. The initial sign of hypothermia is:
  A. shivering.
  B. numbness.
  C. drowsiness and slow breathing.
  D. white, waxy skin.

114. Extreme hypothermia is characterized by:
  A. unconsciousness, absence of discernible vital signs.
  B. shivering, numbness, and drowsiness.
  C. flaccid muscles.
  D. rapid breathing.

115. The emergency care steps for a hypothermic patient who is alert and responding include all of the following except:
  A. keep the patient still.
  B. keep the patient dry.
  C. apply heat to the patient's body.
  D. encourage the patient to walk.

©2009 Pearson Education, Inc.
Emergency Care, 11th Ed.

116. After calming a snakebite victim and treating for shock, you locate the fang marks. Next, you should:
    A. immobilize the affected extremity.
    B. conserve patient body heat.
    C. cleanse the wound site.
    D. apply a tourniquet to the extremity.

117. A patient who was working in a hot environment complains of severe muscle cramps in the legs and feels faint. You should move the patient to a cool place and begin care by:
    A. administering oxygen by nonrebreather.
    B. transporting the patient immediately.
    C. administering oxygen by nasal cannula.
    D. giving the patient water.

118. The first step in caring for a rescued drowning submersion victim is to:
    A. expel water from the patient's lungs.
    B. provide ventilations with oxygen.
    C. establish an airway.
    D. initiate chest compressions.

119. Your first step when called to care for any attempted suicide victim is to:
    A. gain access to the patient.
    B. wait for police assistance.
    C. survey for behavioral changes.
    D. ensure your own safety.

120. You are unable to perform normal assessment and care procedures because the patient is aggressive and hostile. What action should you take?
    A. Restrain the patient immediately.
    B. Ask a family member to assist you.
    C. Seek advice from medical direction.
    D. Call the patient's physician.

121. When is the EMT allowed to use reasonable force?
    A. only when the police are on the scene
    B. to defend against attack by an emotionally disturbed patient
    C. whenever a patient refuses treatment
    D. whenever alcohol abuse is suspected

122. The developing unborn baby is called a:
    A. crowning.
    B. fetus.
    C. placenta previa.
    D. stillborn.

123. The muscular organ in which the fetus develops is the:
    A. umbilical cord.
    B. placenta.
    C. uterus
    D. cervix.

124. The organ of pregnancy in which exchange of oxygen, nutrients, and wastes occurs between mother and fetus is the:
    A. placenta.   C. vagina.
    B. cervix.   D. amniotic.

125. While developing, the fetus is protected by a thin, membranous "bag of waters" called the _____ sac.
    A. uterine   C. amniotic
    B. placental   D. peritoneal

126. When the presenting part of the baby first bulges from the vaginal opening, this is called:
    A. crowning.   C. labor.
    B. dilating.   D. prolapsing.

127. The first stage of labor begins with:
    A. cervical dilation.
    B. perineum thinning.
    C. uterine contractions.
    D. afterbirth.

128. The second stage of labor ends with:
    A. cervical dilation.
    B. infant delivery.
    C. placental delivery.
    D. uterine contractions.

129. The third stage of labor ends with:
    A. full cervical dilation.
    B. perineum tearing.
    C. delivery of the placenta.
    D. delivery of infant.

130. If a woman is having her first baby, the first stage of labor will usually last _____ hours on the average.
    A. 4   C. 12
    B. 8   D. 16

131. During the most active stage of labor, the uterus usually contracts every _____ minutes.
    A. 1 to 2   C. 5 to 9
    B. 2 to 3   D. 10 to 15

132. If the amniotic sac does not break during delivery, the EMT should:
    A. do nothing; it will break after birth.
    B. quickly remove with sterile scissors.
    C. puncture it with a finger.
    D. transport the patient immediately.

133. To assist the mother in delivering the baby, gently:
    A. pull at the baby's shoulders.
    B. support the baby's head.
    C. rotate the baby to the left or right.
    D. push your gloved hand into the vagina.

©2009 Pearson Education, Inc.
Emergency Care, 11th Ed.

134. After the delivery, which of the following should be done first?
    A. Clamp and cut the cord.
    B. Suction the baby's mouth and nose.
    C. Lay the baby on his back.
    D. Lift the baby by the feet and slap the buttocks.

135. Following the delivery, if spontaneous respiration does not begin after suctioning the baby's mouth and nose, the EMT should first:
    A. begin mouth-to-mouth-and-nose resuscitation.
    B. apply mechanical resuscitation with 100% oxygen.
    C. vigorously rub the baby's back.
    D. transport immediately, administering 100% oxygen.

136. The first clamp placed on the umbilical cord should be about _____ inches from the baby.
    A. 2   C. 10
    B. 5   D. 12

137. If bleeding continues from the umbilical cord after clamping and cutting, the EMT should:
    A. clamp the cord again.
    B. unclamp the cord and tie.
    C. apply a sterile dressing.
    D. transport the baby immediately.

138. Which of the following is the maximum amount of time the EMT should wait for the placenta to be delivered before transporting the mother and infant?
    A. 20 minutes   C. 1 hour
    B. 45 minutes   D. 2 hours

139. Delivery of the placenta is usually accompanied by the loss of no more than _____ of blood.
    A. 500 cc   C. 800 cc
    B. 600 cc   D. 1,000 cc

140. The first step to control vaginal bleeding after birth is to:
    A. apply a pressure dressing.
    B. position a sanitary napkin.
    C. massage the uterus.
    D. pack the vagina with sterile gauze.

141. The presenting part of the baby in a breech birth is the:
    A. arms.   C. face.
    B. buttocks or legs. D. head.

142. If, during birth, the umbilical cord presents first, you should:
    A. gently push the cord back into the vagina.
    B. gently push up on the baby's head or buttocks to keep pressure off the cord.
    C. gently push on the cervix.
    D. clamp and cut the cord.

143. If an arm presentation without a prolapsed cord is noted, the EMT should:
    A. reach up the vagina and turn the baby.
    B. do nothing; the delivery will be normal.
    C. transport immediately, providing O_2.
    D. insert gloved hand and push back the vaginal wall.

144. A baby is considered premature if it weighs less than 5 pounds or is born before the _____ week of pregnancy.
    A. 35th   C. 37th
    B. 36th   D. 38th

Interim Exam 2 Answer Sheet

Fill in the correct answer for each item. When scoring, note there are 144 questions valued at 0.666 points each.

1. [ ] A　[ ] B　[ ] C　[ ] D
2. [ ] A　[ ] B　[ ] C　[ ] D
3. [ ] A　[ ] B　[ ] C　[ ] D
4. [ ] A　[ ] B　[ ] C　[ ] D
5. [ ] A　[ ] B　[ ] C　[ ] D
6. [ ] A　[ ] B　[ ] C　[ ] D
7. [ ] A　[ ] B　[ ] C　[ ] D
8. [ ] A　[ ] B　[ ] C　[ ] D
9. [ ] A　[ ] B　[ ] C　[ ] D
10. [ ] A　[ ] B　[ ] C　[ ] D
11. [ ] A　[ ] B　[ ] C　[ ] D
12. [ ] A　[ ] B　[ ] C　[ ] D
13. [ ] A　[ ] B　[ ] C　[ ] D
14. [ ] A　[ ] B　[ ] C　[ ] D
15. [ ] A　[ ] B　[ ] C　[ ] D
16. [ ] A　[ ] B　[ ] C　[ ] D
17. [ ] A　[ ] B　[ ] C　[ ] D
18. [ ] A　[ ] B　[ ] C　[ ] D
19. [ ] A　[ ] B　[ ] C　[ ] D
20. [ ] A　[ ] B　[ ] C　[ ] D
21. [ ] A　[ ] B　[ ] C　[ ] D
22. [ ] A　[ ] B　[ ] C　[ ] D
23. [ ] A　[ ] B　[ ] C　[ ] D
24. [ ] A　[ ] B　[ ] C　[ ] D
25. [ ] A　[ ] B　[ ] C　[ ] D
26. [ ] A　[ ] B　[ ] C　[ ] D
27. [ ] A　[ ] B　[ ] C　[ ] D
28. [ ] A　[ ] B　[ ] C　[ ] D
29. [ ] A　[ ] B　[ ] C　[ ] D
30. [ ] A　[ ] B　[ ] C　[ ] D
31. [ ] A　[ ] B　[ ] C　[ ] D
32. [ ] A　[ ] B　[ ] C　[ ] D
33. [ ] A　[ ] B　[ ] C　[ ] D
34. [ ] A　[ ] B　[ ] C　[ ] D
35. [ ] A　[ ] B　[ ] C　[ ] D
36. [ ] A　[ ] B　[ ] C　[ ] D

37. [ ] A　[ ] B　[ ] C　[ ] D
38. [ ] A　[ ] B　[ ] C　[ ] D
39. [ ] A　[ ] B　[ ] C　[ ] D
40. [ ] A　[ ] B　[ ] C　[ ] D
41. [ ] A　[ ] B　[ ] C　[ ] D
42. [ ] A　[ ] B　[ ] C　[ ] D
43. [ ] A　[ ] B　[ ] C　[ ] D
44. [ ] A　[ ] B　[ ] C　[ ] D
45. [ ] A　[ ] B　[ ] C　[ ] D
46. [ ] A　[ ] B　[ ] C　[ ] D
47. [ ] A　[ ] B　[ ] C　[ ] D
48. [ ] A　[ ] B　[ ] C　[ ] D
49. [ ] A　[ ] B　[ ] C　[ ] D
50. [ ] A　[ ] B　[ ] C　[ ] D
51. [ ] A　[ ] B　[ ] C　[ ] D
52. [ ] A　[ ] B　[ ] C　[ ] D
53. [ ] A　[ ] B　[ ] C　[ ] D
54. [ ] A　[ ] B　[ ] C　[ ] D
55. [ ] A　[ ] B　[ ] C　[ ] D
56. [ ] A　[ ] B　[ ] C　[ ] D
57. [ ] A　[ ] B　[ ] C　[ ] D
58. [ ] A　[ ] B　[ ] C　[ ] D
59. [ ] A　[ ] B　[ ] C　[ ] D
60. [ ] A　[ ] B　[ ] C　[ ] D
61. [ ] A　[ ] B　[ ] C　[ ] D
62. [ ] A　[ ] B　[ ] C　[ ] D
63. [ ] A　[ ] B　[ ] C　[ ] D
64. [ ] A　[ ] B　[ ] C　[ ] D
65. [ ] A　[ ] B　[ ] C　[ ] D
66. [ ] A　[ ] B　[ ] C　[ ] D
67. [ ] A　[ ] B　[ ] C　[ ] D
68. [ ] A　[ ] B　[ ] C　[ ] D
69. [ ] A　[ ] B　[ ] C　[ ] D
70. [ ] A　[ ] B　[ ] C　[ ] D
71. [ ] A　[ ] B　[ ] C　[ ] D
72. [ ] A　[ ] B　[ ] C　[ ] D

73. [ ] A	[ ] B	[ ] C	[ ] D
74. [ ] A	[ ] B	[ ] C	[ ] D
75. [ ] A	[ ] B	[ ] C	[ ] D
76. [ ] A	[ ] B	[ ] C	[ ] D
77. [ ] A	[ ] B	[ ] C	[ ] D
78. [ ] A	[ ] B	[ ] C	[ ] D
79. [ ] A	[ ] B	[ ] C	[ ] D
80. [ ] A	[ ] B	[ ] C	[ ] D
81. [ ] A	[ ] B	[ ] C	[ ] D
82. [ ] A	[ ] B	[ ] C	[ ] D
83. [ ] A	[ ] B	[ ] C	[ ] D
84. [ ] A	[ ] B	[ ] C	[ ] D
85. [ ] A	[ ] B	[ ] C	[ ] D
86. [ ] A	[ ] B	[ ] C	[ ] D
87. [ ] A	[ ] B	[ ] C	[ ] D
88. [ ] A	[ ] B	[ ] C	[ ] D
89. [ ] A	[ ] B	[ ] C	[ ] D
90. [ ] A	[ ] B	[ ] C	[ ] D
91. [ ] A	[ ] B	[ ] C	[ ] D
92. [ ] A	[ ] B	[ ] C	[ ] D
93. [ ] A	[ ] B	[ ] C	[ ] D
94. [ ] A	[ ] B	[ ] C	[ ] D
95. [ ] A	[ ] B	[ ] C	[ ] D
96. [ ] A	[ ] B	[ ] C	[ ] D
97. [ ] A	[ ] B	[ ] C	[ ] D
98. [ ] A	[ ] B	[ ] C	[ ] D
99. [ ] A	[ ] B	[ ] C	[ ] D
100. [ ] A	[ ] B	[ ] C	[ ] D
101. [ ] A	[ ] B	[ ] C	[ ] D
102. [ ] A	[ ] B	[ ] C	[ ] D
103. [ ] A	[ ] B	[ ] C	[ ] D
104. [ ] A	[ ] B	[ ] C	[ ] D
105. [ ] A	[ ] B	[ ] C	[ ] D
106. [ ] A	[ ] B	[ ] C	[ ] D
107. [ ] A	[ ] B	[ ] C	[ ] D
108. [ ] A	[ ] B	[ ] C	[ ] D

109. [ ] A	[ ] B	[ ] C	[ ] D
110. [ ] A	[ ] B	[ ] C	[ ] D
111. [ ] A	[ ] B	[ ] C	[ ] D
112. [ ] A	[ ] B	[ ] C	[ ] D
113. [ ] A	[ ] B	[ ] C	[ ] D
114. [ ] A	[ ] B	[ ] C	[ ] D
115. [ ] A	[ ] B	[ ] C	[ ] D
116. [ ] A	[ ] B	[ ] C	[ ] D
117. [ ] A	[ ] B	[ ] C	[ ] D
118. [ ] A	[ ] B	[ ] C	[ ] D
119. [ ] A	[ ] B	[ ] C	[ ] D
120. [ ] A	[ ] B	[ ] C	[ ] D
121. [ ] A	[ ] B	[ ] C	[ ] D
122. [ ] A	[ ] B	[ ] C	[ ] D
123. [ ] A	[ ] B	[ ] C	[ ] D
124. [ ] A	[ ] B	[ ] C	[ ] D
125. [ ] A	[ ] B	[ ] C	[ ] D
126. [ ] A	[ ] B	[ ] C	[ ] D
127. [ ] A	[ ] B	[ ] C	[ ] D
128. [ ] A	[ ] B	[ ] C	[ ] D
129. [ ] A	[ ] B	[ ] C	[ ] D
130. [ ] A	[ ] B	[ ] C	[ ] D
131. [ ] A	[ ] B	[ ] C	[ ] D
132. [ ] A	[ ] B	[ ] C	[ ] D
133. [ ] A	[ ] B	[ ] C	[ ] D
134. [ ] A	[ ] B	[ ] C	[ ] D
135. [ ] A	[ ] B	[ ] C	[ ] D
136. [ ] A	[ ] B	[ ] C	[ ] D
137. [ ] A	[ ] B	[ ] C	[ ] D
138. [ ] A	[ ] B	[ ] C	[ ] D
139. [ ] A	[ ] B	[ ] C	[ ] D
140. [ ] A	[ ] B	[ ] C	[ ] D
141. [ ] A	[ ] B	[ ] C	[ ] D
142. [ ] A	[ ] B	[ ] C	[ ] D
143. [ ] A	[ ] B	[ ] C	[ ] D
144. [ ] A	[ ] B	[ ] C	[ ] D

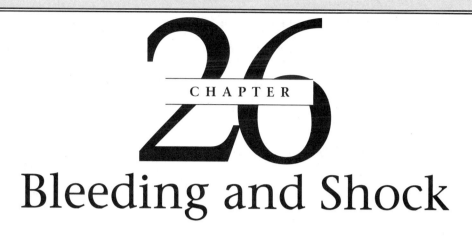

Bleeding and Shock

MATCH TERMINOLOGY/ DEFINITIONS

▶ **PART A**

A. Major artery of the upper arm

B. When the patient is developing shock, but the body is still able to maintain perfusion

C. Bleeding that is characterized by a slow, oozing flow of blood

D. Shock resulting from blood loss

E. Condition that occurs when the body can no longer compensate for low blood volume or lack of perfusion; late signs, such as falling blood pressure, develop.

F. Major artery supplying the thigh

G. Severe bleeding; a major cause of shock

H. Lack of perfusion brought on by inadequate pumping action of the heart

I. Optimum time limit between time of injury and surgery at the hospital; survival rates are best if surgery takes place within this time period.

J. Blood vessel with thick, muscular walls that carries blood away from the heart

_____ **1.** Artery

_____ **2.** Brachial artery

_____ **3.** Capillary bleeding

_____ **4.** Cardiogenic shock

_____ **5.** Compensated shock

_____ **6.** Decompensated shock

_____ **7.** Femoral artery

_____ **8.** Golden hour

_____ **9.** Hemorrhage

_____ **10.** Hemorrhagic shock

A. Device that closes off all blood flow to and from an extremity

B. Blood vessel that has one-way valves and carries blood back to the heart

C. Adequate circulation of blood throughout the body, filling the capillaries and supplying the cells and tissues with oxygen and nutrients

D. Site where a large artery lies near the surface of the body and directly over a bone; pressure on such a location can control profuse bleeding in the extremities.

E. When the body has lost the battle to maintain perfusion to the organ systems; cell damage occurs, especially to the liver and kidneys.

F. Another name for hypoperfusion

G. Bulky dressing held in position with a tightly wrapped bandage to help control bleeding

H. Shock resulting from uncontrolled bleeding or plasma loss

I. Shock resulting from uncontrolled dilation of blood vessels due to nerve paralysis (sometimes caused by spinal cord injuries)

J. Inadequate circulation of the blood in which the body's cells and organs do not receive adequate supplies of oxygen and dangerous waste products build up

_____ **1.** Hypoperfusion

_____ **2.** Hypovolemic shock

_____ **3.** Irreversible shock

_____ **4.** Neurogenic shock

_____ **5.** Perfusion

_____ **6.** Pressure dressing

_____ **7.** Pressure point

_____ **8.** Shock

_____ **9.** Tourniquet

_____ **10.** Vein

MULTIPLE-CHOICE REVIEW

_____ **1.** Blood that has been depleted of oxygen and loaded with carbon dioxide empties into the _____, which carry it back to the heart.
 A. arteries
 B. veins
 C. capillaries
 D. tissues

_____ **2.** Cells and tissues of the brain, spinal cord, and _____ are the <u>most</u> sensitive to inadequate perfusion.
 A. kidneys
 B. lungs
 C. stomach
 D. heart

_____ **3.** The use of _____ is essential whenever bleeding is discovered or anticipated.
 A. full protective gear
 B. Standard Precautions
 C. universal isolation precautions
 D. Tyvek overalls

_____ **4.** Bleeding is classified as all of the following <u>except</u>:
 A. arterial.
 B. venous.
 C. cellular.
 D. capillary.

_____ **5.** Which statement about arterial bleeding is correct?
 A. Clot formation takes place rapidly.
 B. It is often rapid and profuse.
 C. It is the least difficult to control.
 D. It causes the blood pressure to rise.

_____ **6.** A steady flow of dark red or maroon blood is a result of _____ bleeding.
   A. arterial
   B. venous
   C. capillary
   D. pulmonary

_____ **7.** Bleeding described as oozing usually is a result of _____ bleeding.
   A. arterial
   B. venous
   C. capillary
   D. bronchiole

_____ **8.** When a large bleeding vein in the neck sucks in debris or an air bubble, this can cause:
   A. an evisceration.
   B. heart stoppage.
   C. infection.
   D. severe bleeding.

_____ **9.** Sudden blood loss of _____ in an adult is considered serious.
   A. 250 cc
   B. 500 cc
   C. 600 cc
   D. 1,000 cc

_____ **10.** Sudden blood loss of _____ in a child is considered serious.
   A. 200 cc
   B. 300 cc
   C. 400 cc
   D. 500 cc

_____ **11.** Sudden blood loss of _____ in a 1-year-old infant is considered serious.
   A. 25 cc
   B. 50 cc
   C. 100 cc
   D. 150 cc

_____ **12.** The body's natural responses to bleeding is constriction of the injured blood vessel and:
   A. perfusion.
   B. hypoperfusion.
   C. compensation.
   D. clotting.

_____ **13.** The EMT's assessment of external bleeding includes all of the following items except:
   A. estimating the amount of blood lost in order to predict potential shock.
   B. waiting for signs and symptoms of shock to appear before beginning treatment.
   C. triaging, or prioritizing, bleeding patients properly.
   D. identifying bleeding that must be treated during the initial assessment.

_____ **14.** The major methods used to control external bleeding include all of the following except:
   A. direct pressure.
   B. elevation.
   C. pressure points.
   D. vessel clamps.

_____ **15.** Why is administration of supplemental oxygen an important treatment for any trauma patient?
   A. It enhances blood clotting.
   B. It improves oxygenation of the tissues.
   C. It constricts the blood vessels.
   D. All of the above.

_____ **16.** The most common and effective way to control external bleeding is by:
   A. cold application.
   B. elevation.
   C. pressure points.
   D. direct pressure.

_____ **17.** The initial dressing should not be removed from a bleeding wound because it:
   A. can become a biohazard.
   B. takes too long to remove.
   C. is a necessary part of clot formation.
   D. may increase the chance of infection.

_____ **18.** After controlling bleeding from an extremity using a pressure dressing, be sure to:
   A. loosen the tourniquet.
   B. check the distal pulse.
   C. apply a PASG.
   D. administer oxygen by nasal cannula.

_____ **19.** Elevation is used to assist in bleeding control for all of the following reasons except:
   A. it slows bleeding.
   B. it raises the limb above the heart.
   C. it helps to reduce blood pressure in the limb.
   D. it speeds up the pulse rate.

_____ **20.** When is it inappropriate to use elevation to assist in bleeding control?
   A. as you apply direct pressure
   B. while trying to bandage an extremity
   C. if you suspect musculoskeletal injuries
   D. when a patient is found lying down

_____ **21.** A pressure point is a site where:
   A. A main artery lies near the surface of the body directly over the bone.
   B. the blood pressure can be taken by auscultation.
   C. a large vein lies within the outer layer of the skin.
   D. excessive pressure causes the pulse rate to increase rapidly.

_____ **22.** Use of a pressure point may not be effective if the wound:
   A. was caused by an impaled object.
   B. was accompanied by spinal injury.
   C. is at the distal end of a limb.
   D. is bleeding profusely.

_____ **23.** Which of the following is true about the use of an air splint?
   A. It is effective for controlling venous and capillary bleeding.
   B. It should be used only if there is no suspected bone injury.
   C. It is most effective for controlling arterial bleeding.
   D. It should be used before other manual methods of bleeding control.

_____ **24.** Which of the following is not a guideline for supplementing bleeding control with cold application?
   A. Wrap the ice pack in a cloth or towel.
   B. Do not apply directly onto the skin.
   C. Do not leave the cold pack in place for more than 20 minutes.
   D. Insert the ice directly into the wound.

_____ **25.** Many experts agree that the pneumatic antishock garment (PASG) is useful for:
   A. controlling bleeding from head trauma.
   B. controlling bleeding from the areas the garment covers.
   C. penetrating chest trauma.
   D. the patient in cardiogenic shock.

_____ **26.** Bleeding from a clean-edged amputation is usually initially cared for with:
   A. a pressure dressing.   **C.** a tourniquet.
   B. cold application.   **D.** a pneumatic antishock garment.

_____ **27.** Rough-edged amputations, usually produced by crushing or tearing injuries:
   A. are easily controlled by a pressure bandage.
   B. tend to stop bleeding on their own.
   C. often will bleed very heavily.
   D. will constrict quickly to control bleeding.

©2009 Pearson Education, Inc.
Emergency Care, 11th Ed.

_____ **28.** Once a tourniquet is in place, it must:
- **A.** not be removed or loosened unless ordered by medical direction.
- **B.** be covered immediately to prevent accidental removal.
- **C.** be loosened every 15 minutes to dislodge clots.
- **D.** be used under the pneumatic antishock garment.

_____ **29.** A blood pressure cuff:
- **A.** can be used as a tourniquet if inflated to 70 mmHg.
- **B.** should never be used for bleeding control.
- **C.** can be used as a temporary tourniquet if inflated to 150 mmHg.
- **D.** should always be used to control arterial bleeding.

_____ **30.** If a patient has a head injury and you note bleeding or loss of cerebrospinal fluid from the patient's ears or nose, you should:
- **A.** apply direct pressure to the skull.
- **B.** apply direct pressure to the ears and nose.
- **C.** apply cold packs to the ears and nose.
- **D.** allow the drainage to flow freely.

_____ **31.** The medical term for a nosebleed is:
- **A.** hemorrhage.
- **B.** epistaxis.
- **C.** epihemorrhage.
- **D.** nostrium.

_____ **32.** To stop a nosebleed, try each of the following except:
- **A.** place the patient in a sitting position, leaning forward.
- **B.** apply direct pressure by pinching the nostrils.
- **C.** keep the patient calm.
- **D.** apply cold packs to the bridge of the nose.

_____ **33.** The leading cause of internal injuries and bleeding is:
- **A.** blunt trauma.
- **B.** penetrating trauma.
- **C.** auto collisions.
- **D.** large lacerations.

_____ **34.** Which is not an example of a penetrating trauma?
- **A.** blast injury
- **B.** gunshot wound
- **C.** knife wound
- **D.** ice-pick wound

_____ **35.** Signs of internal bleeding include all of the following except:
- **A.** vomiting a coffee-ground-like substance.
- **B.** bradycardia and a flushed face.
- **C.** dark, tarry stools.
- **D.** tender, rigid, or distended abdomen.

_____ **36.** A patient who has internal bleeding may have all of the following except:
- **A.** painful, swollen, or deformed extremities.
- **B.** signs and symptoms of shock.
- **C.** bright red blood in the stool.
- **D.** laceration to the forearm.

_____ **37.** Inadequate tissue perfusion is referred to as:
- **A.** hyperperfusion.
- **B.** hypoxia.
- **C.** hypoperfusion.
- **D.** hypotension.

_____ **38.** Shock may develop as a result of all of the following except:
- **A.** pump failure.
- **B.** lost blood volume.
- **C.** dilated blood vessels.
- **D.** injury to the head.

_____ **39.** The type of shock most commonly seen by EMTs is _____ shock.
- **A.** cardiogenic
- **B.** irreversible
- **C.** neurogenic
- **D.** hypovolemic

_____ **40.** The most common mechanism of shock for a heart attack patient is:
- **A.** vasoconstriction.
- **B.** fluid loss.
- **C.** pump failure.
- **D.** vasodilation.

_____ **41.** Shock caused by the failure of the nervous system to control the diameter of blood vessels is called _____ shock. .
  A. hypovolemic
  B. cardiogenic
  C. neurogenic
  D. reversible

_____ **42.** When a patient is in shock but the body is still able to maintain perfusion to the vital organs, this is called _____ shock.
  A. compensated
  B. decompensated
  C. delayed
  D. irreversible

_____ **43.** Early signs of shock that are actually the body's compensating mechanisms include all of the following except:
  A. increased heart rate.
  B. increased respirations.
  C. pale, cool skin.
  D. decreased capillary refill time.

_____ **44.** When the body has lost the battle to maintain perfusion to the organ systems, this is called _____ shock.
  A. delayed
  B. compensated
  C. decompensated
  D. irreversible

_____ **45.** Why does a patient in shock feel nauseated?
  A. Blood is diverted from the digestive system.
  B. Blood rushes rapidly to the digestive system.
  C. Shock increases the production of digestive juices.
  D. The patient has swallowed a great amount of blood.

_____ **46.** The pulse of a patient in shock will:
  A. decrease.
  B. be absent.
  C. increase.
  D. be irregular.

_____ **47.** A drop in blood pressure is:
  A. an early sign of shock.
  B. an early sign of shock in a child.
  C. always present in shock.
  D. a late sign of shock.

_____ **48.** Additional signs of shock may include any of the following except:
  A. thirst.
  B. dilated pupils.
  C. cyanosis around the lips and nail beds.
  D. flushed, warm skin.

_____ **49.** The EMT should be especially careful when evaluating pediatric patients for shock because they:
  A. cannot be administered oxygen at low flow rates.
  B. may display few signs/symptoms until a large percentage of blood volume is lost.
  C. can decompensate for blood loss very quickly.
  D. may exhibit erratic capillary refill times.

_____ **50.** Which of the following is the best description of the "platinum 10 minutes"?
  A. maximum on-scene time when caring for a trauma or shock patient
  B. optimum time limit from the time of injury until surgery
  C. maximum time limit for controlling arterial bleeding before shock occurs
  D. optimum time limit for applying PASG to the shock patient

©2009 Pearson Education, Inc.
Emergency Care, 11th Ed.

COMPLETE THE FOLLOWING

1. List three major types of shock:

   A. _____

   B. _____

   C. _____

2. List six signs and symptoms of shock.

   A. _____

   B. _____

   C. _____

   D. _____

   E. _____

   F. _____

STREET SCENES DISCUSSION

Review the Street Scene on pp. 640–641 of the textbook. Then answer the questions below.

1. This patient may have broken a rib or two. What abdominal organs are protected by the rib cage?

2. Would an ALS unit be appropriate for this patient?

3. You observed that the patient's mental status was changing. What might this indicate to you?

ON THE WEB

To help you review and practice basic skills, visit the *Emergency Care 11th Ed. Companion Website* at www.prenhall.com/limmer. For Online Test Preparation, visit www.prenhall.com/emtachieve.

EMT SKILL PERFORMANCE CHECKLISTS

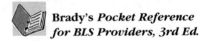

Brady's *Pocket Reference for BLS Providers*, 3rd Ed.

▶ BLEEDING CONTROL/SHOCK MANAGEMENT (P. 622)

❑ Take Standard Precautions.

❑ Apply direct pressure to the wound.

❑ Elevate the extremity.

❑ Apply a dressing to the wound.

❑ If wound continues to bleed, apply an additional dressing to the wound.

❑ If wound continues to bleed, locate and apply pressure to appropriate arterial pressure point.

❑ Administer high-concentration oxygen by nonrebreather mask.

❑ Properly position the patient.

❑ Initiate steps to prevent heat loss from the patient.

❑ Determine need for immediate transportation.

▶ APPLICATION OF PASG (P. 638)

❑ Take Standard Precautions.

❑ Assure patient meets local protocol for PASG.

❑ Check for contraindications (e.g., pulmonary edema or penetrating chest injury).

❑ Remove clothing and check for sharp objects.

❑ Quickly assess areas that will be under the PASG.

❑ Position PASG with top of abdominal section at or below the last set of ribs.

❑ Secure PASG around patient.

❑ Attach hoses.

❑ Check blood pressure.

❑ Begin inflation sequence.

❑ Stop inflation sequence (106 mmHg or pop-off valves release).

❑ Operate PASG to maintain air pressure in device.

❑ Reassess patient's vital signs.

WARNINGS: Do not actually inflate a PASG on a mock victim in a classroom setting. Do not inflate abdominal section if patient is pregnant.

CASE STUDY

▶ **Convenience Store Shooting**

You respond to a local convenience store where there has been an armed robbery. The call was dispatched as a shooting in which the police already have secured the scene. A bystander who pulled up to the store just as the shooter was running out the front door states, "The injured clerk is sitting on the floor, clutching his stomach."

1. What is the importance of a secure scene?

2. As you enter the store, what other scene size-up procedures are important?

You find the 18-year-old male clerk holding the right upper quadrant of his abdomen with a piece of cloth soaked in blood. He is conscious and alert, knows his name, where he is, and the day of the week. His name is Tom. He complains of pain and says he is very thirsty. You reach down and feel for his radial pulse. You can barely feel it because it is so fast and weak.

3. What important information have you just found out about this patient?

4. What phase and what type of shock is your patient in based upon the information you know?

5. What is the relevance of his being thirsty?

When you check Tom's carotid pulse, it is about 120 per minute and thready. His respirations are 24/shallow and regular. You quickly assess his chest and find no entry into the chest and equal breath sounds on both lungs. You immediately search for other injuries, ask him about other complaints, and find he has none. You do a very quick search from head to toe for additional external hemorrhage and an exit bullet wound. Your partner begins to control the bleeding and administer oxygen to the patient. Together, you and your partner carefully lay Tom down on a long spine board.

6. Since Tom was shot in the abdomen, what is the importance of listening to his lungs?

7. What device should be used and at what liter flow rate should the regulator be set for this patient?

8. Should an ALS unit be called for if one was not dispatched with you? If so, should you wait on the scene for ALS or arrange an intercept?

The patient is very pale and sweating profusely. He is beginning to get anxious about dying. You and your partner rapidly move him to the ambulance.

9. On a call like this, what is the maximum time you should spend on the scene? What is this time frame commonly called?

10. To give the surgeons a fighting chance to save Tom's life, what is the maximum time you should spend in assessment and transportation of the patient to the trauma center? What is this time frame commonly called?

©2009 Pearson Education, Inc.
Emergency Care, 11th Ed.

The patient is loaded in the ambulance. His level of responsiveness is reassessed, and he is responding to painful stimuli only. ALS will intercept you en route.

11. Aside from reassessing the vitals, what airway care should be considered at this time?

12. Would the PASG be indicated in this case?

13. Is this patient critical?

You meet up with the ALS unit. They jump aboard your ambulance with their portable equipment. The driver quickly continues to the hospital.

14. What procedures would you suspect an ALS unit might do en route to the hospital?

15. Briefly write down the radio report that you would give to the hospital en route. The patient initially told you he has no allergies, takes no medications, and has been healthy; his last meal was lunch a few hours ago. The paramedics establish two large-bore IVs and prepare to endotracheally intubate the patient. His pulse oximeter reading is 85% and his ECG is sinus tachycardia at a rate of 136.

Radio Report:

_____

_____

_____

_____

_____

CHAPTER 27

Soft-Tissue Injuries

MATCH TERMINOLOGY/ DEFINITIONS

▶ **PART A**

A. Swelling caused by the collection of blood under the skin or in damaged tissues as a result of an injured or broken blood vessel

B. Outer layer of the skin

C. Any material used to hold a dressing in place

D. Cut that can be smooth or jagged

E. Intestine or other internal organ protruding through a wound in the abdomen

F. Internal injury in which there is no open pathway from the outside to the injured site

G. Burn in which all the layers of the skin are damaged; also called a third-degree burn

H. Flap of skin or other tissue torn loose or pulled off completely

I. Any material used to cover a wound in an effort to control bleeding and help prevent additional contamination

J. Injury caused when force is transmitted from the body's exterior to its internal structures

K. Air bubble in the bloodstream

L. Layer of the skin found below the epidermis; it is rich in blood vessels, nerves, and specialized structures such as sweat glands, sebaceous (oil) glands, and hair follicles.

M. Bruise

_____ **1.** Abrasion

_____ **2.** Air embolus

_____ **3.** Amputation

_____ **4.** Avulsion

_____ **5.** Bandage

_____ **6.** Closed wound

_____ **7.** Contusion

_____ **8.** Crush injury

_____ **9.** Dermis

_____ **10.** Dressing

_____ **11.** Epidermis

_____ **12.** Evisceration

_____ **13.** Full thickness burn

_____ **14.** Hematoma

_____ **15.** Laceration

N. Scrape or scratch in which the outer layer of the skin is damaged but all the layers are not penetrated

O. Surgical removal or traumatic severing of a body part, usually an extremity

▶ **PART B**

A. Large bulky dressing

B. Method for estimating the extent of a burn area in which areas on the body are assigned certain percentages of the body's total surface area

C. Open chest wound in which air is drawn into the chest cavity

D. Burn in which the epidermis is burned through and the dermis is damaged; also called a second-degree burn

E. Burn that involves only the epidermis, the outer layer of the skin; also called a first-degree burn

F. Injury in which the skin is interrupted, or broken, exposing the tissue underneath

G. Layers of fat and soft tissues found below the dermis

H. Any dressing that forms an airtight seal

I. Method for estimating the extent of a burn area; palm of patient's hand, which equals about 1% of the body's surface area, is compared to patient's burn to estimate size.

J. Open wound caused by a sharp, pointed object that tears through the skin and destroys underlying tissues

K. Fracture of two or more adjacent ribs in two or more places that allows for free movement of the fractured segment.

L. Movement of ribs in a flail segment that is opposite to the rest of the chest wall

M. Air in the chest cavity

N. A type of pneumothorax in which air that enters the chest cavity is prevented from escaping.

_____ **1.** Occlusive dressing

_____ **2.** Open wound

_____ **3.** Partial thickness burn

_____ **4.** Puncture wound

_____ **5.** Rule of nines

_____ **6.** Rule of palm

_____ **7.** Subcutaneous layers

_____ **8.** Sucking chest wound

_____ **9.** Superficial burn

_____ **10.** Universal dressing

_____ **11.** Flail chest

_____ **12.** Paradoxical motion

_____ **13.** Pneumothorax

_____ **14.** Tension pneumothorax

MULTIPLE-CHOICE REVIEW

_____ **1.** The soft tissues of the body include all of the following <u>except</u>:
  A. skin, fatty tissue, muscles.
  B. blood vessels and fibrous tissues.
  C. teeth, bones, cartilage.
  D. nerves, membranes, glands.

_____ **2.** Which of the following is <u>not</u> a function of the skin?
  A. protection
  B. shock absorption
  C. temperature regulation
  D. blood insulation

_____ **3.** The layers of the skin include all of the following <u>except</u>:
  A. epidermis.
  B. dermis.
  C. subcutaneous.
  D. epithelial.

_____ **4.** The layer of the skin called the _____ is composed of dead cells, which are rubbed off or sloughed off and are replaced continuously.
  A. epidermis
  B. dermis
  C. subcutaneous
  D. epithelial

_____ **5.** Specialized nerve endings in the skin layer called the _____ are involved with the senses of touch, cold, heat, and pain.
  A. epidermis
  B. dermis
  C. subcutaneous layers
  D. epithelial cells

_____ 6. Shock absorption and insulation are major functions of which layer of the skin?
   A. epidermis
   B. dermis
   C. subcutaneous
   D. epithelial

_____ 7. Wounds that usually result from the impact of a blunt object are called:
   A. stabbings.
   B. lacerations.
   C. closed.
   D. perforations.

_____ 8. A closed wound that involves a large amount of tissue damage and a collection of blood at the injury site is called a:
   A. perforation.
   B. hematoma.
   C. contusion.
   D. penetration.

_____ 9. A soft-tissue injury caused by a force that can cause rupture or bleeding of internal organs is called a:
   A. contusion.
   B. hematoma.
   C. crush injury.
   D. force injury.

_____ 10. A(n) _____ is an injury in which the skin is interrupted, exposing the tissues underneath.
   A. hematoma
   B. closed wound
   C. open wound
   D. crush injury

_____ 11. A minor ooze of blood from capillary beds is from an injury called a(n):
   A. amputation.
   B. abrasion.
   C. laceration.
   D. puncture.

_____ 12. A cut caused by a sharp-edged object such as a razor blade or broken glass is called a(n):
   A. abrasion.
   B. puncture.
   C. laceration.
   D. avulsion.

_____ 13. When a sharp, pointed object passes through the skin or other tissue, a(n) _____ wound has occurred.
   A. abrasion
   B. puncture
   C. amputation
   D. crush injury

_____ 14. When the tip of the nose is cut or torn off, this is a(n):
   A. avulsion.
   B. penetration.
   C. crush injury.
   D. amputation.

_____ 15. The priority when treating severe open wounds is to:
   A. control bleeding.
   B. clean the wound.
   C. prevent contamination.
   D. bandage the wound.

_____ 16. Care for a laceration includes:
   A. applying a tourniquet.
   B. applying a butterfly bandage, then releasing the patient.
   C. pulling apart the edges to inspect the wound.
   D. checking the pulse distal to the injury.

_____ 17. Various types of guns fired at close range can cause all of the following except:
   A. burns around the entry wound.
   B. injection of air into the tissues.
   C. large contusion to the tissue.
   D. damage to underlying tissue.

_____ 18. Care in the field for a patient with an impaled object in the leg involves all of the following except:
   A. stabilize the object.
   B. use direct pressure.
   C. leave the object in place.
   D. carefully remove the object.

_____ **19.** Which of the following is <u>not</u> true about an injury caused by an impaled object?
  A. The object may plug bleeding from a major artery.
  B. Removal may cause further injury to the nerves, muscles, and soft tissue.
  C. Pressure should be applied to the object to stabilize it.
  D. All of the above.

_____ **20.** To control profuse bleeding resulting from an injury caused by an impaled object:
  A. position your gloved hands on either side of the object and exert downward pressure.
  B. use a pressure point distal to the injury to control the bleeding.
  C. let the blood flow freely from the wound left by removal of the object.
  D. stabilize the object with gloved hands and then immediately apply a tourniquet.

_____ **21.** Which of the following is <u>untrue</u> of an impaled object in the cheek?
  A. It should never be removed.
  B. It can create an airway obstruction.
  C. It can cause nausea and vomiting.
  D. It is pulled out in the direction it entered.

_____ **22.** If a patient has an impaled object in the eye, your care should include use of a:
  A. pressure bandage placed over the eye.
  B. loose bandage placed over the eye.
  C. combination of 4 × 4s and a paper cup.
  D. combination of 3-inch gauze and a Styrofoam cup.

_____ **23.** When an avulsed flap of tissue has been torn loose but not off, the EMT should do all of the following <u>except</u>:
  A. fold the skin back to its normal position.
  B. control bleeding and dress the wound.
  C. clean the wound surface.
  D. tear off the remainder of the flap and put it on ice.

_____ **24.** Avulsed parts torn from the body should be wrapped and placed in a:
  A. cup of dry ice placed in an airtight container.
  B. plastic bag filled with ice.
  C. plastic bag on top of a sealed bag of ice.
  D. saline and ice solution.

_____ **25.** The most effective treatment for an amputation is to:
  A. apply a tourniquet.
  B. place the amputated part in ice.
  C. place a snug pressure dressing over the stump.
  D. apply ice over the stump.

_____ **26.** When treating an amputation, whenever possible:
  A. place the amputated body part in ice and transport before the patient.
  B. transport the patient and the amputated body part in the same ambulance.
  C. apply a tourniquet after completing a partial amputation.
  D. immerse the amputated part in saline and transport before the patient.

_____ **27.** An air bubble sucked into a large vein in the neck is called a(n):
  A. air embolus.   **C.** occlusion.
  B. blood clot.   **D.** case of the "bends."

_____ **28.** The treatment of neck vein injury is aimed at all of the following <u>except</u> to:
  A. compress the region of injury.   **C.** prevent cardiac arrest.
  B. prevent an embolus.   **D.** stop bleeding.

_____ **29.** To treat a neck laceration, the EMT should use a(n):
    A. pressure bandage.   **C.** ACE bandage.
    B. thin dressing.   **D.** occlusive dressing.

_____ **30.** When applying pressure to a neck wound, be sure you do <u>not</u>:
    A. apply pressure over the laceration.
    B. compress both carotids at the same time.
    C. administer oxygen to the patient.
    D. treat the patient for shock.

_____ **31.** The chest can be injured in a number of ways, including:
    A. blunt trauma.   **C.** compression.
    B. penetrating objects.   **D.** all of the above.

_____ **32.** When the driver of a motor vehicle pitches forward after a head-on collision and strikes the chest on the steering column, this is called:
    A. closed lung injury.   **C.** compression injury.
    B. penetrating trauma.   **D.** puncture trauma.

_____ **33.** All open wounds to the chest should be considered:
    A. potentially infectious.   **C.** a low priority.
    B. life-threatening.   **D.** an indication for PASG.

_____ **34.** An injury that has both an entrance and an exit is called a _____ wound.
    A. puncture   **C.** perforating puncture
    B. penetrating   **D.** compression injury

_____ **35.** When the delicate pressure balance within the chest cavity is compromised, initially the:
    A. diaphragm stops working.
    B. lung on the injured side will collapse.
    C. lung on the uninjured side will collapse.
    D. patient will stop breathing.

_____ **36.** When the chest cavity is open to the atmosphere, this is referred to as a:
    A. flail chest.   **C.** sucking chest wound.
    B. hemothorax.   **D.** rib fracture.

_____ **37.** The treatment for an open chest wound includes all of the following <u>except</u>:
    A. maintaining an open airway.
    B. binding the chest tightly.
    C. administering high-concentration oxygen.
    D. sealing the open wound.

_____ **38.** When air becomes trapped in the chest cavity, it can affect the body in all of the following ways <u>except</u>:
    A. put pressure on the unaffected lung and heart.
    B. reduce cardiac output.
    C. affect oxygenation of the blood.
    D. increase the ventilatory volume of the chest.

_____ **39.** The signs of pneumothorax or tension pneumothorax include all of the following <u>except</u>:
    A. tracheal deviation to the uninjured side.
    B. distended neck veins.
    C. uneven chest wall movement.
    D. increased depth of respiration.

_____ **40.** Which of the following is <u>not</u> a sign of traumatic asphyxia?
    A. distended neck veins
    B. coughed-up frothy blood
    C. head, neck, and shoulders that appear dark blue
    D. bloodshot and bulging eyes

_____ **41.** When taping an occlusive dressing in place:
 A. have the patient inhale as you tape.
 B. have the patient exhale as you tape.
 C. tape between breaths.
 D. have the patient hold his or her breath.

_____ **42.** When an open wound to the abdomen is so large and deep that organs protrude through the opening, this is called an:
 A. impaled object.   **C.** avulsion.
 B. evisceration.   **D.** amputated intestine.

_____ **43.** The signs of an abdominal injury include all the following <u>except</u>:
 A. lacerations and puncture wounds to the lower back.
 B. large bruised area on the abdomen.
 C. indications of developing shock.
 D. contusions over the upper ribs.

_____ **44.** Partially digested blood that is vomited looks like:
 A. black and tarry material.   **C.** stained mucus.
 B. coffee grounds.   **D.** meconium staining.

_____ **45.** Which of the following is <u>not</u> a symptom of an abdominal injury?
 A. cramps   **C.** headache
 B. nausea   **D.** thirst

_____ **46.** Consider positioning the patient with an abdominal injury:
 A. prone, with arms outstretched.
 B. supine, with legs flexed at knees.
 C. left lateral recumbent.
 D. supine, with legs straight.

_____ **47.** The treatment of an evisceration should <u>never</u> include:
 A. using an occlusive dressing.
 B. cutting away the clothing.
 C. replacing or touching the exposed organ.
 D. applying a sterile, saline-soaked dressing.

_____ **48.** When covering an exposed abdominal organ, you should apply a(n) _____ directly over the wound site.
 A. plastic wrap   **C.** saline-moistened dressing
 B. occlusive dressing   **D.** aluminum foil wrap

_____ **49.** Burn injuries often involve structures below the skin, including muscles and:
 A. nerves.   **C.** blood vessels.
 B. bones.   **D.** all of the above.

_____ **50.** In addition to the physical damage caused by burns, patients often suffer:
 A. heart attacks.
 B. emotional and psychological problems.
 C. diabetic emergencies.
 D. delayed reactions such as cancer.

_____ **51.** When caring for a burn patient:
 A. think beyond the burn to possible medical causes and results.
 B. always begin transport before treatment.
 C. obtain the name of the product that caused the burn.
 D. determine the duration of the exposure.

_____ **52.** When caring for a burn patient:
 A. do not neglect assessment to begin burn care.
 B. transport immediately.
 C. take the patient to the closest hospital.
 D. run cold water on the patient for at least 20 minutes.

_____ **53.** Examples of agents causing burns include all of the following <u>except</u>:
- **A.** AC current.
- **B.** hydrochloric acid.
- **C.** dry lime.
- **D.** distilled water.

_____ **54.** A burn that involves only the epidermis is called a _____ burn.
- **A.** superficial
- **B.** partial thickness
- **C.** full thickness
- **D.** epi thickness

_____ **55.** Which of the following burns will result in deep, intense pain, blisters, and mottled skin?
- **A.** superficial
- **B.** partial thickness
- **C.** full thickness
- **D.** medium layer

_____ **56.** To distinguish between a partial thickness burn and a full thickness burn, look for _____, which indicate(s) a full thickness burn.
- **A.** blisters
- **B.** mottled skin
- **C.** dry and white areas
- **D.** swelling

_____ **57.** Electrical burns are of special concern since they:
- **A.** cause respiratory burns if superheated gas is inhaled.
- **B.** pose a great risk of severe internal injuries.
- **C.** may remain on the skin and continue to burn for hours.
- **D.** cause the patient to lose hair over time.

_____ **58.** Chemical burns are of special concern since they:
- **A.** cause respiratory burns if superheated gas is inhaled.
- **B.** pose a great risk of internal injury.
- **C.** may remain on the skin and continue to burn for hours.
- **D.** jump from one extremity to another.

_____ **59.** Burns to the face are of special concern because they:
- **A.** continue to burn for hours.
- **B.** can cause heart irregularities.
- **C.** increase the potential for shock.
- **D.** may involve airway injury.

_____ **60.** Burns that can interrupt circulation to distal tissues are called _____ burns.
- **A.** circulation
- **B.** radiation
- **C.** circumferential
- **D.** distal

_____ **61.** You are treating an adult patient who has partial thickness burns to the entire left arm, chest, face, and neck. Using the rule of nines, approximate the size of the burn area.
- **A.** 18%
- **B.** 22%
- **C.** 27%
- **D.** 32%

_____ **62.** You are treating an adult patient who has partial thickness burns totally covering the legs, chest, and abdomen. Using the rule of nines, approximate the size of the burn area.
- **A.** 18%
- **B.** 36%
- **C.** 45%
- **D.** 54%

_____ **63.** A burn the size of five palms would cover approximately _____ % of the body surface area.
- **A.** 5
- **B.** 10
- **C.** 15
- **D.** 20

_____ **64.** The age of the patient is an important factor in burns. Patients under _____ and over _____ years of age have the most severe body responses to burns.
- **A.** 3, 50
- **B.** 5, 55
- **C.** 10, 65
- **D.** 15, 70

©2009 Pearson Education, Inc.
Emergency Care, 11th Ed.

_____ **65.** A partial thickness burn that involves less than 15% of the body surface is
    classified as:
    A. minor.   **C.** critical.
    B. moderate.   **D.** unnecessary to treat.

_____ **66.** A partial thickness burn that involves between 15% and 30% of the body
    surface area is classified as a _____ burn.
    A. minor   **C.** critical
    B. moderate   **D.** life-threatening

_____ **67.** A partial thickness burn that involves more than 30% of the body surface
    area is classified as a _____ burn.
    A. minor   **C.** critical
    B. moderate   **D.** fatal

_____ **68.** Critical burns include all of the following except:
    A. circumferential burns.
    B. moderate burns in an infant or elderly patient.
    C. burns complicated by musculoskeletal injuries.
    D. partial thickness burns on the wrist.

_____ **69.** A partial thickness burn that involves between 10% and 20% of the body
    surface area of a child under 5 years of age is considered a _____ burn.
    A. minor   **C.** critical
    B. moderate   **D.** fatal

_____ **70.** Which of the following is not considered a critical burn?
    A. entire genitalia area
    B. full thickness burn to the entire chest and abdomen
    C. full thickness burn to the front of the right forearm
    D. partial thickness burn to both the lower extremities

_____ **71.** If a patient has a partial thickness burn to the entire back, the patient
    should be:
    A. wrapped in a dry, sterile burn sheet.
    B. cooled down with ice for 15 minutes.
    C. wrapped in moist sterile dressings.
    D. dried and wrapped in an airtight dressing.

_____ **72.** The primary care for a patient with a chemical burn is to:
    A. wrap the patient in a dry sterile burn sheet.
    B. wash away the chemical with flowing water.
    C. dry the patient and wrap in an airtight dressing.
    D. wrap the patient with moist sterile dressings.

_____ **73.** You are treating a patient who was burned. The patient is having visual
    difficulties, is restless and irritable, and has an irregular pulse rate and
    muscle tenderness. This patient probably has a(n) _____ burn.
    A. chemical   **C.** electrical
    B. thermal   **D.** radiation

_____ **74.** If _____ is the burn agent, brush it from the patient's skin and then flush
    with water.
    A. dry lime   **C.** radiation
    B. electricity   **D.** acid

_____ **75.** An occlusive dressing is used to:
    A. form an airtight seal.   **C.** control severe bleeding.
    B. stabilize an impaled object.   **D.** secure sprain injuries.

COMPLETE THE FOLLOWING

1. List eight signs of abdominal injury.

   A. _____

   B. _____

   C. _____

   D. _____

   E. _____

   F. _____

   G. _____

   H. _____

2. List the parts of the adult body that account for 9% each, using the rule of nines.

   A. _____

   B. _____

   C. _____

   D. _____

   E. _____

   F. _____

   G. _____

   H. _____

3. List five signs and symptoms of an electrical injury.

   A. _____

   B. _____

   C. _____

   D. _____

   E. _____

LABEL THE DIAGRAM

Fill in the name of each type of burn and how the skin is damaged.

1.   2.   3.

Epidermis
Dermis
Fat
Muscle

4.   5.   6.

1. _____

2. _____

3. _____

4. _____

5. _____

6. _____

STREET SCENES DISCUSSION

Review the Street Scene on pp. 691–692 of the textbook. Then answer the questions below.

1. Your patient had a serious laceration, but the bleeding had stopped by the time you arrived. Suppose it was a different situation, and when you uncovered the wound, blood spurted across the room. How should the bleeding be controlled?

2. Suppose that the patient's wound when uncovered was only bleeding slowly but there was a large piece of glass impaled in her arm. How would you manage this?

3. If upon assessment of the patient's vital signs, it is apparent that she already has low blood pressure, how should the patient be managed?

ON THE WEB

To help you review and practice basic skills, visit the *Emergency Care 11th Ed. Companion Website* at www.prenhall.com/limmer. For Online Test Preparation, visit www.prenhall.com/emtachieve.

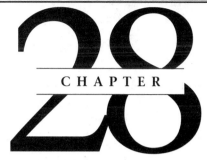

CHAPTER 28

Musculoskeletal Injuries

MATCH TERMINOLOGY/ DEFINITIONS

A. Hard but flexible living structures that provide support for the body and protection for vital organs

B. Disruption or "coming apart" of a joint

C. Extremity injury in which the skin has been broken or torn through from the inside by an injured bone or from the outside by something that has caused a penetrating wound with associated injury to the bone

D. Special splint that applies constant pull along the length of the leg to help stabilize the fractured femur and reduce muscle spasms

E. Grating sensation or sound made when broken bone ends rub together

F. Bands of connective tissue that bind muscles to bones

G. Any break in a bone

H. Portion of the skeleton that includes the clavicles, scapulae, arms, wrists, hands, pelvis, thighs, legs, ankles, and feet

I. Connective tissue that covers the outside of the bone ends and acts as a surface for articulation, allowing for smooth movement at joints

J. Muscle injury caused by overstretching or overexertion of the muscle

K. Process of applying tension to straighten and realign a fractured limb before splinting

L. Places where bones articulate, or meet

M. Stretching and tearing of ligaments

N. Injury to an extremity in which the skin is not broken

O. Connective tissue that supports joints by attaching the bone ends and allowing for a stable range of motion

_____ **1.** Bones

_____ **2.** Cartilage

_____ **3.** Closed extremity injury

_____ **4.** Crepitus

_____ **5.** Dislocation

_____ **6.** Extremities

_____ **7.** Fracture

_____ **8.** Joints

_____ **9.** Ligaments

_____ **10.** Manual traction

_____ **11.** Open extremity injury

_____ **12.** Sprain

_____ **13.** Strain

_____ **14.** Tendons

_____ **15.** Traction splint

MULTIPLE-CHOICE REVIEW

_____ 1. As we age, our bones become:
   A. deficient in magnesium.   C. high in iron.
   B. deficient in calcium.   D. high in potassium.

_____ 2. The strong white fibrous material covering the bones is called the:
   A. perineum.   C. periosteum.
   B. marrow.   D. shell.

_____ 3. In children, the majority of the long bone growth occurs in the:
   A. bone marrow.   C. periosteum.
   B. growth plate.   D. growth shaft.

_____ 4. Musculoskeletal injuries are caused by direct, indirect, and _____ forces.
   A. positive   C. negative
   B. penetrating   D. twisting

_____ 5. Fractures of the femur typically cause a _____ pint blood loss over the first 2 hours.
   A. 1   C. 3
   B. 2   D. 4

_____ 6. The death rate from closed fracture of the femur dropped from 80% to 20% in the post-WWI period due to the invention of the:
   A. PASG.   C. traction splint.
   B. IV bag.   D. tourniquet.

_____ 7. The coming apart of a joint is referred to as a:
   A. dislocation.   C. sprain.
   B. fracture.   D. strain.

_____ 8. The stretching or tearing of ligaments is called a:
   A. dislocation.   C. sprain.
   B. fracture.   D. strain.

_____ 9. A break in the continuity of the skin of a painful, swollen, deformed extremity is considered a(n) _____ bone or joint injury.
   A. simple   C. closed
   B. open   D. grating

_____ 10. Proper splinting of a possible closed fracture is:
   A. done with an air splint and gentle traction.
   B. done with the pneumatic antishock garment.
   C. designed to prevent closed injuries from becoming open ones.
   D. completed in the hospital by a surgeon.

_____ 11. The signs and symptoms of a bone or joint injury include all of the following except:
   A. grating.   C. vomiting.
   B. swelling.   D. bruising.

_____ 12. When a joint is locked into position, the EMT should:
   A. splint the joint in the position found.
   B. pull traction and straighten the joint.
   C. use a long backboard as a full body splint.
   D. disregard splinting and transport immediately.

_____ 13. Which procedure is done at least twice whenever a splint is applied?
   A. elevation of the injured extremity.
   B. manual stabilization of the injured extremity.
   C. assessment for pulses, sensation, and movement distal to the injury.
   D. application of gentle manual traction.

_____ **14.** The treatment of a painful, swollen, deformed extremity includes the steps below:
   1. Take Standard Precautions.
   2. Elevate the extremity.
   3. Splint the injury.
   4. Apply a cold pack.

   What is the correct order of the steps?
   A. 2, 3, 4, 1   **C.** 3, 2, 4, 1
   B. 1, 3, 2, 4   **D.** 1, 4, 2, 3

_____ **15.** Multiple fractures, especially of the _____, can cause life-threatening external and internal bleeding.
   A. radius   **C.** femur
   B. ulna   **D.** tibia

_____ **16.** Applying a cold pack to a possible fracture will
   A. help to reduce the swelling.
   B. stop bleeding from the bone.
   C. eliminate the need for a pressure bandage.
   D. stop all the pain and discomfort.

_____ **17.** If the initial assessment of a patient with a musculoskeletal injury reveals the patient is unstable, care should include all of the following except:
   A. manage the ABCs.
   B. immobilize on a long spine board.
   C. transport immediately.
   D. splint each injury individually.

_____ **18.** A splint properly applied to a closed bone injury should help prevent all of the following except:
   A. damage to muscles, nerves, or blood vessels.
   B. an open bone injury.
   C. motion of bone fragments.
   D. circulation to the extremity.

_____ **19.** Complications of bone injuries include all of the following except:
   A. excessive bleeding.
   B. increased pain from movement.
   C. paralysis of the extremity.
   D. increased distal circulation.

_____ **20.** The objective of realignment is to:
   A. minimize blood loss and reduce pain.
   B. immobilize the bone ends and adjacent joints.
   C. assist in restoring circulation and to fit the extremity into a splint.
   D. prevent incorrect healing and avoid surgery.

_____ **21.** If there is a severe deformity of the distal extremity or it is cyanotic or pulseless, the EMT should:
   A. align with gentle traction before splinting.
   B. apply PASG to align the extremity.
   C. delay splinting until en route to the hospital.
   D. contact medical direction immediately.

_____ **22.** What are the three categories of splints?
   A. rigid, formable, and traction.
   B. PASG, board, and ladder.
   C. padded, soft, and anatomical.
   D. air, cardboard, and vacuum.

_____ 23. Which of the following is a <u>false</u> statement about rigid splints?
  A. They require the limb be moved into anatomical position.
  B. They tend to provide the greatest support.
  C. They are ideally used to splint long bones.
  D. They can immobilize joint injuries in the position found.

_____ 24. Traction splints are used specifically for fractures of the:
  A. pelvis.   C. femur.
  B. humerus.   D. clavicle.

_____ 25. When splinting, the EMT should:
  A. first move the patient to a stretcher.
  B. leave any open wounds exposed so bleeding can be monitored.
  C. replace protruding bones as soon as priorities are arranged.
  D. secure the injury site and the joints above and below.

_____ 26. To ensure proper stabilization and increase patient comfort when using a
      rigid splint:
  A. place the patient on a stretcher before splinting.
  B. place the patient on a long spine board before splinting.
  C. pad the spaces between the body part and the splint.
  D. ensure that the splint conforms to the body curves.

_____ 27. The method of splinting is always dictated by the:
  A. location of the injury and whether it is open or closed.
  B. severity of the patient's condition and the priority decision.
  C. number of available rescuers and the type of splints.
  D. all of the above.

_____ 28. If the patient with a musculoskeletal injury is unstable, the EMT should do all
      of the following <u>except</u>:
  A. care for life-threatening problems first.
  B. align the injuries in an anatomical position.
  C. immobilize the entire body to a long spine board.
  D. apply a fixation splint before securing to a long spine board.

_____ 29. Hazards of improper splinting include:
  A. aggravation of a bone or joint injury.
  B. reduced distal circulation.
  C. delay in transport of patient with life-threatening injury.
  D. all of the above.

_____ 30. If the lower leg is cyanotic or lacks a pulse when a knee joint injury is
      assessed, the EMT should:
  A. splint it in the position it was found.
  B. transport the patient to the hospital immediately.
  C. realign with gentle traction if no resistance is met.
  D. call for assistance from a paramedic unit.

_____ 31. Examples of a bipolar traction splint include all of the following <u>except</u>:
  A. Hare®.   C. Fernotrac®.
  B. Sager®.   D. half-ring.

_____ 32. The amount of traction the EMT should pull when applying a Sager traction
      splint is:
  A. enough until the patient verbalizes relief.
  B. about 10% of the patient's body weight up to 15 pounds.
  C. minimal since it doesn't require traction.
  D. about 15% of the patient's body weight up to 30 pounds.

©2009 Pearson Education, Inc.
Emergency Care, 11th Ed.

_____ **33.** The indications for a traction splint are a painful, swollen, deformed mid-thigh with:
  A. either knee or ankle involvement.
  B. no joint or lower leg injury.
  C. extensive blood loss.
  D. an open fracture.

_____ **34.** Whenever possible, _____ rescuers should be used to apply a traction splint.
  A. two   **C.** four
  B. three   **D.** five

_____ **35.** If the patient has multiple leg fractures and exhibits signs of shock (hypoperfusion), the EMT should:
  A. apply two traction splints and pull tension to 30 pounds.
  B. align in a normal position and transport on a backboard.
  C. apply PASG as a splint and treat for shock.
  D. apply a vacuum splint to each leg and transport quickly.

_____ **36.** Signs and symptoms of a knee injury may include:
  A. pain and tenderness.
  B. swelling.
  C. deformity.
  D. all of the above.

_____ **37.** Elderly patients are more susceptible to _____ fractures because of brittle bones or bones weakened by disease.
  A. hip   **C.** heel
  B. tibia   **D.** spine

_____ **38.** When a patient has a fractured hip, the injured limb:
  A. will rarely be swollen.
  B. may appear shorter.
  C. often is lengthened.
  D. will have all of the above.

_____ **39.** When a patient who was involved in a serious fall has an unexplained sensation of having to empty her bladder, the patient may have a _____ fracture.
  A. femur   **C.** pelvic
  B. hip   **D.** none of the above

_____ **40.** When stabilizing a patient who has a pelvic injury, you should do all of the following <u>except</u>:
  A. assume there is a spinal injury.
  B. determine distal function.
  C. apply PASG if the patient is hypotensive.
  D. raise the lower legs.

COMPLETE THE FOLLOWING

1. List eight signs and symptoms of musculoskeletal injury.

   A. _____

   B. _____

   C. _____

   D. _____

   E. _____

   F. _____

   G. _____

   H. _____

2. List eight signs and symptoms of a hip fracture.

   A. _____

   B. _____

   C. _____

   D. _____

   E. _____

   F. _____

   G. _____

   H. _____

©2009 Pearson Education, Inc.
Emergency Care, 11th Ed.

LABEL THE DIAGRAM

Fill in the name of each bone on the line provided.

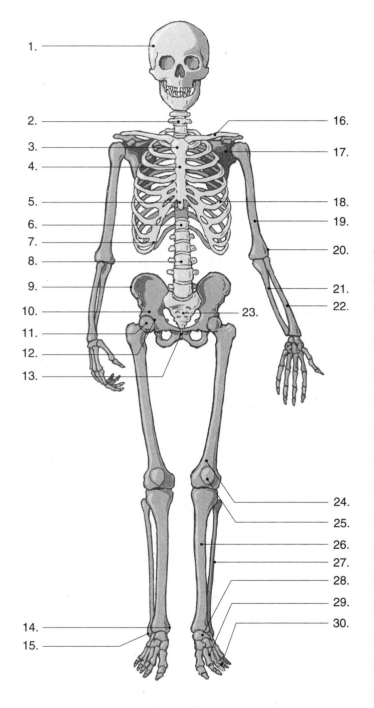

1. _____

2. _____

3. _____

4. _____

5. _____

6. _____

7. _____

8. _____

9. _____

10. _____

11. _____

12. _____

13. _____

14. _____

15. _____

16. _____

17. _____

18. _____

19. _____

20. _____

21. _____

22. _____

23. _____

24. _____

25. _____

26. _____

27. _____

28. _____

29. _____

30. _____

STREET SCENES DISCUSSION

Review the Street Scene on pp. 745–746 of the textbook. Then answer the questions below.

1. When the injured leg was examined, it was found to be swollen. If it had been an open fracture, what would you have observed?

2. Imagine that the patient is found lying on the ground with the injured leg grossly deformed in the mid-shaft area. Should you attempt to straighten it? Explain.

3. Suppose the patient does not have a distal pulse in the injured leg. What can you do?

4. Should you have called for ALS in this case?

ON THE WEB

To help you review and practice basic skills, visit the *Emergency Care 11th Ed. Companion Website* at www.prenhall.com/limmer. For Online Test Preparation, visit www.prenhall.com/emtachieve.

EMT SKILLS PERFORMANCE CHECKLISTS

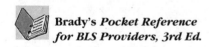

Brady's *Pocket Reference for BLS Providers, 3rd Ed.*

▶ REALIGNING AN EXTREMITY (PP. 705–706)

❑ Take Standard Precautions.

❑ Assess distal pulse, motor function, and sensation (PMS).

❑ One EMT grasps the distal extremity while a partner places one hand above and one hand below the injury site.

©2009 Pearson Education, Inc.
Emergency Care, 11th Ed.

- The partner supports the injury site while the first EMT pulls gentle manual traction in the direction of the long axis of the body. If resistance is felt or if it appears that bone ends will come through the skin, stop realignment and splint the extremity in the position found.

- If no resistance is felt, maintain gentle traction until the extremity is properly splinted.

- Reassess distal pulse, motor function, and sensation (PMS).

▶ IMMOBILIZATION: LONG BONE (PP. 708–709)

- Take Standard Precautions.
- Direct application of manual stabilization.
- Assess distal pulse, motor function, and sensation (PMS).
- Measure splint.
- Apply splint.
- Immobilize joints above and below the injury.
- Secure entire injured extremity from distal to proximal direction.
- Immobilize hand/foot in functional position.
- Reassess distal pulse, motor function, and sensation (PMS).

▶ IMMOBILIZATION: JOINT INJURY (P. 710)

- Take Standard Precautions.
- Direct application of manual stabilization of injured extremity.
- Assess distal pulse, motor function, and sensation (PMS).
- Select proper splinting device.
- Immobilize the site of injury and bones above and below.
- Reassess distal pulse, motor function, and sensation (PMS).

▶ IMMOBILIZATION: TRACTION SPLINTING (PP. 712–713)

- Take Standard Precautions.
- Direct manual stabilization of injured leg.
- Assess distal pulse, motor function, and sensation (PMS).
- Direct application of manual traction.
- Adjust and position splint at the injured leg.
- Apply proximal securing device (e.g., ischial strap).
- Apply distal securing device (e.g., ankle hitch).
- Apply mechanical traction.
- Position and secure support straps.
- Reassess distal pulse, motor function, and sensation (PMS).
- Secure patient's torso and traction splint to long backboard for transport.

CHAPTER 29

Injuries to the Head and Spine

MATCH TERMINOLOGY/ DEFINITIONS

A. Pairs of nerves that enter and exit the spinal cord between the vertebrae, 12 pairs of cranial nerves that travel between the brain and organs without passing through the spinal cord, and all of the body's other motor and sensory nerves

B. Mild closed head injury without detectable damage to the brain

C. Body system that is divided into two subsystems and that provides overall control of thought, sensation, and the voluntary and involuntary motor functions of the body

D. Cheek bone; also called the zygomatic bone

E. Bony bump on a vertebra that you can feel on a person's back

F. Bones of the spinal column

G. Movable joint formed between the mandible and the temporal bones; also called the TM joint

H. Bony structure making up the forehead, top, back, and upper sides of the skull

I. Fluid that surrounds the brain and spinal cord

J. Bruised brain caused when the force of a blow to the head is great enough to rupture blood vessels

K. The brain and the spinal cord

L. Bones that form part of the sides of the skull and floor of the cranial cavity

M. Bones that form the upper third, or bridge, of the nose

N. Bony structures, or sockets, around the eyes

O. Nervous system that consists of nerves that control involuntary functions such as the heartbeat and breathing

_____ **1.** Autonomic nervous system

_____ **2.** Central nervous system

_____ **3.** Cerebrospinal fluid (CSF)

_____ **4.** Concussion

_____ **5.** Contusion

_____ **6.** Cranium

_____ **7.** Malar

_____ **8.** Nasal bones

_____ **9.** Nervous system

_____ **10.** Orbits

_____ **11.** Peripheral nervous system

_____ **12.** Spinous process

_____ **13.** Temporal bones

_____ **14.** Temporomandibular joint

_____ **15.** Vertebrae

©2009 Pearson Education, Inc.
Emergency Care, 11th Ed.

MULTIPLE-CHOICE REVIEW

_____ 1. The function of the spinal column is to:
   A. produce cerebrospinal fluid.
   B. protect the spinal cord.
   C. allow for back movement in all directions.
   D. manufacture platelets.

_____ 2. The spine is made up of _____ vertebrae.
   A. 35   C. 33
   B. 23   D. 38

_____ 3. When a patient has a scalp injury:
   A. expect minimal bleeding.   C. expect profuse bleeding.
   B. determine the wound depth. D. palpate the site with fingertips.

_____ 4. A bruise behind the ear is called:
   A. Cushing's syndrome.   C. Battle's sign.
   B. raccoon's eyes.   D. posturing syndrome.

_____ 5. Discoloration of the soft tissues under both eyes is called:
   A. Cushing syndrome.   C. Battle's sign.
   B. raccoon's eyes.   D. posturing syndrome.

_____ 6. The signs and symptoms of a skull or brain injury include:
   A. blood or fluid flowing from the ears and/or nose.
   B. yellow discoloration in the eyes.
   C. bruising around the base of the nose.
   D. pain at the base of the neck.

_____ 7. Skull or brain injury may result in:
   A. airway swelling and dizziness.
   B. altered mental status and unequal pupils.
   C. difficulty moving below the waist.
   D. headache and hypoperfusion.

_____ 8. Which of the following is a late sign of brain or skull injury?
   A. temperature increase   C. irregular breathing patterns
   B. raccoon's eyes   D. Battle's sign

_____ 9. Which of the following is generally <u>not</u> a sign of head injury except in infants?
   A. bleeding from the nose and ears   C. hypoperfusion
   B. unequal pupils   D. seizures

_____ 10. What is the significance of an increase in carbon dioxide in the injured brain?
   A. It decreases the blood pressure. C. It raises the heart rate.
   B. It causes brain tissue swelling. D. It causes brain tissue shrinkage.

_____ 11. In most EMS systems, a patient with a Glasgow Coma Scale (GCS) of less than _____ is taken to a trauma center.
   A. 8   C. 12
   B. 10   D. 15

_____ 12. If an object has penetrated a patient's skull, the EMT should:
   A. shorten lengthy objects, using any available tools.
   B. elevate the patient's legs immediately.
   C. remove the object and quickly control the bleeding.
   D. stabilize the object with bulky dressings.

_____ 13. The primary concern for emergency care of a facial fracture or jaw injury is the:
   A. external bleeding.   C. loss of teeth.
   B. patient's airway.   D. basilar skull fracture.

_____ 14. The vertebrae that are most frequently injured are the:
    A. lumbar and sacral.   **C.** coccygeal and thoracic.
    B. thoracic and cervical.   **D.** cervical and lumbar.

_____ 15. When the spine is excessively pulled, which commonly occurs during a
    hanging, this is called a(n) _____ injury.
    A. excessive rotation   **C.** distraction
    B. lateral bending   **D.** compression

_____ 16. On your size-up of an automobile collision, you notice that both
    sides of the windshield have a spider-web crack. It is wise to call
    for a backup ambulance because:
    A. every collision should have a two-ambulance response.
    B. patients hitting their heads on the windshield will be critical.
    C. both the driver and the passenger require spinal injury treatment.
    D. It takes four EMS personnel to properly immobilize one patient.

_____ 17. Which of the following would <u>not</u> create a high index of suspicion of
    a spine injury?
    A. motor vehicle or motorcycle collisions
    B. falls that cause open fractures to the ankles
    C. trauma patients who are found unconscious
    D. a fall from two times the patient's height

_____ 18. All of the following are examples of cervical-spine injuries that can result
    from a diving accident <u>except</u>:
    A. excessive extension.   **C.** excessive flexion.
    B. compression.   **D.** lateral bending.

_____ 19. The unconscious trauma patient should be:
    A. treated as if he has a spine injury.
    B. rolled immediately to check for back injuries.
    C. placed in the recovery position.
    D. placed in a prone position for fluid to drain.

_____ 20. The most reliable sign of spinal-cord injury in the conscious patient is:
    A. pain with movement.   **C.** tenderness on the spine.
    B. impaired breathing.   **D.** paralysis of the extremities.

_____ 21. A lack of spinal pain does not rule out the possibility of spinal-cord injury
    because:
    A. spinal injuries seldom cause pain.
    B. other painful injuries may mask it.
    C. spinal injuries are not painful until shock sets in.
    D. a patient may feel the pain but cannot verbalize it.

_____ 22. When assessing a suspected spine-injured patient, you note a reversal of the
    normal breathing pattern. This is likely a result of damage to the nerves that
    control the:
    A. rib cage.   **C.** abdomen.
    B. diaphragm.   **D.** lungs.

_____ 23. If a patient is found on her back with arms extended above the head,
    this may indicate a _____ spine injury.
    A. thoracic   **C.** sacral
    B. lumbar   **D.** cervical

_____ 24. If a patient is up and walking around at the scene of a high-speed collision,
    the EMT should:
    A. assess for a potential spinal injury.
    B. check with medical direction for orders.
    C. check with bystanders about the patient's mental status.
    D. assume that the patient is uninjured.

©2009 Pearson Education, Inc.
Emergency Care, 11th Ed.

_____ **25.** If a responsive patient has the mechanism of injury for a spinal injury, the EMT should do all of the following <u>except</u>:
   A. assess for spinal pain by asking the patient to move.
   B. keep the patient still while asking him or her questions.
   C. assess for equality of strength in the extremities.
   D. assess for tingling in the extremities.

_____ **26.** After performing the initial assessment and rapid trauma exam on a spine-injured patient, your next step is to:
   A. determine the patient's priority.
   B. administer high-concentration oxygen.
   C. immobilize the patient on a long spine board.
   D. determine the mechanism of injury.

_____ **27.** If a suspected spine-injured patient complains of pain when you attempt to place the head in a neutral in-line position:
   A. pad the neck before immobilizing.
   B. steady the head in the position found.
   C. continue with the stabilization procedure.
   D. contact medical direction immediately.

_____ **28.** When treating a patient with a spine injury, one EMT should:
   A. strap the patient's head, then the torso, to the long spine board.
   B. maintain constant manual in-line immobilization until the patient is secured to a backboard.
   C. assess for range of cervical spine motion.
   D. pad the neck before stabilizing.

_____ **29.** Which of the following statements about the rigid cervical collar is <u>false</u>?
   A. A wrong-sized collar can hyperextend the neck.
   B. Maintain manual stabilization when applying.
   C. The collar completely eliminates neck movement.
   D. The collar should never obstruct the airway.

_____ **30.** If a stable patient is found in a sitting position on the ground and is complaining about back pain, the EMT should:
   A. apply a cervical collar and rapidly transport the patient.
   B. ask the patient to lie down, then immobilize.
   C. immobilize with a short spine board or extrication vest.
   D. perform a rapid take-down procedure with a long spine board.

_____ **31.** The rapid extrication technique is used in all of the following situations <u>except</u>:
   A. to rapidly move a patient from an unsafe scene.
   B. when a stable, low-priority patient must be immobilized.
   C. when more seriously injured patients must be accessed.
   D. to move a high-priority patient.

_____ **32.** When immobilizing a 6-year-old or younger child on a long backboard:
   A. provide padding beneath the shoulder blades.
   B. it is unnecessary to apply a cervical collar.
   C. place a chin cup or chin strap on the patient.
   D. secure the head first, then secure the torso.

_____ **33.** Do <u>not</u> remove an injured patient's helmet:
   A. if it interferes with breathing management.
   B. if it has a snug fit that allows no head movement.
   C. by using a two-rescuer procedure.
   D. if it hinders immobilization.

_____ **34.** Which is the correct order of steps for applying a short spine immobilization device?
   1) Secure the device to the patient's torso.
   2) Secure the patient's head to the device.
   3) Position device behind the patient.
   4) Evaluate torso fixation and pad behind neck as necessary.
   A. 3, 2, 1, 4   **C.** 4, 3, 1, 2
   B. 3, 1, 4, 2   **D.** 3, 4, 1, 2

_____ **35.** Prior to and after immobilization, the EMT should assess:
   A. pulses in all extremities.   **C.** sensation in all extremities.
   B. motor function in all extremities.   **D.** all of the above.

COMPLETE THE FOLLOWING

1. List six signs of a skull fracture or brain injury.

   A. _____   **D.** _____

   B. _____   **E.** _____

   C. _____   **F.** _____

2. List three types of brain injuries.

   A. _____

   B. _____

   C. _____

LABEL THE DIAGRAM

Fill in the name of each division of the spine on the line provided.

   1. _____

   2. _____

   3. _____

   4. _____

   5. _____

©2009 Pearson Education, Inc.
Emergency Care, 11th Ed.

STREET SCENES DISCUSSION

Review the Street Scene on pp. 790–791 of the textbook. Then answer the questions below.

1. Suppose that this patient had a lucid interval followed by decreasing mental status. What would be your highest priority in the treatment of this patient?

2. If the patient tells you he has no neck pain, why is it necessary to continue to immobilize him?

3. If the patient has a serious head injury, what would you expect to happen with his vital signs (provided he had no other injury)?

ON THE WEB

To help you review and practice basic skills, visit the *Emergency Care 11th Ed. Companion Website* at www.prenhall.com/limmer. For Online Test Preparation, visit www.prenhall.com/emtachieve.

EMT SKILLS PERFORMANCE CHECKLISTS

Brady's *Pocket Reference for BLS Providers, 3rd Ed.*

▶ SPINAL IMMOBILIZATION: SUPINE PATIENT (PP. 774–775)

❑ Take Standard Precautions.

❑ Direct assistant to place/maintain head in neutral, in-line position and maintain manual stabilization until the patient is completely immobilized.

❑ Assess distal pulses, motor function, and sensory response (PMS).

❑ Apply a properly sized rigid extrication collar.

❑ Position the immobilization device appropriately.

❑ Move patient onto device without compromising the integrity of the spine. Apply padding to voids between torso and board as necessary.

❑ Immobilize patient's torso to the device.

(continued on next page)

- ❑ Evaluate and pad behind the patient's head as necessary or behind shoulders with patients age 6 and under.

- ❑ Pad and immobilize patient's head.

- ❑ Secure patient's arms and legs to board.

- ❑ Reassesses distal pulses, motor function, and sensory response (PMS).

▶ SPINAL IMMOBILIZATION: SEATED PATIENT (PP. 767–768)

- ❑ Take Standard Precautions.

- ❑ Direct assistant to manually stabilize head in neutral, in-line position.

- ❑ Assess distal pulses, motor function, and sensory response (PMS).

- ❑ Apply a properly sized rigid extrication collar.

- ❑ Position immobilization device behind the patient.

- ❑ Secure device to the patient's torso.

- ❑ Evaluate and pad behind the patient's head as needed.

- ❑ Secure patient's head to the device.

- ❑ Evaluate and adjust straps.

- ❑ Secure patient's wrists and legs and transfer to a long spine board.

- ❑ Reassess distal pulses, motor function, and sensory response (PMS).

▶ RAPID TAKEDOWN OF STANDING PATIENT (PP. 778–780)

Step 1: Rescuers get in position.

- ❑ Rescuer A: Get in position behind patient and hold manual in-line stabilization of head and neck. Maintain manual stabilization until the patient is completely immobilized on a long backboard.

- ❑ Rescuer B: Get in position in front of patient. Explain procedure so patient does not move.

Step 2: Assess PMS and apply a cervical collar.

- ❑ Rescuer B: Quickly assess pulses, motor function, and sensory response (PMS) in all four extremities.

- ❑ Rescuer B: Apply a properly sized rigid extrication collar.

Step 3: Position the long backboard.

- ❑ Rescuers B or C: Position long backboard behind patient, being careful not to disturb manual stabilization in any way.

- ❑ Rescuers B and C: Standing in front of patient to each side, reach under the patient's armpit and grasp backboard handhold at level of the armpit or higher. Both rescuers must hold same level.

- ❑ Rescuers B and C: Then place your other hand on patient's upper arm, securing patient to backboard by holding it on board.

Step 4: Slowly lower the patient.

- ❑ Rescuers B and C: Slowly lower patient backwards, communicating with Rescuer A behind board so it is clear when the scapulae are beginning to rest on the board. Remember to lift with your legs, bending at knees, not at waist. Rescuer A gently allows the head to come back to the board as shoulders come back.

❑ Once patient's head is on the board, it never is lifted off the board again as Rescuer A kneels down at patient's head.

❑ Reassess PMS when the patient is finally down.

Step 5: Secure patient to backboard.

▶ **RAPID EXTRICATION PROCEDURE FOR HIGH-PRIORITY PATIENTS (PP. 769–770)**

Step 1: Perform an initial assessment.

❑ Rescuer A: Maintain manual stabilization of patient's head and neck.

❑ Rescuer B: Conduct initial assessment of patient and determine need for rapid extrication based on patient status. Assess pulses, motor ability, and sensory response (PMS) in four extremities.

Step 2: Apply a cervical collar.

❑ Rescuer B: Apply a properly sized cervical rigid collar.

❑ Rescuer A: Continue to maintain manual stabilization before, during, and after application of collar.

Step 3: Lift patient and position the long backboard.

❑ Rescuer B: Hold patient's armpit, and join hands with Rescuer C under patient's thighs.

❑ Rescuer A: Call for a lift, while maintaining manual stabilization.

❑ Rescuer B: Lift patient approximately 1.5 to 2 inches (just enough) off seat with Rescuer C.

❑ Bystander (or 4th Rescuer): Insert long backboard under patient on seat.

Step 4: Begin to position patient for extrication.

❑ Rescuer B: Reach across patient's chest and support by both armpits.

❑ Rescuer A: While maintaining manual stabilization, call for one-fourth turn, so patient is moved perpendicular to steering wheel, ready to exit car head-first.

❑ Rescuer C: Free patient's lower legs from any obstructions.

❑ Rescuer B: Begin to turn patient's back toward door until Rescuer A says "stop turn."

❑ Rescuer A: Turn patient. Call for "stop turn" just before being unable to hold patient's head anymore.

❑ Rescuer C: Begin to turn patient's back toward door, freeing legs, then sliding up to thighs until Rescuer A says "stop."

Step 5: Complete another one-quarter turn.

❑ Rescuer B: Stop move and wait for Rescuer C. Then take over manual stabilization of head and neck from Rescuer A.

❑ Rescuer A: Maintain head/neck stabilization until Rescuer B takes over, allowing him or her to either exit car and work from outside or reach over seat from inside if there is room or if the roof has been removed.

❑ Rescuer C: Move hands from thighs to patient's armpits. Then replace Rescuer B.

❑ Rescuers A, B, and C: Complete another one-quarter turn.

Step 6: Lower patient onto the long backboard.

❑ Rescuer B: Lower patient onto long backboard.

❑ Rescuer A: Call for move to lower patient's torso into a supine position onto long backboard.

(continued on next page)

- ❑ Rescuer C: Lower patient onto long backboard.
- ❑ Bystander (or 4th Rescuer): Stabilize the board.

Step 7: Position patient on the backboard.

- ❑ Rescuer B: Slide patient as a unit.
- ❑ Rescuer A: Call for move to slide patient toward head end of backboard. Once in position, tell partners to "stop." Slide the chest as a unit.
- ❑ Rescuer C: Slide pelvis as a unit until Rescuer A says "stop."
- ❑ Bystander (or 4th Rescuer): Stabilize the head end of long backboard.

Step 8: Secure patient to the backboard.

- ❑ Crew carefully straps patient's torso first, head last, and then moves backboard to stretcher.
- ❑ Reassess PMS.

▶ CHILD SAFETY SEAT IMMOBILIZATION: ASSESSMENT (P. 784)

- ❑ Take Standard Precautions.
- ❑ EMT #1 gets in position or positions himself behind patient and holds manual in-line stabilization of the head/neck. This remains his job throughout the procedure.
- ❑ Based on the initial assessment and the patient's status, determine if the infant/toddler should be immobilized in the child safety seat or rapidly extricated from the seat.
- ❑ EMT #2 assesses distal pulses, motor function, and sensation (PMS) in all four extremities before and after the immobilization.

▶ IMMOBILIZING PATIENT IN A CHILD SAFETY SEAT* (PP. 784–786)

- ❑ Take Standard Precautions.
- ❑ EMT #1: Stabilize child safety seat in an upright position. Maintain manual head/neck stabilization of head and neck throughout procedure until patient is completely immobile.
- ❑ EMT #2: Prepare equipment. Apply rigid extrication collar or improvise with rolled hand towel for the newborn/infant.
- ❑ EMT #2: Place a small blanket or bath towel on the child's lap. Either strap or use wide tape to secure the pelvis and chest area to the seat.
- ❑ EMT #2: Place a towel roll on either side of the head to fill the voids. Tape the forehead in place. Then place tape across collar or maxilla. Avoid taping the chin, which would place pressure on the child's neck.
- ❑ EMT #1: Carry child and seat to ambulance and strap onto the stretcher with the stretcher head raised.
- ❑ Reassess distal pulses, motor function, and sensation (PMS).

*NOTE: As long as the seat is not damaged.

▶ RAPID EXTRICATION FROM A CHILD SAFETY SEAT (PP. 785–786)

- ❑ Take Standard Precautions.
- ❑ EMT #1: Stabilize the child safety seat in upright position. Maintain manual stabilization of head and neck throughout procedure until patient is completely immobilized.

- ❑ EMT #2: Prepare the equipment. Loosen or cut the seat straps and raise the front guard.

- ❑ Apply the rigid extrication collar or improvise with a rolled hand towel in the newborn/infant.

- ❑ EMT #2: Place the child safety seat on the center of the long backboard and slowly tilt it back into a supine position, being careful not to allow the child to slide out of the chair. If the child has a large head, it is helpful to place a towel under the area where his shoulders will end up on the board.

- ❑ EMT #1: Call for a coordinated long-axis move onto the board.

- ❑ EMT #2: Grasp the chest and armpits with each hand and do a coordinated long-axis move onto the board. Make sure the child is positioned at the end of the board and not in the middle.

- ❑ EMT #2: Place a rolled blanket on each side of the patient.

- ❑ EMT #2: Strap the pelvis and upper chest to the board. Do not strap abdomen down. Tape the lower legs to the board with wide tape.

- ❑ EMT #2: Place a towel roll on each side of the head to fill the voids. Tape the forehead in place. Then place tape across the collar or the maxilla. Do not tape across the chin to avoid pressure on the child's neck.

CASE STUDY

▶ DEEP DIVE IN A SHALLOW POOL

You respond to a call for an injury in a pool at a private residence in your district. The EMS dispatcher tells you they have received numerous 911 calls on this incident and they are trying to calm someone down to obtain better information. Fortunately, your EMS station is about a mile from the location. As you pull up in front, you see there are lots of cars parked outside. A bystander runs up to the ambulance and says, "Please come quickly. He is still in the swimming pool. Can I help you carry anything?" Hearing this, you notify the dispatcher to continue the ALS unit and have the police respond also.

Both you and your partner are experienced swimmers. As you enter the backyard with your equipment, you ask her quickly, "Wet or dry?" She says, "Go. I'll take care of coordinating the poolside activities."

When you first see the patient, he is face up and being assisted in floating on his back by one other person in the pool, who states his name is Bill. He says he was a lifeguard 20 years ago. The patient is an adult male about 40 years old, and in about 5 feet of water. There is some blood in the pool from a large laceration to the patient's forehead.

You quickly empty your pockets, remove your shoes, hand the radio to your partner, and carefully enter the shallow end of the pool without making any waves. You also happen to notice that everyone has a soccer team shirt on.

1. What would you want to know about the patient from Bill right away?

2. How would you move the patient from the deep water to the shallow end of the pool?

Seeing that most of the adults are a bit intoxicated and most of the children at poolside are a bit small, you ask your partner to get an ETA on the backup unit. Just then they come walking into the backyard. There are two paramedics and an EMT who is a student in the paramedic course. You ask them to assist with the patient removal (if they are good swimmers).

3. What equipment will be needed?

In talking with Bill, you find that the party is a celebration for the children winning the soccer tournament. The patient, whose name is Tom, is the coach and apparently is not a drinker, so after two beers he did something he never would have done normally. Apparently, they were horsing around near the edge of the pool and he flipped head-first into the shallow end. The laceration was from striking his head. He was initially unconscious. Bill had entered the pool and carefully turned him over, as he was trained years ago to do, and Tom regained consciousness after a moment or two. Bill said that he did not believe Tom swallowed any water.

4. What other information should you obtain?

As one of the medics and the student enter the water with a long backboard and a rigid collar, you instruct Bill to continue to stabilize the patient's head and neck in a neutral position. You assist the patient in floating. The patient is very scared because he is unable to feel his arms or legs.

5. When the patient asks you what are you going to do, what should you tell him?

©2009 Pearson Education, Inc.
Emergency Care, 11th Ed.

You carefully float the patient to the shallow end of the pool and do the immobilization there. The voids are padded, and the patient is strapped to the board. By this time, the police have arrived and have asked the soccer team and their parents to move up to the deck area and watch from there. Your partner has found two more helpers who are not intoxicated to assist in the lifting at poolside. Your in-water team lifts the immobilized patient onto the edge of the pool, and the out-of-water team carefully lifts the patient and backboard onto a stretcher.

6. What are some of the initial management steps your partner should take while you get out of the pool?

Once it is clear that your patient does not have any movement of his arms and legs, your partner and the paramedic call for a helicopter and ask the police to set up a landing zone. Fortunately, there is an elementary school with a large field about two blocks away. The patient will be going directly to the Regional Trauma Center and a paramedic will be going along.

When the patient is loaded into your ambulance, the paramedic inserts an IV, the patient's clothing is cut off and he is covered with a blanket, the pulse oximeter is attached, and ECG electrodes are placed on him. His vital signs are still within normal range at this time.

After the patient and paramedic fly off in the helicopter, you look at your partner and say, "Can you imagine? Forty years old. Life can change so fast!" You talk about the call as you clean up back at the station. Although the situation is very sad, and life will change dramatically for the patient and his family, you are satisfied that the response, assessment, management, and teamwork went well. You and your partner agree that you will both stop at the hospital tomorrow to visit the patient. The report that was relayed back to you from the helicopter team was that the patient sustained a fracture of C-4, which severed his spinal cord.

7. Before handing in your PCR, is there anything that you should make sure is clearly documented? If so, what?

Putting It All Together for the Trauma Patient

MATCH TERMINOLOGY/ DEFINITIONS

A. Optimum limit of time between the moment of injury and surgery at the hospital

B. Quick assessment of the head, neck, chest, abdomen, pelvis, extremities, and posterior of the body to detect signs and symptoms of injury

C. Cooperation of crew members, each knowing their role and working together to manage the serious patient

D. Patient with more than one serious injury

E. Action or forces that may have caused or contributed to the injury

F. Swelling caused by a collection of blood under the skin or in damaged tissues as a result of an injured or broken blood vessel

G. Inability of the body to adequately circulate blood to the body's cells to supply them with oxygen and nutrients

H. A procedure designed to move a patient in a hurry when the situation of safety warrants it

_____ **1.** Multiple-trauma patient

_____ **2.** Teamwork

_____ **3.** Rapid trauma assessment

_____ **4.** Hypoperfusion

_____ **5.** Golden hour

_____ **6.** Emergency move

_____ **7.** Hematoma

_____ **8.** Mechanism of injury

©2009 Pearson Education, Inc.
Emergency Care, 11th Ed.

MULTIPLE-CHOICE REVIEW

_____ 1. The patient with a fractured right leg and a crushed pelvis is called a _____ patient.
   A. lower extremity
   B. multiple-trauma
   C. shock
   D. stable

_____ 2. When a patient has an obvious angulated forearm and is unresponsive, what is the priority?
   A. splinting
   B. immobilization
   C. the airway
   D. distal pulses

_____ 3. At what point is the multiple-trauma patient most likely stabilized?
   A. at the emergency department
   B. once splints have been provided
   C. in the surgical suite
   D. once the PASG is applied

_____ 4. The three "Ts" involved in the management of a multiple-trauma patient are timing, transport, and:
   A. teamwork.
   B. trauma.
   C. treatment.
   D. thorax.

_____ 5. A reasonable goal for scene time when dealing with a critical trauma patient is _____ minutes.
   A. 60
   B. 45
   C. 10
   D. 2

_____ 6. When a trauma patient is making gurgling sounds as he breathes, what should you do?
   A. Ventilate him.
   B. Suction the airway.
   C. Hyperextend the neck.
   D. Apply high-concentration oxygen.

_____ 7. Sometimes a _____ can act as a full-body splint when the critical patient must be immobilized quickly.
   A. wheeled stretcher
   B. short KED
   C. warm blanket
   D. long backboard

_____ 8. When a patient has two fractured femurs, a crushed pelvis, and a possible abdominal injury, you should:
   A. not apply a traction splint.
   B. consider the PASG.
   C. set up an ALS intercept en route to the hospital.
   D. do all of the above.

_____ 9. When you must minimize the scene care of a multiple-trauma patient, you can perform any of the following except:
   A. suction the airway.
   B. ventilate with a BVM.
   C. bandage all the lacerations.
   D. immobilize the cervical spine.

_____ 10. Even when you are trying to cut scene time for a multiple-trauma patient, the one thing you do not cut out is:
   A. applying a traction splint if needed.
   B. the detailed physical exam.
   C. scene safety.
   D. immobilization.

COMPLETE THE FOLLOWING

1. List the five treatments that would be appropriate on the scene of a critical trauma patient.

   A. _____

   B. _____

   C. _____

   D. _____

   E. _____

STREET SCENES DISCUSSION

Review the Street Scene on pp. 802–803 of the textbook. Then answer the questions below.

1. In this case, the use of rapid extrication seems appropriate, considering the mechanism of injury and the patient findings. But suppose the patient was alert, obviously pregnant, lying supine on the seat, and complaining of dizziness. Would rapid extrication still be appropriate? Explain.

2. Imagine that after immobilizing the patient on a long backboard, she developed breathing difficulty due to blood in the airway. What might you consider doing to help her?

3. If the patient has a fractured femur, would a traction splint be appropriate?

4. What should be your concern for the other patients on the scene?

ON THE WEB

To help you review and practice basic skills, visit the *Emergency Care 11th Ed. Companion Website* at www.prenhall.com/limmer. For Online Test Preparation, visit www.prenhall.com/emtachieve.

CHAPTER

31

Infants and Children

MATCH TERMINOLOGY/ DEFINITIONS

A. Child from 12 to 18 years of age

B. "Soft spot" at the front of an infant's skull where bones have not yet fused together

C. Flowing oxygen over the face of a small child so it will be inhaled

D. Child from 6 to 12 years of age

E. Child from 1 to 3 years of age

F. Feeding tube placed through the abdominal wall directly into the stomach

G. Child between birth and 1 year of age

H. Child from 3 to 6 years of age

I. Bacterial infection that produces swelling of the epiglottis and partial airway obstruction

J. Sudden unexplained death during sleep of an apparently healthy baby in its first year of life

K. Complication of a rapidly rising temperature

L. Group of viral illnesses that cause inflammation of the larynx, trachea, and bronchi

M. Tube placed through the neck into the trachea to create an open airway

N. Intravenous line that is placed close to the heart

O. Drainage device that runs from the brain to the abdomen to relieve excess cerebrospinal fluid

_____ **1.** Adolescent

_____ **2.** Blow-by oxygen

_____ **3.** Central line

_____ **4.** Croup

_____ **5.** Epiglottitis

_____ **6.** Febrile seizure

_____ **7.** Fontanelle

_____ **8.** Gastrostomy tube

_____ **9.** Newborn or infant

_____ **10.** Preschooler

_____ **11.** School-aged child

_____ **12.** Shunt

_____ **13.** SIDS

_____ **14.** Toddler

_____ **15.** Tracheostomy tube

MULTIPLE-CHOICE REVIEW

_____ **1.** When a child is considered a toddler, his age group is between _____ year(s).
  A. birth and 1   **C.** 3 and 6
  B. 1 and 3   **D.** 6 and 12

_____ **2.** When a child is considered school age, his age group is between _____ years.
  A. 1 and 3   **C.** 6 and 12
  B. 3 and 6   **D.** 12 and 18

_____ **3.** Which of the following is <u>not</u> appropriate when assessing the toddler?
  A. Have the child sit on the parent's lap.
  B. Avoid lying to the patient.
  C. Explain what you are doing.
  D. Perform the head exam first.

_____ **4.** Until about age 4, a child's head is proportionately _____ than the adult's.
  A. smaller and lighter   **C.** larger and heavier
  B. smaller and heavier   **D.** larger and lighter

_____ **5.** The soft spot on an infant's skull is called a:
  A. croup.   **C.** depression.
  B. fontanelle.   **D.** shunt.

_____ **6.** A sunken fontanelle may indicate:
  A. dehydration.   **C.** external hemorrhage.
  B. rising intracranial pressure.   **D.** hypertension.

_____ **7.** A bulging fontanelle may indicate:
  A. dehydration.   **C.** external hemorrhage.
  B. elevated intracranial pressure.   **D.** hypertension.

_____ **8.** Newborns usually breathe:
  A. over 60 times a minute.   **C.** through their mouths.
  B. less than 8 times a minute.   **D.** through their noses.

_____ **9.** In an infant, hyperextension of the neck:
  A. is necessary to open the airway.
  B. may result in airway obstruction.
  C. is necessary if trauma is suspected.
  D. is a procedure reserved for respiratory distress.

_____ **10.** If the EMT suctions the unresponsive child's airway for longer than a few seconds at a time, this is most likely to lead to:
  A. gag reflex activation.   **C.** airway blockage.
  B. vagus nerve stimulation.   **D.** cardiac arrest.

_____ **11.** The tongues of infants and children are more likely than an adult's to fall back into and block the airway because their tongues are:
  A. proportionately larger than an adult's.
  B. larger than an adult's.
  C. proportionately smaller than an adult's.
  D. smaller than an adult's.

_____ **12.** The insertion procedure for an oropharyngeal airway in an infant or a child is performed:
  A. much more quickly than in an adult.
  B. with the tip pointing toward the tongue and throat.
  C. the same way it is done for adults.
  D. without inserting a tongue depressor.

©2009 Pearson Education, Inc.
Emergency Care, 11th Ed.

_____ **13.** When assessing the capillary refill of a child 5 years old or younger, peripheral perfusion is considered satisfactory if the color returns in less than _____ seconds.

A. 2

B. 3

C. 4

D. 5

_____ **14.** Which of the following is <u>not</u> a sign of a partial airway obstruction in an infant or a child?

A. pink skin

B. adequate peripheral perfusion

C. stridor and crowing

D. loss of consciousness

_____ **15.** Signs of a severe partial airway obstruction or complete airway obstruction in an infant or a child include all of the following <u>except</u>:

A. cyanosis.

B. altered mental status.

C. crying or coughing.

D. inability to speak.

_____ **16.** The effects of hypoxia on an infant or a child are:

A. slowed heart rate and improved mental status.

B. increased heart rate and decreased mental status.

C. slowed heart rate and altered mental status.

D. increased heart rate and coma.

_____ **17.** All of the following are appropriate guidelines to follow when ventilating the infant or child <u>except</u>:

A. avoid breathing too hard through the pocket face mask.

B. avoid using excessive bag pressure and volume.

C. use a properly sized mask to assure a good mask seal.

D. omit the use of infection control barriers.

_____ **18.** The flow-restricted, oxygen-powered ventilation device (FROPVD) is:

A. used with caution in an infant.

B. contraindicated in infants and children.

C. preferred during the resuscitation of a child.

D. only used with the pop-off valve engaged in children.

_____ **19.** Common causes of shock in children include infection, trauma, blood loss, and:

A. meningitis.

B. heart failure.

C. dehydration.

D. lack of insulin.

_____ **20.** Less common causes of shock in a child include all of the following <u>except</u>:

A. allergic reactions.

B. cardiac events.

C. poisoning.

D. croup.

_____ **21.** The blood volume of infants and children is approximately _____ of the total body weight.

A. 6%

B. 8%

C. 10%

D. 12%

_____ **22.** When children are in shock, they do all of the following <u>except</u>:

A. compensate for a long time.

B. appear better than they actually are.

C. decompensate very rapidly.

D. decompensate very slowly.

_____ **23.** When a child is bleeding internally, the EMT should avoid:

A. administering too much oxygen.

B. transporting too quickly.

C. waiting for signs of decompensated shock before treating for shock.

D. placing the child in the Trendelenburg position if respiratory distress is not evident.

_____ 24. Decreased urine output and absence of tears are signs of _____ in infants and children.
  A. epiglottitis
  B. shock
  C. hypothermia
  D. croup

_____ 25. When treating a child in shock, unless there are injuries that would contraindicate it, the EMT should:
  A. lower the patient's legs.
  B. elevate the patient's legs.
  C. have the patient sit up.
  D. have the patient lie supine.

_____ 26. Because children have a large skin surface area in proportion to their body mass, they can easily become victims of:
  A. hypothermia.
  B. high fever.
  C. airway obstruction.
  D. hypovolemia.

_____ 27. If a child has an airway respiratory disease, it is very important that the EMT avoid:
  A. opening the airway.
  B. inserting a tongue blade into the mouth.
  C. positioning the child in the parent's lap.
  D. administering blow-by oxygen.

_____ 28. A child with signs of an airway disease should be transported as quickly as possible. The signs include all of the following except:
  A. stridor on inspiration.
  B. breathing effort on exhalation.
  C. rapid breathing.
  D. wheezing.

_____ 29. A viral illness that causes inflammation of the upper airway and bronchi, which is often accompanied by a "seal bark" cough, is called:
  A. bronchitis.
  B. asthma.
  C. croup.
  D. epiglottitis.

_____ 30. About _____ of all pediatric trauma deaths are related to airway mismanagement.
  A. one-fifth
  B. one-fourth
  C. one-third
  D. one-half

_____ 31. Causes of fever in children include all of the following except:
  A. upper respiratory infection.
  B. hypothermia.
  C. pneumonia.
  D. infection.

_____ 32. In the prehospital setting, which of the following is used to determine an infant's skin temperature?
  A. ungloved hand
  B. rectal thermometer
  C. oral thermometer
  D. pulse oximeter

_____ 33. When treating an infant or a child with a high fever:
  A. submerge the patient in cold water.
  B. use rubbing alcohol to cool the patient.
  C. monitor for shivering while cooling with tepid water.
  D. cover the patient with a towel soaked in ice water.

_____ 34. Infants are more susceptible to _____ because, compared to adults, a greater percentage of their body is water.
  A. shock
  B. dehydration
  C. high fever
  D. all of the above

_____ 35. Which of the following is not true of seizures in the pediatric patient?
  A. Seizures require medical evaluation.
  B. Seizures should be considered life-threatening.
  C. Seizures are rarely caused by fever.
  D. Seizures may be a sign of an underlying condition.

©2009 Pearson Education, Inc.
Emergency Care, 11th Ed.

_____ **36.** Severe aspirin poisoning in children can cause all of the following <u>except</u>:
   A. seizures.   **C.** coma.
   B. dehydration.   **D.** shock.

_____ **37.** A common cause of lead poisoning in children is:
   A. ingesting or licking chips of lead-based paint.
   B. chewing on pencils.
   C. drinking water from a well.
   D. eating fish from fresh water lakes.

_____ **38.** You are treating a child who accidentally ingested a handful of her mother's vitamin tablets. Should you be concerned?
   A. No. The body eliminates excess vitamins.
   B. No. The child will just have diarrhea for a few days.
   C. Yes. Many vitamin pills contain iron, which can be fatal to a child.
   D. Yes. Adult vitamins are too concentrated for children.

_____ **39.** The majority of meningitis cases occur between the ages of 1 month and:
   A. 6 months.   **C.** 3 years.
   B. 1 year.   **D.** 5 years.

_____ **40.** In cases of sudden infant death syndrome, the EMT should:
   A. not deliver care and transport immediately.
   B. pronounce the infant's death.
   C. look for evidence of child neglect.
   D. provide resuscitation and transport.

_____ **41.** The number one cause of death in infants and children is:
   A. respiratory arrest.
   B. trauma.
   C. cardiac arrest.
   D. child abuse.

_____ **42.** The child who has been struck by a vehicle may present with a triad of injuries that include head injury, lower extremity injury, and _____ injury.
   A. chest   **C.** abdominal
   B. neck   **D.** upper extremity

_____ **43.** Which of the following is <u>true</u> of a head-injury child?
   A. The most frequent sign is altered mental status.
   B. Respiratory arrest is a common secondary effect.
   C. Suspect internal injuries whenever the patient presents with shock.
   D. All of the above.

_____ **44.** Because the musculoskeletal structures of the chest are less developed in infants and children:
   A. they are able to maintain rapid respiratory rates for a long time.
   B. they are more likely than adults to fracture their ribs.
   C. the chest is less easily deformed.
   D. they are more likely to incur injury to structures beneath the ribs.

_____ **45.** Because the abdominal muscles of infants and small children are immature:
   A. they have less visible signs of breathing difficulty.
   B. they use their chest muscles for breathing.
   C. there is less protection for underlying organs.
   D. they rarely have distention of the abdomen.

_____ **46.** When using a PASG on a pediatric patient, the EMT should remember:
   A. to place the infant in the leg of an adult garment.
   B. the abdominal section is not generally used on children.
   C. it is contraindicated with pelvic instability.
   D. it is contraindicated in children younger than 12 years old.

_____ **47.** Guidelines for managing pediatric burn patients include all of the following
<u>except</u>:
  A. use the rule of nines to estimate the extent of burns.
  B. identify candidates for transportation to burn centers.
  C. cover the burn with sterile dressing.
  D. keep the patient cool to reduce pain.

_____ **48.** Indications that child abuse may be occurring include all of the following
<u>except</u>:
  A. repeated responses to provide care for the same child or family.
  B. poorly healing wounds or improperly healed fractures.
  C. indications of past injuries.
  D. a parent who seems concerned about the child's injuries.

_____ **49.** When you respond to the home of a person that you think may be a child
abuser, observe for all of the following <u>except</u>:
  A. a family member who has trouble controlling anger.
  B. indications of alcohol and drug abuse.
  C. torn clothing on the child.
  D. any adult who appears in a state of depression.

_____ **50.** Which of the following is <u>not</u> a role of the EMT when child abuse is
suspected?
  A. Control your emotions and hold back accusations.
  B. Gather information from parents/caregiver away from the child.
  C. Talk to the child separately and ask her if she has been abused.
  D. Report your suspicions of abuse to the emergency department.

_____ **51.** When treating a child who you suspect is suffering from epiglottitis, it is
important to:
  A. immediately transport the child.
  B. not place anything in the child's mouth.
  C. constantly monitor the respiratory status.
  D. all of the above.

_____ **52.** The primary cause of cardiac arrest in children is:
  A. electrocution.
  B. drowning.
  C. respiratory disorders.
  D. meningitis.

_____ **53.** When managing a child who had a febrile seizure, the EMT should be careful
not to:
  A. rub the child down with rubbing alcohol.
  B. monitor for shivering.
  C. remove any clothing.
  D. all of the above.

_____ **54.** An example of a poisoning that is not typically associated with adults but
considered to be common to children is ingestion of:
  A. morphine.
  B. acetaminophen.
  C. sleeping pills.
  D. codeine.

_____ **55.** When a young child runs out into the street and is struck by a car, the EMT
should expect to see:
  A. head injury.
  B. chest and abdomen injuries.
  C. leg injuries.
  D. all of the above.

©2009 Pearson Education, Inc.
Emergency Care, 11th Ed.

COMPLETE THE FOLLOWING

List ten signs of respiratory distress in a child.

A. _____   F. _____

B. _____   G. _____

C. _____   H. _____

D. _____   I. _____

E. _____   J. _____

COMPLETE THE CHART

Fill in each numbered box to complete the chart.

Artificial Ventilation (Rescue Breathing)

	Child with signs of puberty (adult)	Child without signs of puberty	Infant (birth to 1 year)
Ventilation duration	1.	2.	3.
Ventilation rate	4.	5.	6.

STREET SCENES DISCUSSION

Review the Street Scene on pp. 862–863 in the textbook. Then answer the questions below.

1. The mother reported seeing her child "shake." What do you suppose happened to this child?

2. This child's mental status improved. Suppose it had not improved and the child was warm to the touch and had a rash. What Standard Precautions would be appropriate?

3. Why would it be important for you to follow up on the hospital admission of this child?

ON THE WEB

To help you review and practice basic skills, visit the *Emergency Care 11th Ed. Companion Website* at www.prenhall.com/limmer. For Online Test Preparation, visit www.prenhall.com/emtachieve.

CASE STUDY

▶ THE CASE OF THE POISONED JUICE

You are dispatched to a community child care center that called 911 because a number of the children suddenly became ill after lunch. Upon arrival, you determine the scene is safe to enter and size up the situation. There are at least six children of different ages, ranging from infant to 6 years old, who have become nauseated after drinking apple juice that was left over from a few days ago. They are vomiting and complaining of stomach cramps. You have decided to call for an ALS unit and another BLS unit for backup at this time.

1. What Standard Precautions should you take?

2. How could you prepare for additional patients with the assistance of the day-care workers?

As your crew begins to evaluate each of the children, the day-care supervisor notifies you that all the parents of the sick children have been called. It appears that all of the children are in various stages of vomiting and most also have diarrhea. Initial assessment doesn't reveal any patients who are high priority except one infant who normally requires special care.

3. What can be a complication of children vomiting and having diarrhea?

4. The infant who receives special care is normally healthy except she is closely watched because she has had a shunt installed since birth. What is a shunt and why are they used frequently in infants?

The other ambulances arrive and the decision is made to immediately transport the infant with the shunt as a high priority and call for an additional ambulance to respond to the scene. Each of the EMTs begins obtaining complete sets of vital signs on the remaining children. Most of the 60 children in the day-care center are being evaluated for complaints and a full set of vitals; a prehospital care report has been completed on each child. Most of the children are not sick; however, you are noticing a trend of "sympathy" pains from children who could not possibly have had a drink from the contaminated can of juice.

5. What would be the normal vital signs to expect from the infants?

6. What would be the normal vital signs to expect from the toddlers?

7. What would be the normal vital signs to expect from the preschoolers?

8. As you examine the infants, are there any assessment strategies that would be helpful?

9. As you examine the toddlers, are there any assessment strategies that would be helpful?

10. As you examine the preschoolers, are there any assessment strategies that would be helpful?

When the parents arrive, some of them decide to sign the appropriate documentation and to take their children to their pediatricians. Eight other parents have agreed to be transported with their children to the local hospital so the children can be examined further in the emergency department.

11. For the infants and toddlers who are being transported by ambulance, what is the safest way to transport them provided they are not unstable and their parents are nearby to assist?

12. For the infants being transported by ambulance, what is the best way to determine their level of responsiveness with the assistance of their parents?

13. One of the paramedics suggests taking a sample of the juice that all the children drank. Why might this be helpful?

▶ **ABUSER OR LOVING PARENT?**

You respond to a call for a motor vehicle collision at an intersection. A police officer explains that two cars were involved and that car #1 did not stop at the stop sign and broadsided car #2. The driver of car #1, a middle-aged man, is limping around outside of his vehicle. He says he has no injury but appears to be very anxious about the damage to the side of his new car. The driver of car #2 is sitting in the front seat of her car, consoling her toddler who is still crying. Both the mother, who appears to be approximately 20 years old, and her young son have lacerations to the front of their heads and blood stains on the front of their clothing. As you approach the vehicle, you note that there are two "spider-web" cracks in the windshield, one in front of the driver's seat and the other in front of the passenger seat.

1. At the scene of an automobile collision in an intersection, what is your greatest scene safety hazard?

2. Is there a need for another ambulance at the scene? Why or why not?

After taking Standard Precautions, you approach car #2 and begin your assessment of the mother and child. You notice there is no car seat in the vehicle. After introducing yourself, you explain to the mother she should keep her head and neck still and that your partner would like to do the same for her child. She cooperates as she is concerned that her son has become a little "confused" since he smashed his head on the windshield.

3. Aside from manual stabilization of the head and neck, what are your initial concerns for the assessment of the child?

4. You note that the child is no longer crying and does not seem to care that you are evaluating him. Is this a significant finding? Explain.

5. Aside from AVPU, how else can you determine if the child's mental status is "normal" for this toddler?

6. What is the significance of the cracks in the car's windshield to the patient assessment process?

7. When you ask the mother if the child was restrained, she says, "He does not like the belt and there is no way I can keep him still enough to sit in a special seat." What is the significance of this statement in relation to the child's current mental status?

During your assessment, you note that the inside of the vehicle smells like "cheap wine" and the mother is acting as if she is intoxicated. When you assess the mother, you ask if she has eaten this afternoon or had anything to drink. She says she was upset today and had a few glasses of wine, but, "Please don't tell the cops!" By this time, her child has been immobilized and is being placed into the ambulance by your partner and the First Responders. You proceed to immobilize the mother in the seated position with a vest-style immobilization device since her baseline vital signs are all normal and her other injuries are minor. The child, on the other hand, is being closely monitored since he has already vomited twice. You and your partner decide to go to the hospital as soon as the mother is loaded.

8. Should oxygen be administered to the child?

9. Would it be appropriate to set up an ALS intercept en route to the hospital?

10. After arrival at the hospital, while you are cleaning up your equipment, the emergency department physician comes out to talk to you. He says that the child did not have a spine injury but the head trauma was serious. What should you say if he asks you how this incident and the child's injuries could have been prevented?

EMT SKILL PERFORMANCE CHECKLISTS

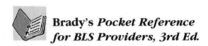

Brady's *Pocket Reference for BLS Providers*, 3rd Ed.

▶ THE PEDIATRIC PHYSICAL EXAMINATION* (PP. 823–825)

☐ Examine the head for D-CAP-BTLS. Look for blood or clear fluid draining from the nose and ears. Palpate gently for soft or spongy areas, skull irregularities, or crepitus. Check the fontanelle in infants.

☐ Check the eyes. The pupils should be equal in size and reactivity to light.

☐ Examine the neck. Check for D-CAP-BTLS, equal chest rise and fall, crepitus.

☐ Examine the chest. Check for D-CAP-BTLS, equal chest rise and fall, crepitus. Watch for signs of difficulty breathing.

☐ Auscultate for breath sounds over all lung fields. While examining the chest, be aware of the contents of the thorax.

☐ Examine the abdomen. Check for D-CAP-BTLS and guarding. Look for swelling that may indicate swallowed air. Divide the abdomen into quadrants and examine each one, while remembering which organs are located in each quadrant.

☐ Examine the pelvis for D-CAP-BTLS and crepitus. If the patient complains of pain, injury, or other problems in the genital area, access that area for bruising, swelling, or tenderness.

☐ Examine the extremities for D-CAP-BTLS and crepitus. Evaluate for distal pulses, motor function, and sensory function (PMS) and warmth. Look for unequal movement.

☐ If you have immobilized an extremity, check capillary refill and peripheral pulses, comparing them with the opposite arm or leg.

☐ Examine the back and buttocks for D-CAP-BTLS and crepitus. If the child requires immobilization, the back can be checked while the child is being log-rolled onto the long backboard.

*Conduct toe-to-head on toddlers.

©2009 Pearson Education, Inc.
Emergency Care, 11th Ed.

CHAPTER

Special Needs Patients

MATCH TERMINOLOGY/ DEFINITIONS

A. A disease or condition that is present at birth

B. A device that breathes for a patient

C. A battery-powered mechanical pump implanted in the body to assist a failing left ventricle in pumping blood to the body

D. A device implanted under the skin that can detect life-threatening cardiac dysrhythmias and respond by delivering one or more high-energy shocks to correct the rhythm

E. A tube used to provide delivery of nutrients of the stomach; a nasogastric feeding tube is inserted through the nose and into the stomach; a gastric feeding tube is surgically implanted through the abdominal wall and into the stomach

F. A surgical opening in the neck into the trachea

G. A surgically created opening into the body, as with a tracheostomy, colonostomy, or ileostomy

H. A tube inserted into the bladder through the urethra to drain urine from the bladder

I. The process of filtering the blood to remove toxic or unwanted wastes and fluids

J. A catheter surgically inserted for long-term delivery of medications or fluids into the central circulation

K. An external pouch that collects fecal matter diverted from the colon or ileum

_____ **1.** Central IV catheter

_____ **2.** Ventilator

_____ **3.** Congenital disease/condition

_____ **4.** Pacemaker

_____ **5.** Stoma

_____ **6.** Acquired disease/condition

_____ **7.** Automatic implanted cardiac defibrillator (AICD)

_____ **8.** Left ventricular assist device (LVAD)

_____ **9.** Continuous positive airway pressure (CPAP)

_____ **10.** Ostomy bag

_____ **11.** Dialysis

_____ **12.** Urinary catheter

_____ **13.** Tracheostomy

_____ **14.** Feeding tube

L. A device that exerts constant pressure through a tube and mask worn by a patient to keep airway passages from collapsing at the end of a breath

M. A disease or condition that occurs after birth

N. A device that uses electrical impulses to regulate rhythms of the heart, usually implanted under the skin

MULTIPLE-CHOICE REVIEW

_____ 1. To ensure proper care for the patient with special needs, the EMT must be able to _____ the patient's specific special health care needs in addition to the chief complaint.
  A. recognize
  B. understand
  C. evaluate
  D. all of the above

_____ 2. The EMT may find patients with special care needs when responding to calls in any of the following locations, <u>except:</u>
  A. the emergency department.
  B. nursing homes.
  C. specialty rehabilitation centers.
  D. specialized care facilities.

_____ 3. One of the best resources to help you when confronted with a special needs patient who is on a specific device would be to use the:
  A. instruction manual for the device.
  B. website for the product.
  C. family member with the patient.
  D. medical direction physician over the radio.

_____ 4. A condition that is present at birth of the special needs patient is considered:
  A. acquired.
  B. adopted.
  C. congenital.
  D. inflamed.

_____ 5. A device designed to keep the air passages from collapsing at the end of a breath is called a:
  A. positive-pressure ventilator.
  B. CPAP.
  C. bag-mask device.
  D. endotracheal tube.

_____ 6. A patient who has a tracheostomy tube may need to be suctioned occasionally. This is especially common:
  A. during times of distress.
  B. within the first few weeks after the tube insertion.
  C. if the patient has an infection.
  D. if any of the above conditions exists.

_____ 7. A device that is programmed to take over the functions of timing and rate of the patient's breathing is called a:
  A. inhalator.
  B. exhalator.
  C. ventilator.
  D. CPAP device.

_____ 8. If the patient on the device in question 7 has an electrical or battery failure, the EMT will need to begin:
  A. CPAP.
  B. using a nonrebreather mask.
  C. bag-mask ventilation.
  D. attaching the AED.

_____ 9. A cardiac device that is occasionally implanted in the patient's left upper abdominal quadrant is called a/an:
  A. pacemaker.
  B. AED.
  C. heart valve.
  D. AICD.

_____ **10.** Your patient is a special needs heart patient whose family member describes that he has a cardiac chamber that pumps blood through the aorta to the body; this is called a/an:

    A. pacemaker.
    C. left ventricular assist device.

    B. bypass machine.
    D. AICD.

_____ **11.** A tube that is inserted into a patient who has lost the ability to regulate his urine is called a/an:

    A. colostomy.
    C. ileostomy.

    B. urinary catheter.
    D. stoma.

_____ **12.** When a patient tells you he needs to go for dialysis every other day, this is done to:

    A. detoxify the blood.
    C. remove excess fecal material.

    B. increase the blood sugar.
    D. all of the above.

_____ **13.** Examples of devices commercially available as a Groshong@, Hickman®, and a Broviac® are called:

    A. peripherally inserted central catheters.

    B. angiocaths.

    C. central venous lines.

    D. implanted port devices.

_____ **14.** A special needle is required to access a device called a/an:

    A. implanted port.
    C. Mediport®.

    B. Port-a-Cath®.
    D. all of the above.

STREET SCENES DISCUSSION

Review the Street Scene on pp. 879–880 in the textbook. Then answer the questions below.

1. The ambulance was called because Amber was experiencing a fever and beginning to look gray. What is most likely wrong with the patient?

2. Why is it necessary to suction Amber's trach tube?

3. What do you suppose was causing the gurgling sounds when Amber was breathing?

ON THE WEB

To help you review and practice basic skills, visit the *Emergency Care 11th Ed. Companion Website* at www.prenhall.com/limmer. For Online Test Preparation, visit www.prenhall.com/emtachieve.

Geriatric Patients

MATCH TERMINOLOGY/ DEFINITIONS

A. Elderly person, generally considered 65 years of age or older

B. Chronic disorder resulting in dementia

C. When an elderly person replaces lost circumstances with imaginary ones

D. An abnormal heart rhythm

E. Abnormally low body temperature

F. An inflammation in the tissue of the lung

G. A separation of the layers of the artery described as a tearing sensation

H. An outpouching of the intestine provides a sac where food can lodge and cause inflammation

_____ **1.** Alzheimer's disease

_____ **2.** Confabulation

_____ **3.** Hypothermia

_____ **4.** Pneumonia

_____ **5.** Aortic dissection

_____ **6.** Geriatric

_____ **7.** Dysrhythmia

_____ **8.** Diverticulosis

MULTIPLE-CHOICE REVIEW

_____ 1. Starting at age _____, our organ systems lose about _____ function each year.
  A. 20, 1%   C. 30, 1%
  B. 20, 2%   D. 40, 2%

_____ 2. Older patients are at least twice as likely to use EMS as younger patients. Older patients' traumatic complaints are often due to:
  A. a medical problem.
  B. sporting events.
  C. a car crash or fall.
  D. none of the above.

_____ 3. Assessing the airway of an older patient is often difficult because of dentures and because:
  A. large, poorly chewed pieces of food are often found.
  B. dysrhythmias occur frequently.
  C. an older person's trachea is usually narrower.
  D. of arthritic changes in the bones of the neck.

_____ 4. Since older patients are less likely to show severe symptoms in certain conditions, it can be difficult to:
  A. find a radial pulse.
  B. determine a patient's priority.
  C. assess for foreign body obstruction.
  D. note sudden onset of weakness.

_____ 5. After interviewing an elderly patient, the family tells you that some of the patient's responses were incorrect. This is sometimes the result of neurological problems as well as:
  A. paranoia.   C. medications.
  B. depression.   D. all of the above.

_____ 6. When a patient replaces lost circumstances with imaginary ones, this is known as:
  A. depression.   C. flustering.
  B. confabulation.   D. dysrhythmia.

_____ 7. Many older people have a _____ threshold for pain.
  A. high   C. decreased sensitivity
  B. low   D. all of the above

_____ 8. As a person ages, the systolic blood pressure has a tendency to:
  A. decrease.   C. become erratic.
  B. increase.   D. stay constant.

_____ 9. Hip fractures are common in elderly patients, especially women, due to:
  A. women's shorter legs.
  B. motor vehicle collisions.
  C. abnormal curvature of the hip.
  D. loss of calcium.

_____ 10. An EMT should consider that any injury of an elderly person could be a sign of:
  A. a severe fall.
  B. Alzheimer's disease.
  C. abuse or neglect.
  D. depression.

COMPLETE THE FOLLOWING

The Physiological Effects of Aging and Implications for Assessment

Change	Result	Implications for Assessment
Depositing of cholesterol on arterial walls that have become thicker	(1)	Heart attack and stroke more likely
Decreased cardiac output	(2)	More prone to falls
Decreased elasticity of lungs and decreased activity of cilia	(3)	Higher risk of pneumonia and other respiratory infections
Fewer taste buds, less saliva; less acid production and slower movement in digestive system	(4)	Weight loss; abdominal pain common
Diminished liver and kidney function	(5)	Need for reduced doses of medication; bleeding tendencies
Diminished function of thyroid	(6)	Increased risk of hypothermia and hyperthermia
Diminished muscle mass, loss of minerals from bones	(7)	Falls more likely; minor falls more likely to cause fractures
Multiple medical conditions	(8)	Increased risk of medication error; potentially harmful medication interactions common
Death of friends and family	(9)	Increased risk of suicide
Loss of skin elasticity, shrinking of sweat glands	(10)	Increased risk of injury (The EMT must handle the patient gently to avoid injuring skin and subcutaneous tissues.)

1. _____

2. _____

3. _____

4. _____

5. _____

6. _____

7. _____

8. _____

9. _____

10. _____

STREET SCENES DISCUSSION

Review the Street Scene on pp. 896–897 of the textbook. Then answer the questions below.

1. Should an ALS unit be called for an intercept en route to the hospital?

2. Imagine you found that it was very cold in the apartment and the patient had on many layers of clothing. Why is it not uncommon for elderly people to do that? What might you expect as a consequence?

3. Unlike the patient in the Street Scenes, some elderly patients become very anxious about going in the ambulance to the hospital. Why do you think that is true? What can you do about it?

ON THE WEB

To help you review and practice basic skills, visit the *Emergency Care 11th Ed. Companion Website* at www.prenhall.com/limmer. For Online Test Preparation, visit www.prenhall.com/emtachieve.

CHAPTER 34

Ambulance Operations

MATCH TERMINOLOGY/ DEFINITIONS

A. Legal term, which appears in most states' driving laws, referring to the responsibility of the emergency vehicle operator to drive safely and keep the safety of all others in mind at all times

B. Emergency Medical Dispatcher

C. Call in which the driver of the emergency vehicle responds with lights and siren because he or she is of the understanding that loss or life or limb is possible

D. Large, flat area without aerial obstruction in which a helicopter can land to pick up a patient

E. Special thermometer that is designed to go down to 82°F

F. Traction splint for the immobilization of a painful, swollen, deformed thigh

G. Automated external defibrillator

H. Cervical immobilization device

I. Automatic transport ventilator

J. Mechanical compressor for performing CPR that is especially helpful to services with transport time to the hospital greater than 15 minutes

_____ **1.** AED

_____ **2.** ATV

_____ **3.** CID

_____ **4.** Due regard

_____ **5.** EMD

_____ **6.** Hypothermia thermometer

_____ **7.** Landing zone (LZ)

_____ **8.** Sager

_____ **9.** Thumper

_____ **10.** True emergency

MULTIPLE-CHOICE REVIEW

_____ 1. The federal agency that develops specifications for ambulance vehicle designs is the:
A. U.S. Department of Motor Vehicles.
B. Food and Drug Administration.
C. U.S. Department of Transportation.
D. U.S. Department of Health, Education, and Welfare.

_____ 2. The purpose(s) for carrying an EPA-registered, intermediate-level disinfectant on the ambulance is to:
A. clean up blood spills.
B. destroy mycobacterium tuberculosis.
C. disinfect patient wounds.
D. do all of the above.

_____ 3. Which of the following is not a piece of equipment that should be in the portable first-in kit, which is taken directly to a patient's side?
A. suction unit   C. blood pressure cuff
B. rigid cervical collar   D. telemetry repeater

_____ 4. Supplies used for the "C" step of the initial assessment of a trauma victim include all of the following except:
A. disposable gloves.   C. the AED.
B. occlusive dressings.   D. a suction unit.

_____ 5. Each of the following is a piece of equipment used to obtain vital signs except:
A. rubber bulb syringe.   C. sphygmomanometer kit.
B. adult and pediatric stethoscope. D. penlight.

_____ 6. A device used to carry patients over long distances is called a:
A. Stokes basket.   C. Reeves stretcher.
B. scoop stretcher.   D. wheeled ambulance stretcher.

_____ 7. Which one of the following pieces of patient transfer equipment is incorrectly matched with its function?
A. wheeled ambulance stretcher: transporting patients in sitting, supine, or Trendelenburg position
B. folding stair chair: moving patients down stairs in a sitting position
C. Reeves stretcher: carrying patients from a high-angle rescue
D. scoop stretcher: picking up patients found in tight spaces

_____ 8. Components of a typical fixed oxygen delivery system include:
A. 3,000-liter reservoir.
B. a two-stage regulator.
C. the necessary reducing valve and yokes.
D. all of the above.

_____ 9. Of the following devices carried on the ambulance for prehospital respiratory care, which is an optional item?
A. six adult and four pediatric nasal cannula
B. flow-restricted, oxygen-powered ventilation device (FROPVD)
C. automatic transport ventilator (ATV)
D. plastic cup for blow-by oxygen

_____ 10. The fixed suction unit in the ambulance should:
A. provide an airflow of over 15 liters per minute.
B. be usable by a person seated beside the patient.
C. have a current hydrostat test date.
D. reach a vacuum of at least 300 mmHg within 4 seconds.

©2009 Pearson Education, Inc.
Emergency Care, 11th Ed.

_____ **11.** Which of the following pieces of equipment carried on ambulances for defibrillation or assisting with cardiopulmonary resuscitation is optional?
   A. short or long spine board
   B. mechanical CPR compressor
   C. automated external defibrillator
   D. kit with oral and nasal airways

_____ **12.** Equipment that is carried on an ambulance for immobilization includes all of the following except:
   A. a Hare traction splint.
   B. triangular bandages.
   C. padded aluminum splints.
   D. a burn sheet.

_____ **13.** Chemical cold packs are carried on an ambulance primarily for use with _____ injuries.
   A. musculoskeletal
   B. abdominal
   C. respiratory
   D. cardiac

_____ **14.** Supplies used for wound care should include all of the following except:
   A. sterile burn sheets.
   B. 5 × 9-inch combine dressings.
   C. self-adhering roller bandages.
   D. Hare traction device.

_____ **15.** What is the purpose of carrying sterilized aluminum foil on the ambulance?
   A. to wrap body parts in
   B. to maintain body heat
   C. to make a shield over an avulsed eye
   D. for warming minor abrasions

_____ **16.** The supplies for childbirth include all the following except:
   A. a rubber bulb syringe.
   B. sanitary napkins.
   C. large safety pins.
   D. sterile surgical gloves.

_____ **17.** Every shift, both you and your partner should:
   A. wash and wax the ambulance.
   B. change the oil on the ambulance.
   C. complete the equipment checklist.
   D. do preventative maintenance on the ambulance.

_____ **18.** Of the following items checked on the ambulance, which is checked with the engine off?
   A. dash-mounted gauges
   B. battery
   C. windshield wiper operation
   D. vehicle's warning lights

_____ **19.** The responsibilities of the Emergency Medical Dispatcher include all of the following except:
   A. dispatching and coordinating EMS resources.
   B. interrogating the caller and prioritizing the call.
   C. coordinating with other public safety agencies.
   D. advising the caller that an ambulance is not needed.

_____ **20.** When an Emergency Medical Dispatcher questions a patient or caller, which of the following is not routinely asked?
   A. What is the exact location of the patient?
   B. What's the problem?
   C. Has the patient been in the hospital recently?
   D. How old is the patient?

_____ **21.** When speaking with a caller who is at the scene of a traffic collision, the Emergency Medical Dispatcher should ask all the following except:
   A. Is traffic moving?
   B. What brand vehicle was involved in the collision?
   C. How many lanes of traffic are open?
   D. Are any of the vehicles on fire?

_____ **22.** To be a safe ambulance operator, the EMT should:
  A. be tolerant of other drivers.
  B. always wear glasses or contact lenses if required.
  C. have a positive attitude about his or her ability as a driver.
  D. do all of the above.

_____ **23.** Every state has statutes that regulate the operation of emergency vehicles. Under certain circumstances, vehicle operators can do all of the following except:
  A. park the vehicle anywhere so long as it does not damage personal property.
  B. proceed past red stop signals, flashing red stop signals, and stop signs.
  C. exceed the posted speed limit as long as life and property are not endangered.
  D. pass a school bus that has its red lights blinking.

_____ **24.** At the scene of a collision, you examine a patient and find that he is stable. This situation is no longer a:
  A. true emergency.   **C.** cold response.
  B. due regard.   **D.** priority-one response.

_____ **25.** Which guideline for the use of the ambulance siren is inappropriate?
  A. Use the siren sparingly.
  B. Never assume that all motorists will hear your signal.
  C. Be prepared for erratic movements of motorists.
  D. Keep it on until the call is completed.

_____ **26.** Which of the following is true about the use of lights and sirens?
  A. Motorists are more inclined to give way to ambulances when sirens are continually sounded.
  B. The decision about their use should be based on the patient's medical condition.
  C. The use of the siren has little effect on the ambulance operator.
  D. Four-way flashers should be used in addition to emergency lights.

_____ **27.** Use of escorts or multivehicle responses is a:
  A. very quick and successful means of response.
  B. very dangerous means of response.
  C. means of decreasing the chance of collision.
  D. standard operating procedure in most communities.

_____ **28.** Factors that can affect ambulance response include all of the following except:
  A. time of the day.
  B. weather.
  C. road maintenance and construction.
  D. type of emergency.

_____ **29.** You are the first vehicle on the scene of an auto collision in which one of the automobiles is on fire. You should park your vehicle _____ the wreckage.
  A. 50 feet from   **C.** beyond
  B. in front of   **D.** downwind from

_____ **30.** A sequence of operations to ready a patient for transfer is called:
  A. stabilization.   **C.** transport.
  B. packaging.   **D.** removal.

_____ **31.** An unconscious patient who has no potential spine injury and no signs of impending shock should be positioned in the ambulance:
  A. in the recovery position.   **C.** in the supine position.
  B. with legs raised 8 to 12 inches.   **D.** in a sitting-up position.

_____ **32.** Which of the following is an action you would <u>not</u> perform en route to the hospital?
  A. Recheck the patient's bandages and splints.
  B. Form a general impression of the patient.
  C. Perform ongoing assessment and continue to monitor vital signs.
  D. Notify the receiving facility of your estimated time of arrival.

_____ **33.** If a patient develops cardiac arrest en route to the hospital, the EMT's <u>first</u> action should be to:
  A. apply and operate the AED.
  B. begin cardiopulmonary resuscitation.
  C. notify the emergency department.
  D. tell the operator to stop the ambulance.

_____ **34.** When delivering the patient to the hospital, the EMT should <u>never</u>:
  A. complete the prehospital care report at the hospital.
  B. move a patient onto the hospital stretcher and leave.
  C. transfer the patient's personal effects.
  D. obtain a release from the hospital.

_____ **35.** When approaching a helicopter, first wait for the pilot or medic to wave you in. Then approach from the _____ of the craft.
  A. rear   **C.** front or side
  B. uphill slope side   **D.** downhill slope rear

_____ **36.** Of the following patients, which is the <u>least</u> likely to be transported in a helicopter?
  A. carbon monoxide poisoning victim   **C.** cardiac arrest patient
  B. patient with a suspected stroke   **D.** patient with a critical burn

COMPLETE THE FOLLOWING

1. List the seven questions an EMD should ask a caller who is reporting a medical emergency.

  A. _____   **E.** _____

  B. _____   **F.** _____

  C. _____   **G.** _____

  D. _____

2. List seven factors that can affect an ambulance response.

  A. _____   **E.** _____

  B. _____   **F.** _____

  C. _____   **G.** _____

  D. _____

3. List the four major ways the EMT on the scene of a collision should describe the landing zone to the air rescue service.

A. _____

B. _____

C. _____

D. _____

LABEL THE PHOTOGRAPHS

Fill in the name of each level of disinfecting shown in the photo on the line provided.

1. _____

2. _____

3. _____

4. _____

STREET SCENES DISCUSSION

Review the Street Scene on pp. 936–937 of the textbook. Then answer the questions below.

1. Imagine that the ambulance had gone through a red light and had a collision en route to the call. What should you do right away?

2. If the collision involved another motorist, whose fault would it be?

3. Why is it an unsafe practice to drive an ambulance through a red light?

ON THE WEB

To help you review and practice basic skills, visit the *Emergency Care 11th Ed. Companion Website* at www.prenhall.com/limmer. For Online Test Preparation, visit www.prenhall.com/emtachieve.

EMT SKILLS PERFORMANCE CHECKLISTS

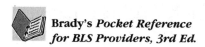

Brady's *Pocket Reference for BLS Providers, 3rd Ed.*

▶ TRANSFERRING THE PATIENT (P. 924)

❑ Take Standard Precautions.

❑ Transfer the patient as soon as possible. In a routine admission or when an illness or injury is not life-threatening, first check to see what is to be done with the patient.

❑ An EMT should remain with the patient until transfer is complete.

❑ Assist the emergency department staff as required.

❑ Give a complete verbal report of the patient's condition and treatment administered.

(continued next page)

- ❑ Complete your prehospital care report and turn a copy over to the hospital staff.
- ❑ Transfer the patient's personal effects.
- ❑ Obtain your release from the hospital if required in your region.

▶ ACTIVITIES AT THE HOSPITAL (P. 926)

- ❑ Take BSI precautions.
- ❑ Clean the ambulance interior as required by your service exposure control plan.
- ❑ Replace respiratory equipment as required.
- ❑ Replace disposable items according to local policies.
- ❑ Exchange equipment according to local policies.
- ❑ Make up the ambulance stretcher.

▶ CHECKING THE AED

- ❑ Check the AED for the following:

  - Unit, cables, and connectors for cleanliness.
  - Supplies carried with the AED.
  - Power supply and its operation.
  - Indicators on the ECG display.
  - ECG recorder operation.
  - Charge display cycle with a simulator.
  - Pacemaker feature if applicable.

- ❑ File a written report on the status of the AED.

NOTE: The specifics can be found on the FDA Automated Defibrillator: Operator's Shift Checklist.

CASE STUDY

▶ THE AMBULANCE COLLISION

You are notified by dispatch to respond to the neighboring district for a mutual aid call—an ambulance has collided with a passenger vehicle at an intersection. Responding with emergency lights and siren, the ambulance had approached the red light and had attempted to pass through it without stopping. The other vehicle's occupants are an elderly couple who were on their way to the store.

As you arrive on the scene, it is obvious that there are a number of very seriously injured patients due to the speed and size of the ambulance that broadsided the car. You are assigned to look after the ambulance operator who has minor cuts and scrapes. Fortunately for him, he was wearing his seat belt. His EMT-B partner was not as fortunate; another ambulance had already removed her from the scene with serious head and neck injuries from being ejected through the windshield of the ambulance. She had not been wearing her shoulder harness. Two other ambulance crews are in the process of removing the elderly man, who is in critical condition, and his wife, who has sustained leg fractures and is having a heart attack from the stress of the incident.

©2009 Pearson Education, Inc.
Emergency Care, 11th Ed.

1. Was this a preventable collision?

2. Could the serious injuries to the female EMT-B have been prevented?

3. What happened to the patient to whom the ambulance was responding?

4. What is the first rule of medicine?

The next day, the headlines in the local newspaper are: "Ambulance Kills Two En Route to Third." The story goes on to say how the initial patient had basically minor medical problems and was taken by an ambulance to the local hospital for the flu and released within three hours. The newspaper concludes with "The driver was suspended. The district attorney requests that a grand jury inquiry be conducted."

5. Aside from the reputation of the EMT-B who was driving, what might this "negative publicity" cost the service and other EMT-Bs who work there?

6. Why can the district attorney request a grand jury for this incident?

7. Is the operator of an emergency vehicle held to a higher standard than other motorists?

8. Who pays for the court defense of the EMT who was driving?

9. Could the EMT be personally sued for the injuries (deaths) that occurred?

10. How can an ambulance service prevent a collision like this from happening in its community?

CHAPTER
35
Gaining Access and Rescue Operations

MATCH TERMINOLOGY/ DEFINITIONS

A. When moving toward the rear of the vehicle, the second post you see, which supports the roof

B. Glass used in an automobile's side and rear windows designed to break into small rounded pieces rather than sharp fragments

C. Named after a well-known consumer advocate, this case-hardened pin is held by the cams of an automobile's door locking system

D. Decreasing circles of voltage on the ground surrounding a point where a charged wire is down

E. When a patient is pinned and requires assistance, sometimes mechanical, to free him

F. Cribbing or blocking a vehicle or structure to prevent further unintended, uncontrolled movement

G. Gear designed to prevent the rescuer from being injured while working in the inner circle

H. Post in front of the driver's compartment that supports the roof and windshield

I. Safety glass used in the windshields of automobiles, made of two sheets of plate glass bonded to a sheet of tough plastic

J. Blocks of hardwood, usually 4 × 4 × 18-inch or 2 × 4 × 18-inch used to stabilize a vehicle

K. Area immediately around and including the wrecked vehicle

_____ **1.** A Post

_____ **2.** B Post

_____ **3.** Complex access

_____ **4.** Cribbing

_____ **5.** Disentanglement

_____ **6.** Entrapment

_____ **7.** Extrication

_____ **8.** Glas-Master

_____ **9.** Ground gradient

_____ **10.** Inner circle

_____ **11.** Laminated glass

_____ **12.** Nader pin

_____ **13.** Personal protective equipment

_____ **14.** Stabilization

_____ **15.** Tempered glass

L. Access that requires tools or special equipment to reach the patient

M. Three-part procedure used by rescue personnel to free a patient trapped in a vehicle

N. Process by which entrapped patients are rescued from vehicles, buildings, tunnels, or other places

O. Saw that is designed to cut laminated windshield glass

MULTIPLE-CHOICE REVIEW

_____ 1. Trench, dive, ice, and high-angle rescue is frequently carried out by:
   A. industrial rescue teams.
   B. specialty rescue teams.
   C. police rescue services.
   D. commercial rescue services.

_____ 2. The phases of extrication include all of the following except:
   A. gaining access to the patient.
   B. defining patient care.
   C. disentangling the patient.
   D. sizing up the situation.

_____ 3. An important part of a rescue scene size-up is:
   A. determining the extent of entrapment.
   B. starting IVs on the patient.
   C. removing shattered glass from around the patient.
   D. informing the patient about the extent of vehicle damage.

_____ 4. During size-up of a collision, you must be able to "read" a collision and develop an action plan based on your knowledge of rescue operations and your:
   A. previous experience at collision scenes.
   B. judgment of the extent of vehicle damage.
   C. estimate of the patient's condition and priority.
   D. evaluation of the resources available.

_____ 5. When developing an action plan for patient extrication, always keep in mind the:
   A. potential for observation by bystanders.
   B. "golden hour" concept of trauma management.
   C. cost of further damage to the vehicle.
   D. type of vehicle that is involved in the incident.

_____ 6. If a vehicle has an airbag that deployed, the manufacturer recommends:
   A. airing out the car for 15 minutes prior to treating the patient.
   B. placing masks on patients before treating.
   C. lifting the bag and examining the steering wheel and dash.
   D. using HEPA masks before gaining access.

_____ 7. The unsafe act that contributes most to collision scene injuries is failure to:
   A. eliminate or control hazards during operations.
   B. wear protective gear during rescue operations.
   C. recognize mechanisms of injury early on.
   D. select the proper tool for the task.

_____ 8. Factors that may contribute to injuries of rescuers at a collision include all of the following except:
   A. careless attitude toward personal safety.
   B. a lack of skill in tool and equipment use.
   C. physical problems that impede strenuous effort.
   D. limiting the inner circle to rescuers who are in protective gear.

_____ 9. Good protective gear at the scene of a collision includes all of the following except:
   A. firefighter or leather gloves.
   B. fire-resistant trousers or turnout pants.
   C. steel toe, high-top work shoes.
   D. plastic "bump caps."

_____ 10. To ensure adequate eye protection at the collision scene, the EMT should wear:
   A. safety goggles with a soft vinyl frame.
   B. a hinged plastic helmet shield.
   C. a thermal mask or shield.
   D. safety glasses with small lenses.

_____ 11. During an extrication, an aluminized rescue blanket may be used to:
   A. maintain the rescuer's body heat.
   B. smother fire in the engine compartment.
   C. protect the patient from poor weather and flying particles.
   D. none of the above.

_____ 12. When using flares, the EMT should:
   A. watch for spilled fuel or other combustibles prior to igniting.
   B. throw them out of the moving vehicle to save time.
   C. use them as a traffic wand to divert traffic.
   D. always walk with oncoming traffic while positioning them.

_____ 13. When there is an electrical hazard, the safe zone:
   A. should be established as soon as the power company arrives.
   B. does not exist due to the numerous dangers of an electrical hazard.
   C. should be far enough away to assure an arcing wire does not cause injury.
   D. is located at least 10 feet from the ground gradient.

_____ 14. A material or object that will carry electricity is:
   A. dangerous to stand near.   **C.** always energized.
   B. not a hazard unless it is arcing. **D.** called a conductor.

_____ 15. If a vehicle collides with a broken utility pole with wires down, you should:
   A. ignore it since the vehicle will not conduct electricity.
   B. tell the vehicle's occupants to stay in the vehicle.
   C. immediately shut off the vehicle's ignition switch.
   D. don full protective gear and remove downed wires.

_____ 16. In wet weather, a phenomenon known as _____ may provide your first clue that a wire is down.
   A. an arc   **C.** lightning
   B. ground gradient   **D.** flash point

_____ 17. As you approach a scene with an electrical hazard, you feel a tingling sensation in your legs and lower torso. Which action should you take?
   A. Turn 180 degrees and shuffle with both feet together to safety.
   B. Turn 90 degrees and walk as quickly as possible to safety.
   C. Ask your partner for his hand and have him pull you to safety.
   D. Turn 180 degrees and crawl to safety.

_____ 18. If there is a fire in the car's engine compartment and people are trapped in the vehicle, you should do all of the following except:
   A. quickly and carefully remove the patients.
   B. assure that the fire department has been called.
   C. don protective gear and use your fire extinguisher.
   D. apply a short spine board to the driver right away.

_____ 19. When a vehicle's hood is closed and there is an engine fire, you should do all of the following except:
  A. use emergency moves to remove occupants.
  B. let the fire department extinguish the fire.
  C. fully open the hood to extinguish the fire.
  D. let the fire burn under the closed hood.

_____ 20. When a vehicle rolls off the roadway into a field of dried grass, it is possible that a fire may be caused by the:
  A. catalytic converter.
  B. leaking radiator fluid.
  C. ground gradient.
  D. airbag deployment.

_____ 21. "Try Before You Pry" is the foundation for the _____ procedure.
  A. disentanglement
  B. stabilization
  C. simple access
  D. entanglement

_____ 22. Once a vehicle is stabilized and an entry point is gained, the EMT should immediately do all of the following except:
  A. begin the initial assessment.
  B. crawl inside the vehicle.
  C. provide manual cervical stabilization.
  D. pull the patient out of the access hole.

_____ 23. If an unconscious patient is in a sitting position behind the wheel with legs pinned by the vehicle, which is the best approach to disentanglement?
  A. Displace the doors, cut the roof, then displace the dash.
  B. Pull the dash, cut the doors, then push the seat.
  C. Cut the roof, displace the doors, and then displace the dash.
  D. Cut the roof, displace the dash, then displace the doors.

_____ 24. Which of the following is not a reason for disposing of the roof to access a patient?
  A. It makes the entire interior of the vehicle accessible.
  B. It creates a large exitway through which to remove a patient.
  C. It provides fresh air and helps cool off the patient.
  D. It helps to quickly stabilize the vehicle.

_____ 25. An extrication involves displacing the dash or steering wheel but the airbag has not yet deployed. What should you do?
  A. Apply heat to the steering wheel.
  B. Drill a hole into the airbag module.
  C. Disconnect the battery cable.
  D. Displace the steering column.

COMPLETE THE FOLLOWING

1. List the ten phases of the rescue process.

A. _____ F. _____

B. _____ G. _____

C. _____ H. _____

D. _____ I. _____

E. _____ J. _____

©2009 Pearson Education, Inc.
Emergency Care, 11th Ed.

2. List six factors that can increase the potential for an injury at a collision site.

A. _____

B. _____

C. _____

D. _____

E. _____

F. _____

LABEL THE PHOTOGRAPHS

Label each procedure on the lines provided.

1. _____

2. _____

3. _____

4. _____

5. _____

6. _____

©2009 Pearson Education, Inc.
Emergency Care, 11th Ed.

Chapter 35 • *Gaining Access and Rescue Operations*   **289**

STREET SCENES DISCUSSION

Review the Street Scene on pp. 961–962 of the textbook. Then answer the questions below.

1. Suppose the patient had been trapped under the dashboard. Would it make more sense to pop open the doors and then take off the roof? Or should the roof come off first?

2. What is the significance of a vehicle with 10 feet of intrusion?

3. Should ALS be requested for this patient?

ON THE WEB

To help you review and practice basic skills, visit the *Emergency Care 11th Ed. Companion Website* at www.prenhall.com/limmer. For Online Test Preparation, visit www.prenhall.com/emtachieve.

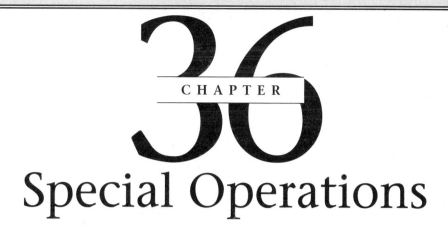

CHAPTER 36
Special Operations

MATCH TERMINOLOGY/ DEFINITIONS

A. Color-coded tag indicating the priority group to which a patient has been assigned

B. Area in which secondary triage takes place at a multiple-casualty incident

C. Process of quickly assessing patients in a multiple-casualty incident and assigning each a priority for receiving emergency care or transportation to definitive care

D. Person responsible for overseeing triage at a multiple-casualty incident

E. Area in which patient care is delivered at a multiple-casualty incident

F. Person responsible for overseeing treatment of patients who have been triaged at a multiple-casualty incident

G. Person responsible for communicating with sector officers and hospitals to manage transportation of patients to hospitals from the scene of a multiple-casualty incident

H. Area in which ambulances are parked and other resources are held until needed

I. Person responsible for overseeing and keeping track of ambulances and ambulance personnel at a multiple-casualty incident and who directs ambulances to treatment areas at the request of the transportation officer/supervisor

J. Any medical or trauma event involving three or more patients that places a great demand on EMS equipment and personnel

_____ **1.** Cold zone

_____ **2.** EMS Command

_____ **3.** Hazardous material

_____ **4.** Hot zone

_____ **5.** National Incident Management System

_____ **6.** Multiple-casualty incident (MCI)

_____ **7.** Staging supervisor

_____ **8.** Staging area

_____ **9.** Transportation supervisor

_____ **10.** Treatment supervisor

_____ **11.** Treatment area

_____ **12.** Triage

_____ **13.** Triage supervisor

_____ **14.** Triage area

_____ **15.** Triage tag

K. System used for the management of a large-scale multiple-casualty incident, involving assumption of responsibility for command and designation and coordination of such elements as triage, treatment, transport, and staging

L. Senior EMS person on the scene who establishes an EMS command post and oversees the medical aspects of a multiple-casualty incident

M. Any substance or material in a form that poses an unreasonable risk to health, safety, and property when transported in commerce

N. Area immediately surrounding a dangerous goods incident that extends far enough to prevent adverse effects from released dangerous goods to personnel outside the zone

O. Area in which the command post and support functions that are necessary to control the incident are located

MULTIPLE-CHOICE REVIEW

_____ **1.** Using the *North American Emergency Response Guidebook,* the EMT would find that ethyl acetate is a chemical that:
  A. irritates the eyes and respiratory tract.
  B. destroys the bone marrow.
  C. damages internal organs.
  D. is extremely explosive.

_____ **2.** Using the *North American Emergency Response Guidebook,* the EMT would find that Benzene (benzol) is a chemical that:
  A. damages the eyes by eliminating moisture.
  B. has toxic vapors that can be absorbed through the skin.
  C. is used as an industrial blasting agent.
  D. is used in surgical techniques to control pain.

_____ **3.** The regulations that require training in hazardous materials for responders to hazmat incidents are found in the:
  A. Ryan White CARE Act.   **C.** FEMA 1910.1030.
  B. NFPA 1200.   **D.** OSHA 1910.120

_____ **4.** The level of training for those who initially respond to releases or potential releases of hazardous materials in order to protect people, property, and the environment is called:
  A. First Responder Awareness.   **C.** Hazardous Materials Technician.
  B. First Responder Operations. **D.** Hazardous Materials Specialist.

_____ **5.** The level of training for those who are likely to witness or discover a hazardous substance release is called:
  A. First Responder Awareness.   **C.** Hazardous Materials Technician.
  B. First Responder Operations. **D.** Hazardous Materials Specialist.

_____ **6.** The standard that deals with competencies for EMS personnel at a hazardous material incident is called:
  A. OSHA 1910.1030.   **C.** NFPA 473.
  B. NFPA 472.   **D.** OSHA 1910.1200.

_____ **7.** Which of the following is <u>not</u> likely to be a potential hazardous material location?
  A. garden center   **C.** trucking terminal
  B. chemical plant   **D.** pet store

©2009 Pearson Education, Inc.
Emergency Care, 11th Ed.

8. Unless EMS personnel are trained to the level of _____, they must remain in the cold zone.
  A. First Responder Awareness
  B. First Responder Operations
  C. Hazardous Materials Technician
  D. Hazardous Materials Specialist

9. All victims leaving the _____ zone should be considered contaminated until proven otherwise.
  A. cold
  B. warm
  C. hot
  D. decontamination

10. What is the primary concern at the scene of a hazardous material incident?
  A. the safety of the EMT and crew, patients, and the public
  B. stabilizing the incident as fast as possible
  C. quickly removing all exposed patients from the scene
  D. determining the extent and cost of the damage

11. Upon arrival at a tanker truck crash where the vehicle has overturned and is rapidly leaking its contents onto the street, the EMT should:
  A. quickly apply a short spine board to the truck driver in the tanker.
  B. isolate the area and call for the appropriate backup assistance.
  C. try to stop or seal the leak as quickly as possible.
  D. send the least-senior EMT in to assess the patient.

12. The "safe zone" of a hazardous materials incident should be established in a _____ location.
  A. downwind/downhill
  B. upwind/same level
  C. downwind/same level
  D. upwind/downhill

13. The role of EMS Command at a hazardous material incident is to delegate responsibility for all the following <u>except</u>:
  A. directing bystanders to a safe area.
  B. establishing a perimeter.
  C. immediately initiating rescue attempts.
  D. evacuating people if necessary.

14. When a contaminated victim of a hazardous material incident comes in contact with other people who are not contaminated, this is referred to as _____ contamination.
  A. secondary
  B. chemical
  C. contact
  D. clone

15. The designations on the sides of tanker trucks are called hazardous material:
  A. license plates.
  B. waybills.
  C. placards.
  D. shipping papers.

16. The commonly used placard system for fixed facilities is called the:
  A. MSDS.
  B. NFPA 704.
  C. CHEM 369 System.
  D. UN Classification System.

17. All employers are required to post in an obvious spot the information about all the chemicals in the workplace on a form called a(n):
  A. NFPA 704.
  B. MSDS.
  C. OSHA Chemical listing.
  D. fair trade posting.

18. Resources that the EMT should use at a hazardous materials incident include all of the following <u>except</u>:
  A. copies of NFPA rules.
  B. the local hazmat team.
  C. the *North American Emergency Response Guidebook*.
  D. CHEM-TEL.

_____ **19.** What is CHEMTREC?
  A. 24-hour service for identifying hazardous materials
  B. oil refinery and manufacturer
  C. national hazmat response team
  D. round-the-clock special rescue teams

_____ **20.** EMS personnel at the scene of a hazardous material incident are responsible for taking care of the injured and:
  A. identifying and controlling the substance involved.
  B. monitoring and rehabilitating hazmat team members.
  C. decontaminating patients exiting the hot zone.
  D. moving patients from the hot zone to the warm zone.

_____ **21.** Which of the following is <u>not</u> a characteristic of the rehab sector at a hazardous material incident?
  A. located in the warm zone
  B. protected from the weather
  C. easily accessible to EMS
  D. free from exhaust fumes

_____ **22.** As soon as possible after a hazmat team member exits the hot zone, the EMT should:
  A. have him drink a pint of water.
  B. remove his protective clothing.
  C. begin the decontamination process.
  D. reassess his vital signs.

_____ **23.** You are confronted with a patient at risk for causing secondary contamination in which treatment calls for irrigation with water. The hazmat team has not yet arrived. Which of the following actions is <u>not</u> recommended?
  A. Cut the patient's clothes off.
  B. Irrigate the patient with tepid water.
  C. Flush runoff water down the nearest drain.
  D. Use disposable equipment for treatment.

_____ **24.** Which of the following is <u>not</u> a feature of a good local disaster plan?
  A. All emergency responders should be familiar with the plan.
  B. The plan must be based on the actual availability of resources.
  C. The plan must be rehearsed to ensure it works correctly.
  D. The plan should be generic and meet national standards.

_____ **25.** Upon arrival of the first EMS unit at the scene of an MCI, the crew leader should do all of the following <u>except</u>:
  A. assume command.
  B. conduct a scene walk-through.
  C. call for backup.
  D. begin patient treatment.

_____ **26.** Which of the following is <u>not</u> a principle of good communication at an MCI?
  A. The person responsible for incident management should have a unique Command name.
  B. Responding units should be informed that a disaster plan is in effect.
  C. The majority of communications should be done via radio transmission.
  D. Communications between Command and sector officers should be face-to-face.

_____ **27.** If an MCI involves hazardous materials, an additional _____ sector would be needed.
  A. hazmat
  B. extrication
  C. rehabilitation
  D. decontamination

_____ **28.** The individual at an MCI who is responsible for the sorting and prioritizing of the patients is the _____ supervisor.
  A. triage
  B. treatment
  C. transportation
  D. extrication

©2009 Pearson Education, Inc.
Emergency Care, 11th Ed.

_____ **29.** Patients who are assessed to have decreased mental status at an MCI are considered Priority-:

A. 1.   **C.** 3.

B. 2.   **D.** 4.

_____ **30.** Patients who are assessed to have shock (hypoperfusion) at an MCI are considered Priority-:

A. 1.   **C.** 3.

B. 2.   **D.** 4.

_____ **31.** Patients who are assessed to have multiple-bone or joint injuries at an MCI are usually considered Priority-:

A. 1.   **C.** 3.

B. 2.   **D.** 4.

_____ **32.** Patients who are assessed to have died at the MCI scene are considered Priority-:

A. 1.   **C.** 3.

B. 2.   **D.** 4.

_____ **33.** The individual at an MCI who is responsible for maintaining a supply of vehicles and personnel at a location away from the incident site is the _____ supervisor.

A. extrication   **C.** staging

B. transportation   **D.** triage

_____ **34.** The individual at an MCI who is responsible for determining patient destinations and notifying the hospitals of the incoming patients is the _____ supervisor.

A. triage   **C.** transportation

B. treatment   **D.** extrication

_____ **35.** Patient transport decisions at an MCI are based upon all of the following except:

A. priority.   **C.** transportation resources.

B. destination facilities.   **D.** patient's family preferences.

COMPLETE THE FOLLOWING

1. List the information you should be prepared to give when you call for assistance from CHEMTREC.

_____

_____

_____

_____

_____

2. List four characteristics of the rehab area at a hazardous material incident.

A. _____

B. _____

C. _____

D. _____

COMPLETE THE CHART

Fill in the blanks to complete the chart.

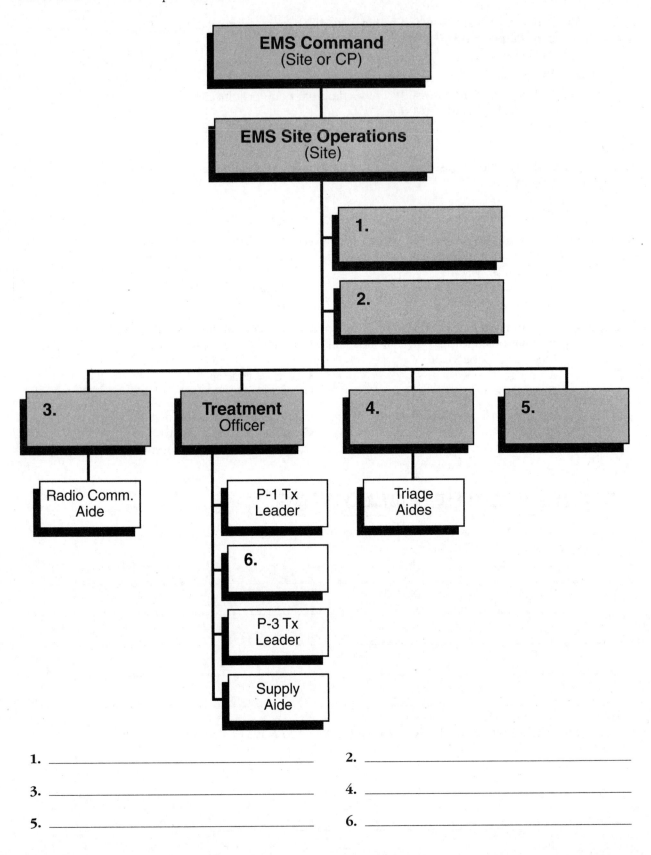

1. _____   2. _____

3. _____   4. _____

5. _____   6. _____

STREET SCENES DISCUSSION

Review the Street Scene on pp. 993–994 of the textbook. Then answer the questions below.

1. For this call, would it have been appropriate to request a helicopter if it were available?

2. How could you find enough additional ambulances?

3. Suppose there was a bus involved at this scene and there were 20 low-priority patients. How could you transport them?

ON THE WEB

To help you review and practice basic skills, visit the *Emergency Care 11th Ed. Companion Website* at www.prenhall.com/limmer. For Online Test Preparation, visit www.prenhall.com/emtachieve.

EMT SKILLS
PERFORMANCE CHECKLIST

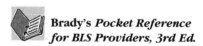

Brady's *Pocket Reference for BLS Providers, 3rd Ed.*

▶ **ESTABLISHING COMMAND AT A MULTIPLE-CASUALTY INCIDENT (MCI) (PP. 977–979)**

❑ Perform a scene size-up.

❑ Locate the police and fire officers and establish a unified command post.

❑ Don the command vest.

❑ Notify the EMS dispatcher:

- Designate EMS Operations Officer (as needed).
- Declare an MCI.
- Describe extent of incident.
- Characterize it as ongoing or contained.
- Give approximate number of patients.
- Give the location of the command posts.
- Request number of BLS and ALS units.

▶ DESIGNATE A TRIAGE SUPERVISOR

❑ Designate a staging supervisor and a location for staging, and notify dispatcher to have all additional ambulances respond to staging.

❑ Request the dispatcher roll call the local hospitals for bed availability.

❑ Designate treatment supervisor and location for this area (as needed).

❑ Designate transportation supervisor and location for this area (as needed).

❑ Consider the need for aeromedical evacuation and appropriate landing zone nearby the scene.

❑ Consider the usefulness of a school bus to transport the "walking wounded" low-priority patients. Make sure everyone on the bus is medically examined and that medical personnel also ride the bus.

❑ Consider the need for extrication area (if not already established).

❑ Consider the need for a safety supervisor (as needed).

❑ Consider the need for rehab of personnel.

❑ Keep the dispatcher and other service chiefs in close contact throughout the incident.

❑ Along with the police and fire officers, consider the need for a public information supervisor to work with the arriving media representatives.

CASE STUDY

▶ THE SCHOOL BUS MCI

You are dispatched to a school bus collision in a major intersection in town. En route the dispatcher notifies you that he has received numerous calls on the collision, and the police as well as the fire department are en route. Callers state that a large truck collided with the bus in an intersection at a high rate of speed, overturning the bus full of schoolchildren. As you near the center of town, the traffic is backed up in both directions for about five blocks. The police have arrived on the scene and are beginning to reroute the traffic after confirming that there are many injured children on and near the bus.

1. What would be your initial role as the crew leader of the first arriving ambulance at the scene?

2. **(A)** Which vest from the MCI kit should you wear and, **(B)** what are your responsibilities?

After declaring the MCI, confirming the incident with dispatch, and establishing contact with the police and fire officers, you begin to estimate the number of patients with the assistance of your two crew members.

©2009 Pearson Education, Inc.
Emergency Care, 11th Ed.

3. What would be the most likely job to designate to one of your partners?

4. What are his or her specific functions?

Upon size-up of the situation, it is determined that there were 40 children on the bus, half of whom have numerous contusions and cuts and who are walking around the scene crying. You decide to designate a nearby store as the location for the P-3 patients. You have one of your partners make a PA announcement that the walking wounded should go to that location. In addition, you call for 10 ambulances and another school bus to respond.

5. Where would be the best place to stage the ambulances?

6. What should be the role of the crew leader on the first ambulance arriving at the staging area?

7. Should any ambulances report directly to the scene?

8. Are there any other sector supervisors needed at this time?

The fire department has cleared the bus for entry now that it is stabilized and no longer leaking any fuel. Inside there are 15 patients who need to be removed from the bus. Many of the patients have head injuries, fractures, contusions, and glass cuts.

9. How should these patients be removed from the bus if it is possible?

10. Once removed from the bus, where should the patients be taken?

Prioritize the patients described below into the following categories: P-1 (critical and unstable), P-2 (potentially unstable), P-3 (stable walking wounded), P-4 (dead).

11. A 7-year-old female who complains of a swollen deformed right lower arm and a contusion to the head with no loss of consciousness. She is alert and has vital signs that are normal for her age.

12. A 9-year-old male who has a seizure disorder who has been unconscious since the collision and has already had two observed grand-mal seizures without a lucid interval.

13. A 10-year-old male who was thrown through the front window of the bus because he was standing up talking to the bus driver. He was ejected from the vehicle, was found approximately 50 feet from the bus, and has a large contusion, depressed skull fracture, and no vital signs.

14. An 8-year-old female who has a bruise on the left upper quadrant and the forehead. She denies any loss of consciousness but is pale, clammy, and has a rapid heart rate for her age.

©2009 Pearson Education, Inc.
Emergency Care, 11th Ed.

The treatment supervisor has set up a treatment area across the street from the collision in the gas station parking lot. He has set out a large yellow and a large red tarp. There is also a smaller black tarp inside the gas station for the P-4 patients. As the incident proceeds, you are able to obtain additional assistance from the firefighters at the scene for lifting the patients being removed from the bus and carried on backboards to the treatment area. Also, the area is becoming quite congested because a number of parents are arriving at the scene.

15. What is the best thing to do with the parents?

16. As a smooth flow of ambulances begins to arrive from the staging area, who should coordinate the destinations of the patient transports and communicate with the hospitals?

17. What might this person want to know immediately from the local hospitals?

18. Other than the bus that was ordered for the P-3 patients, is there any other form of transportation that should be considered for this incident?

19. How should the decision be made as to who rides on the bus to a hospital?

20. As the incident is wrapped up, how could you, as Command, deal with the media and the emotional and physical needs of your personnel?

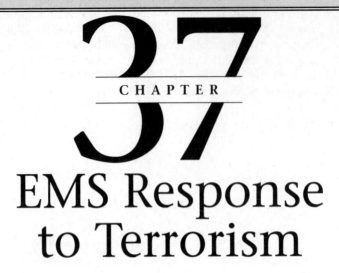

CHAPTER 37

EMS Response to Terrorism

MATCH TERMINOLOGY/DEFINITIONS

A. Contact with or presence of a material where it does not belong and that is somehow harmful to persons, animals, or the environment

B. A chemical and/or physical process used to remove and prevent the spread of a contaminant

C. Spreading

D. The dose or concentration of an agent multiplied by the time, or duration

E. The movement of a substance through a surface or, on a molecular level, through intact materials

F. Pathways into the body, generally by absorption, ingestion, injection, or inhalation

G. Destructive devices, such as bombs, placed to be activated after an initial attack and timed to injure emergency responders who rush in to help care for those targeted by an initial attack

H. Specific operational actions to accomplish assigned tasks

_____ **1.** Permeation

_____ **2.** Dissemination

_____ **3.** Tactics

_____ **4.** Contamination

_____ **5.** Secondary devices

_____ **6.** Decontamination

_____ **7.** Exposure

_____ **8.** Routes of entry

MULTIPLE-CHOICE REVIEW

_____ **1.** In addition to armed attacks, types of incidents of terrorism may be remembered by the EMT using the acronym:
  A. OPQRST.
  B. CBRNE.
  C. CUPS.
  D. AVPU.

_____ **2.** Environmental terrorists, survivalists, militias, and racial-hate groups are examples of:
  A. international terrorists.
  B. state-sponsored terrorist groups.
  C. domestic terrorists.
  D. religious freedom fighters.

_____ **3.** The EMT should be alert to clues when on the scene of a suspicious incident. An acronym designed to help with this process is:
  A. CBRNE.
  B. TRACEM-P.
  C. SAMPLE.
  D. OTTO.

_____ **4.** Potential high-risk targets of terrorists typically include:
  A. controversial businesses.
  B. infrastructure systems.
  C. public buildings.
  D. any of the above.

_____ **5.** Why is April 19th a day the U.S. government stands at heightened security awareness for government facilities?
  A. It is the anniversary of the Pearl Harbor attack.
  B. It is the anniversary of the Murrah building bombing in Oklahoma City.
  C. It is the anniversary of the birth of the FBI.
  D. It is the anniversary of the Bay of Pigs incident.

_____ **6.** Responding EMTs who arrive on the scene of an incident should watch for signs that they may be dealing with a suspicious incident. Examples of unexplained patterns of illness or deaths may include each of the following except:
  A. car crashes involving more than two patients with serious traumatic injuries.
  B. unexplained symptoms of skin or eye irritation.
  C. unexplained vapor clouds, mists, and plumes.
  D. unexplained signs of airway irritation.

_____ **7.** The acronym "TRACEM-P" is designed to help rescuers understand the types of harm to which they can be exposed. What does the letter "E" refer to?
  A. emergency
  B. environmental
  C. biological/etiological
  D. essential

_____ **8.** Danger from alpha particles, beta particles, or gamma rays is caused by _____ harm.
  A. chemical
  B. radiological
  C. biological/etiological
  D. mechanical

_____ **9.** The major routes through which WMD agents can enter the body include each of the following except:
  A. absorption.
  B. ingestion.
  C. osmosis.
  D. inhalation.

_____ **10.** The types of harm from radiological/nuclear incidents would include radiological, chemical, and _____ harm.
  A. psychological
  B. mechanical
  C. thermal
  D. all of the above

_____ 11. The primary harm from a nuclear explosion would involve _____ harm.
   A. chemical
   B. mechanical
   C. psychological
   D. radiological

_____ 12. The mainstays of self-protection at a radiological incident include all of the following except:
   A. time.
   B. Standard Precautions.
   C. distance.
   D. shielding.

_____ 13. Which is the most lethal route of exposure to anthrax?
   A. skin contact
   B. ingestion
   C. inhalation
   D. injection

_____ 14. The _____ route of exposure is very effective with vesicants but less effective with many of the biological agents.
   A. dermal
   B. vector
   C. airborne
   D. bloodborne

_____ 15. Features that influence the potential for a biological agent's use as a weapon may include:
   A. infectivity and virulence.
   B. toxicity and incubation period.
   C. transmissibility and lethality.
   D. any of the above.

_____ 16. The quality of being poisonous, especially the degree of strength of a toxic microbe or of a poison, is referred to as the:
   A. infectivity.
   B. toxicity.
   C. virulence.
   D. transmissibility.

_____ 17. The relative ease with which an agent causes death in a susceptible population is referred to as the:
   A. stability of the product.
   B. infectivity of the agent.
   C. lethality of the agent.
   D. virulence of the virus.

_____ 18. Which virus did the World Health Organization declare eradicated worldwide through immunization efforts in 1980?
   A. polio
   B. encephalitis
   C. viral hemorrhagic fever
   D. smallpox

_____ 19. Which of the following is not a common mechanism for performing decontamination?
   A. demulsification
   B. chemical reaction
   C. disinfection
   D. absorption and adsorption

_____ 20. A process that simply reduces the concentration of the contaminant is called:
   A. removal.
   B. disposal.
   C. dilution.
   D. emulsification.

©2009 Pearson Education, Inc.
Emergency Care, 11th Ed.

COMPLETE THE FOLLOWING

Decontamination for Responders Wearing PPE

1. This is a limited list that may not require personal showers since the responders were wearing PPE. List six items that would be found on the equipment list for decontamination:

   A. _____

   B. _____

   C. _____

   D. _____

   E. _____

   F. _____

2. List six objectives of the responders assigned to decontamination:

   A. _____

   B. _____

   C. _____

   D. _____

   E. _____

   F. _____

STREET SCENES DISCUSSION

Review the Street Scene on pp. 1027–1028 of the textbook. Then answer the questions below.

1. Why would you consider the organization a potential threat to emergency service personnel?

2. Is it unusual to find a motor vehicle collision in an isolated location such as the one in this scenario?

3. Is it an acceptable practice to stop and not proceed if the emergency services personnel feel they are in imminent danger?

4. What are some other examples of groups or types of domestic terrorists that have been identified?

ON THE WEB

To help you review and practice basic skills, visit the *Emergency Care 11th Ed. Companion Website* at www.prenhall.com/limmer. For Online Test Preparation, visit www.prenhall.com/emtachieve.

CHAPTER 38

Advanced Airway Management

MATCH TERMINOLOGY/ DEFINITIONS

▶ **PART A**

A. Fork at the lower end of the trachea where the two mainstem bronchi branch

B. Insertion of a tube

C. Tube designed to be inserted into the trachea; oxygen, medication, or a suction catheter can be directed into the trachea through an endotracheal tube.

D. Area directly above the openings of both the trachea and the esophagus

E. Inadequate oxygenation, or oxygen starvation

F. Opening to the trachea

G. Tube that leads from the pharynx to the stomach

H. To provide ventilations at a higher rate to compensate for oxygen not delivered during intubation or suctioning

I. Leaf-shaped structure that acts as covering to the opening of the trachea and that prevents food and foreign matter from entering it

J. Ring-shaped structure that circles the trachea at the lower portion of the larynx

K. Two large sets of branches that come off the trachea and enter the lungs

L. Voicebox

_____ **1.** Alveoli

_____ **2.** Bronchi

_____ **3.** Carina

_____ **4.** Cricoid cartilage

_____ **5.** EIDD

_____ **6.** Endotracheal tube

_____ **7.** Epiglottis

_____ **8.** Esophagus

_____ **9.** Glottic opening

_____ **10.** Ventilate

_____ **11.** Hypopharynx

_____ **12.** Hypoxia

_____ **13.** Intubation

_____ **14.** Laryngoscope

_____ **15.** Larynx

M. Microscopic sacs of the lungs where exchange of oxygen and carbon dioxide takes place

N. Illuminating instrument that is inserted into the pharynx to permit visualization of the pharynx and larynx

O. Esophageal intubation detector device that may be used to detect incorrect placement (or to verify correct placement) of the endotracheal tube

▶ PART B

A. Placement of an endotracheal tube through the mouth and into the trachea

B. "Windpipe"; structure that connects the pharynx to the lungs

C. Two thin folds of tissue within the larynx that vibrate as air passes between them, producing sounds

D. Long, thin, flexible metal probe

E. Either of the two (right or left) large sets of branches that come off the trachea and enter the lungs

F. Groove-like structure anterior to the epiglottis

G. Tube designed to be passed through the nose, nasopharynx, and esophagus. It is used to relieve distention of the stomach in an infant or child patient.

H. Area directly posterior to the nose

I. Area directly posterior to the mouth

J. Pressure applied to the cricoid cartilage to suppress vomiting and bring the vocal cords into view; also called cricoid pressure

_____ **1.** Mainstem bronchi

_____ **2.** Nasogastric tube (NG tube)

_____ **3.** Nasopharynx

_____ **4.** Oropharynx

_____ **5.** Orotracheal intubation

_____ **6.** Cricoid pressure

_____ **7.** Stylet

_____ **8.** Trachea

_____ **9.** Vallecula

_____ **10.** Vocal cords

MULTIPLE-CHOICE REVIEW

_____ **1.** The area directly above the openings of both the trachea and the esophagus is called the:
A. vallecula.
B. larynx.
C. hypopharynx.
D. oropharynx.

_____ **2.** The groove-like structure anterior to the epiglottis is called the:
A. carina.
B. vallecula.
C. epiglottis.
D. vocal cord.

_____ **3.** Why is food more apt to be aspirated into the right mainstem bronchus rather than the left mainstem bronchus?
A. It splits off the carina at more of an angle than the left.
B. It splits off the carina at less of an angle than the left.
C. It is much larger in diameter than the left.
D. It is much smaller in diameter than the left.

_____ **4.** The brain's center for respiratory control is located in the:
A. brainstem.
B. cerebellum.
C. pons.
D. cerebrum.

©2009 Pearson Education, Inc.
Emergency Care, 11th Ed.

_____ **5.** The endotracheal tube is primarily intended to:
  A. be placed into the esophagus.
  B. provide a medication route.
  C. be inserted into the trachea.
  D. be used as a means of suctioning the hypopharynx.

_____ **6.** Orotracheal intubation allows direct ventilation of the lungs, bypassing the:
  A. entire upper airway.   **C.** vocal cords.
  B. entire lower airway.   **D.** oropharynx.

_____ **7.** When placing the endotracheal tube, EMTs use:
  A. a rapid-sequence technique.   **C.** direct visualization.
  B. a blind technique.   **D.** a surgical technique.

_____ **8.** The advantage of orotracheal intubation is that it offers complete control of the airway and it:
  A. minimizes the risk of aspiration.
  B. allows for better oxygen delivery.
  C. allows for deeper suctioning of the airway.
  D. all of the above.

_____ **9.** All of the following are complications of orotracheal intubation <u>except</u>:
  A. hypoxia from prolonged intubation attempts.
  B. soft tissue trauma to the lips, gums, or airway structures.
  C. increased heart rate from vagal stimulation.
  D. gagging and vomiting from airway stimulation.

_____ **10.** When the endotracheal tube is advanced too deeply, this commonly results in:
  A. vallecula injury.
  B. right-mainstem intubation.
  C. esophageal intubation.
  D. left-mainstem intubation.

_____ **11.** The most serious complication of endotracheal intubation is:
  A. left-mainstem intubation.
  B. bradycardia from airway stimulation.
  C. esophageal intubation.
  D. airway trauma.

_____ **12.** The EMT should reassess endotracheal tube placement each time the patient is moved to prevent disastrous complications from:
  A. accidental extubation.   **C.** right-mainstem intubation.
  B. vomiting.   **D.** occlusion of the ET tube.

_____ **13.** Most adult patients can be intubated using a size _____ straight blade or size _____ curved blade.
  A. 0 or 1; 1   **C.** 2 or 3; 3
  B. 1 or 2; 2   **D.** 3 or 4; 4

_____ **14.** The straight blade is designed so that the tip of the blade is placed:
  A. into the vallecula.   **C.** under the epiglottis.
  B. into the carina.   **D.** behind the epiglottis.

_____ **15.** The curved blade is designed so the tip of the blade is inserted:
  A. into the carina.   **C.** into the glottis.
  B. under the epiglottis.   **D.** into the vallecula.

_____ **16.** The cuff at the distal end of the endotracheal tube:
  A. usually seals with 8 to 10 cc of air.
  B. is called the pilot balloon.
  C. has a standard 15-millimeter adapter.
  D. holds 5 cc of air in an infant tube.

_____ **17.** When using an endotracheal tube on an infant or child less than 8 years of age, do not expect to see:
  A. the child's vocal cords.   **C.** a cuff on the tube.
  B. a Murphy eye.   **D.** a variety of tube sizes.

_____ **18.** No matter what the internal diameter of the endotracheal tube, it:
  A. will always fit into a large adult.
  B. has a standard 15-millimeter adapter.
  C. will have an inflation valve.
  D. will have a pilot balloon.

_____ **19.** It is generally accepted that the adult male should receive either a(n) _____ mm tube.
  A. 6.0 or 6.5   **C.** 8.0 or 8.5
  B. 7.0 or 7.5   **D.** 9.0 or 9.5

_____ **20.** In an adult, the properly placed tube will have the _____-cm mark at the teeth.
  A. 18   **C.** 22
  B. 20   **D.** 24

_____ **21.** Once the lubricated stylet is inserted, the endotracheal tube should be shaped like a:
  A. hairpin.   **C.** "C".
  B. horseshoe.   **D.** hockey stick.

_____ **22.** Prior to securing an endotracheal tube, do all of the following <u>except</u>:
  A. insert an oral airway as a bite block.
  B. listen to both lungs.
  C. listen over the epigastrium.
  D. suction down the tube.

_____ **23.** Items that should be checked prior to an intubation attempt include all of the following <u>except</u> the:
  A. laryngoscope light bulb.   **C.** length of the tube.
  B. cuff on the tube.   **D.** shape of the tube and stylet.

_____ **24.** The laryngoscope is designed to be:
  A. used as a fulcrum, pivoting on the teeth.
  B. placed in the left corner of the patient's mouth.
  C. held in the left hand.
  D. held in the right hand.

_____ **25.** Application of cricoid pressure is designed to help:
  A. reduce the risk of vomiting.   **C.** move the carina into view.
  B. move the vallecula into view.   **D.** compress the trachea.

_____ **26.** The correct order for verifying tube placement by auscultation is:
  A. right, then left, then epigastrium.   **C.** epigastrium, then right, then left.
  B. epigastrium, then left, then right.   **D.** left, then right, then epigastrium.

_____ **27.** If the breath sounds are diminished or absent on the left but present on the right, it is likely the tube has advanced into the:
  A. esophagus.   **C.** right-mainstem bronchus.
  B. left lung.   **D.** carina.

_____ **28.** It is recommended that the EMT make no more than _____ attempt(s) at orotracheal intubation.
  A. one   **C.** three
  B. two   **D.** four

_____ **29.** The narrowest point of the infant's or small child's airway is the:
  A. glottic opening.   **C.** epiglottis.
  B. carina.   **D.** cricoid ring.

_____ **30.** The preferred laryngoscope blade size for infants and small children is:
  A. #2 straight.   **C.** #5 curved.
  B. #1 straight.   **D.** #2 curved.

_____ **31.** A nasogastric tube is commonly used in an infant or child patient to:
  A. suction out the esophagus.
  B. perform deep and extensive suctioning.
  C. decompress the stomach and proximal bowel.
  D. provide a means of ventilating the patient.

_____ **32.** When you are unable to adequately ventilate the pediatric patient due to distention of the stomach, you should consider the use of a:
  A. nasotracheal tube.   **C.** shunt.
  B. nasogastric tube.   **D.** tracheal tube.

_____ **33.** The major contraindication for a nasogastric tube placement in the infant or child is:
  A. pulmonary edema.   **C.** trauma to the chest.
  B. an inflated stomach.   **D.** head or major facial trauma.

_____ **34.** The nasogastric tube should be measured from the:
  A. tip of the nose around the ear to below the xiphoid process.
  B. bottom of the earlobe to the stomach.
  C. tip of the nose and directly to the xiphoid process.
  D. nose to the angle of the jaw and then to the umbilicus.

_____ **35.** Once the nasogastric tube is passed gently downward along the nasal floor, the EMT should do all of the following <u>except</u>:
  A. confirm tube placement by aspirating stomach contents.
  B. secure the tube in place with tape.
  C. confirm placement by auscultating the epigastrium while injecting 10–20 cc of air.
  D. hook the tube up to the suction unit.

COMPLETE THE FOLLOWING

1. List four indications for performing orotracheal intubation.

A. _____

B. _____

C. _____

D. _____

2. List six complications of deep suctioning that can be avoided by proper ventilation technique.

A. _____

B. _____

C. _____

D. _____

E. _____

F. _____

STREET SCENES DISCUSSION

Review the Street Scene on pp. 1067–1068 of the textbook. Then answer the questions below.

1. What would you have done if the patient regained consciousness and started to gag on the tube?

2. Should ALS be requested for this patient?

3. Imagine that when you pull back on the EIDD, the tube fills with stomach contents. What should you do?

4. Suppose your patient had experienced neck trauma. Would your technique be any different?

ON THE WEB

To help you review and practice basic skills, visit the *Emergency Care 11th Ed. Companion Website* at www.prenhall.com/limmer. For Online Test Preparation, visit www.prenhall.com/emtachieve.

EMT SKILL
PERFORMANCE CHECKLISTS

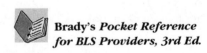

Brady's *Pocket Reference for BLS Providers, 3rd Ed.*

▶ **VENTILATORY MANAGEMENT AND ENDOTRACHEAL INTUBATION**

❑ Take Standard Precautions.

❑ Open airway manually.

❑ Elevate tongue and insert airway adjunct (oropharyngeal or nasopharyngeal airway).

❑ Ventilate the patient immediately using a BVM device attached to high-concentration oxygen at the proper rate and volume.

©2009 Pearson Education, Inc.
Emergency Care, 11th Ed.

▶ ET INTUBATION AND MANAGEMENT

❑ Take Standard Precautions.

❑ Open airway manually.

❑ Elevate tongue and insert airway adjunct (oropharyngeal or nasopharyngeal airway).

❑ Ventilate patient immediately using a BVM device attached to high-concentration oxygen at the proper rate and volume.

❑ Direct assistant to oxygenate patient.

❑ Identify and select proper equipment for intubation.

❑ Check equipment (cuff for leaks, laryngoscope batteries, and bulb for tightness).

❑ Position the head properly (sniffing position).

❑ Insert laryngoscope blade with left hand while displacing tongue to the left.

❑ Elevate mandible with laryngoscope and visualize the vocal cords.

❑ Insert the ET and advance it to proper depth (until cuff is past vocal cords).

❑ Inflate cuff to proper pressure (5 cc to 10 cc of air) and disconnect syringe.

❑ Continue to hold onto the ET until it is secured in place.

❑ Direct ventilation of the patient.

❑ Confirm proper placement by auscultation bilaterally over epigastrium.*

❑ Secure the ET tube with a commercial tube restraint.

*NOTE: Most medical directors also require the use of one or more of the following to confirm proper tube placement: an esophageal intubation detector device, pulse oximeter, colormetric end-tidal CO_2 device, or capnography.

▶ INSERTION OF THE NASOGASTRIC TUBE (OPTIONAL EMT SKILL)

❑ Take Standard Precautions.

❑ Prepare and assemble the equipment.

❑ Oxygenate the patient.

❑ Measure tube from the tip of nose, over ear, to below xiphoid process.

❑ Lubricate end of tube and pass tube gently downward along the nasal floor into the stomach.

❑ To confirm correct placement, auscultate over epigastrium. Listen for bubbling while injecting 10 to 20 cc of air into tube.

❑ Use suction to aspirate stomach contents.

❑ Secure tube in place.

▶ INSERTION OF THE LARYNGEAL MASK AIRWAY (LMA)® (OPTIONAL EMT SKILL)

❑ Ensure that AHA BLS airway maneuvers are being attempted while preparing equipment.

❑ Take Standard Precautions.

(continued on next page)

❑ Select and assemble correct equipment:

- An LMA® properly sized for patient.
- BVM with reservoir.
- 30-cc syringe.
- Suction unit and rigid Yankauer tip.
- Test cuff by inflation and deflation.
- Water-based lubricant gel for mask tip.
- Gloves, mask, and protective eyewear.

❑ Have another rescuer hyperoxygenate the patient with a bag-valve mask device.

❑ Place LMA®.

- Gently introduce into oropharyx, following curvature of tube.
- Swing mask into place in a single circular movement, ensuring pressure is maintained against palate and posterior pharynx.
- Inflate mask without holding the tube.
- Oxygenate the patient with the BVM.

❑ Confirm LMA® placement.

- Visually confirm chest rise.
- Auscultate epigastrium for absence of breath sounds.
- Auscultate lung fields for presence of bilateral breath sounds.
- Monitor EtCO$_2$.

❑ Properly secure the LMA® with tape and a bite block.

❑ Reassess the patient.

- Confirm placement after LMA® is secured.
- Reassess the ventilations for adequacy and depth.

❑ Document the procedure for PCR, confirming placement of the LMA® and the number of attempts.

▶ **INSERTION OF THE ESOPHAGEAL TRACHEAL COMBITUBE®
(OPTIONAL EMT SKILL)**

❑ Take Standard Precautions.

❑ Position yourself at the patient's head.

❑ Assemble equipment.

❑ Insert the device blindly, watching for two black rings used for measuring depth of insertion. The teeth or their bony cavities, if teeth are missing, should be positioned between these rings.

❑ Use the large syringe to inflate the pharyngeal cuff with 100 cc of air. On inflation, the device will seat itself in the posterior pharynx behind the hard palate.

❑ Use the smaller syringe to fill the distal cuff with 10 cc to 15 cc of air.

❑ Usually (90%–95% of the time), the tube will have been placed in the esophagus. On this assumption, ventilate through the esophageal connector (the external tube that is the longer of the two and is marked #1). You must listen for the presence of breath sounds in the lungs and the absence of sounds from the epigastrium in order to be sure that the tube is, in fact, placed in the esophagus.

❑ If there is an absence of lung sounds and presence of sounds in the epigastrium, the tube has been placed in the trachea. In this case, change the ventilator to the shorter tracheal connector, which is marked #2.

❑ Listen again to be sure of proper placement of the tube.

©2009 Pearson Education, Inc.
Emergency Care, 11th Ed.

Interim Exam 3

Use the answer sheet on pages 325–326 to complete this exam. It is perforated so it can be easily removed from this workbook.

1. The circulation of blood throughout the body, filling the capillaries and supplying the cells and tissues with oxygen and nutrients, is called:
   A. physiology.
   B. perfusion.
   C. bleeding.
   D. metabolism.

2. With one exception, arteries carry _____ blood _____ the heart.
   A. deoxygenated, back to
   B. deoxygenated, away from
   C. oxygenated, back to
   D. oxygenated, away from

3. With one exception, veins carry _____ blood _____ the heart.
   A. deoxygenated, back to
   B. deoxygenated, away from
   C. oxygenated, back to
   D. oxygenated, away from

4. Once an adult loses approximately a _____ of blood, his or her condition is considered serious.
   A. pint
   B. gallon
   C. milliliter
   D. liter

5. Once a child loses approximately _____ of blood, his or her condition is considered serious.
   A. a milliliter
   B. 250 cc
   C. 500 ml
   D. 1 liter

6. Once an infant loses approximately _____ of blood volume, his or her condition is considered serious.
   A. 75 cc
   B. 150 cc
   C. 250 cc
   D. 500 cc

7. Since internal bleeding is not visible, you must base severity of blood loss on:
   A. signs and symptoms exhibited.
   B. what the patient tells you.
   C. the size of the contusion.
   D. advice from medical direction.

8. The factors on which severity of bleeding depends include all of the following <u>except</u>:
   A. rate of bleeding and the amount of blood loss.
   B. patient's age and weight.
   C. ability of the patient's body to respond and defend against blood loss.
   D. the patient's history of diabetes.

9. Blood that oozes and is dark red is most likely from a:
   A. vein.
   B. capillary.
   C. artery.
   D. lymphatic vessel.

10. You are treating a patient who has a slashed wrist, which is spurting bright red blood. After trying direct pressure and elevation to control the bleeding, the next step would be to:
    A. apply a tourniquet to the arm.
    B. apply an air splint to the arm.
    C. press on the brachial artery.
    D. press on the femoral artery.

11. When all other methods have failed to control bleeding, the EMT should:
    A. apply the PASG.
    B. apply an air splint.
    C. press harder on the pressure point.
    D. apply a tourniquet.

12. Signs of internal bleeding include all of the following <u>except</u>:
    A. painful, swollen, or deformed extremities.
    B. a tender rigid abdomen.
    C. vomiting bile.
    D. bruising.

13. Examples of penetrating trauma include all of the following <u>except</u>:
    A. handgun bullet wound.
    B. carving-knife wound.
    C. fall from a height.
    D. screwdriver stab wound.

14. Examples of blunt trauma include all of the following <u>except</u>:
    A. blast injuries.
    B. auto-pedestrian collisions.
    C. gunshot wounds.
    D. falls.

15. The signs and symptoms of internal bleeding are:
    A. the same as those of shock.
    B. identical to those of external bleeding.
    C. usually not present in elderly patients.
    D. easy to stabilize in the field.

16. Which is <u>not</u> considered a type of shock?
    A. hypovolemic
    B. hydrophobic
    C. cardiogenic
    D. neurogenic

17. At a point when the body can no longer compensate for the low blood volume, _____ shock begins.
    A. compensated
    B. anaphylactic
    C. decompensated
    D. terminal

18. What are the major components of the central nervous system?
    A. cranial nerves
    B. peripheral nerves
    C. brain and spinal cord
    D. vessels and support tissue

19. Which of the following is not a division of the nervous system?
    A. central
    B. peripheral
    C. autonomic
    D. voluntary

20. The skull is made up of the cranium and the facial bones. The cranium consists of the _____ areas of the skull.
    A. temporal, mandible, and maxilla
    B. frontal, parietal, and distal
    C. anterior, forehead, and lateral
    D. forehead, top, back, and upper sides

21. The bones forming the face include all of the following except:
    A. vertebrae.
    B. zygomatic.
    C. mandible.
    D. maxillae.

22. The brain and spinal cord are bathed in:
    A. cerebrospinal fluid.
    B. lymphatic fluid.
    C. synovial fluid.
    D. mucous secretion.

23. The spine is divided into sections called:
    A. joints.
    B. vertebrae.
    C. coccygeal.
    D. compartments.

24. The lumbar area of the spine includes _____ vertebrae.
    A. 3
    B. 5
    C. 8
    D. 12

25. A bacterial disease, which could be used in an act of biological terrorism to inflict serious illness, severe diarrhea, dehydration, and electrolyte imbalances in its victims, is:
    A. plague.
    B. anthrax.
    C. ricin.
    D. cholera.

26. When a patient strikes her head and states she feels groggy and has a headache, she most likely has a(n):
    A. abrasion.
    B. concussion.
    C. contrecoup.
    D. none of the above.

27. A 50-year-old male driver who was involved in an automobile collision states he did not lose consciousness. However, a bystander says he ran to the car after the collision and tried to talk to the driver, but said the driver "just sat there staring off into space for a few minutes." This patient may have any of the following except:
    A. contusion.
    B. concussion.
    C. coup injury.
    D. attention deficit.

28. When a patient has some memory loss after a head injury, this is referred to as:
    A. bruising.
    B. amnesia.
    C. verbally responsive.
    D. "seeing stars."

29. When a bruising of the brain occurs on the side of the injury, this is referred to as a _____ injury.
    A. contrecoup
    B. hematoma
    C. coup
    D. epidural

30. A collection of blood within the skull or the brain is called a _____ hematoma.
    A. subdural
    B. epidural
    C. intracerebral
    D. any of the above

31. All of the following make a head injury worse except:
    A. limited room for expansion inside the skull.
    B. increased pressure in the skull.
    C. increased carbon dioxide level in the brain.
    D. decreased respiration leading to increased cellular perfusion.

32. An assessment strategy used to check an extremity for injury or paralysis in a conscious patient is:
    A. checking for a proximal pulse.
    B. assessing equality of strength.
    C. checking for foot wave.
    D. confirming sensitivity.

33. The time between exposure and the appearance of symptoms is referred to as the:
    A. toxicity period.
    B. incubation period.
    C. transmissibility time frame.
    D. infectivity window.

34. If a patient has a brain injury with skull fracture, the patient's pupils will tend to be:
    A. equal.
    B. dilated.
    C. constricted.
    D. unequal.

35. Which of the following describes the blood pressure and pulse for a patient with a brain injury?
    A. decreased blood pressure, increased pulse
    B. decreased blood pressure, decreased pulse
    C. increased blood pressure, increased pulse
    D. increased blood pressure, decreased pulse

36. Consider the possibility of a cranial fracture whenever you note:
    A. deep lacerations or severe bruises to the scalp or forehead.
    B. a deformed femur.
    C. facial deformity.
    D. blood or other fluids in the airway.

37. The spinal column is made up of _____ shaped bones.
    A. 33 regularly   C. 12 regularly
    B. 33 irregularly   D. 12 irregularly

38. Any blunt trauma above the clavicles may damage the _____ vertebrae.
    A. lumbar   C. sacral
    B. cervical   D. thoracic

39. Priapism is:
    A. a persistent erection of the penis.
    B. spasms of the hands and feet.
    C. apparent only in unconscious patients.
    D. uncontrolled muscle twitches of the thighs.

40. Often with a cervical-spine injury, the patient in a supine position may have his arms:
    A. straight out at his side.
    B. stretched out above his head.
    C. down at his side.
    D. across his chest.

41. The EMT should consider that any injury of an elderly person could be a sign of:
    A. a severe fall.
    B. Alzheimer's disease.
    C. abuse or neglect.
    D. depression.

42. Geriatric patients usually have decreased elasticity of the lungs and decreased activity of cilia that results in:
    A. increased risk of heart attack.
    B. diminished activity and tolerance of physical stress.
    C. decreased ability to clear foreign substances from the lungs.
    D. decreased energy and tolerance of hot and cold.

43. Loss of skin elasticity and shrinking of sweat glands in a geriatric patient causes:
    A. diminished activity and tolerance of physical stress.
    B. decreased ability to clear foreign substances from the lungs.
    C. decreased energy and tolerance of hot and cold.
    D. thin, dry, wrinkled skin.

44. Diminished function of the thyroid gland is one of the effects of aging. This results in:
    A. thin, dry, wrinkled skin.
    B. decreased energy and tolerance of heat and cold.
    C. depression and loss of social support.
    D. decreased strength.

45. When an elderly patient falls, this may be an indication of a more serious problem, such as:
    A. viral pneumonia.
    B. acute alcoholism.
    C. abnormal heart rhythm.
    D. severe depression.

46. An unstable object impaled in the cheek wall should be:
    A. stabilized from the outside.
    B. stabilized from the inside.
    C. pulled out if easily done.
    D. stabilized from the inside and the outside.

47. If possible, a patient with facial fractures should be transported on a long spine board in the _____ position.
    A. supine
    B. Trendelenburg
    C. head-elevated
    D. prone

48. The pressure point for controlling bleeding from the leg is the:
    A. carotid artery.
    B. brachial artery.
    C. subclavian vein.
    D. femoral artery.

49. Care for an open wound includes all of the following except:
    A. pick embedded particles out of the cut.
    B. control bleeding.
    C. bandage the dressing in place.
    D. clean the wound surface.

50. The best method for control of nasal bleeding is:
    A. packing the nose with cotton.
    B. pinching the nostrils together.
    C. packing the nose with gauze.
    D. applying pressure to the facial artery.

©2009 Pearson Education, Inc.
Emergency Care, 11th Ed.

51. The first step in caring for possible internal bleeding after ensuring respiration and circulation and controlling life-threatening external bleeding is:
    A. administering liquids by mouth to the patient.
    B. applying a bulky dressing.
    C. treating for shock.
    D. placing the patient in a sitting position.

52. A razor blade cut is an example of a(n):
    A. incision.
    B. abrasion.
    C. contusion.
    D. laceration.

53. The injury in which flaps of skin and tissues are torn loose or pulled off completely is called a(n):
    A. laceration.
    B. amputation.
    C. incision.
    D. avulsion.

54. If a patient has an object impaled in the forearm, after the control of profuse bleeding, you should:
    A. remove the object.
    B. place a pressure dressing over the site.
    C. stabilize the object.
    D. apply firm pressure to a pressure point.

55. Which of the following is a sign of shock?
    A. high blood pressure
    B. constricted pupils
    C. slowed pulse rate
    D. pale, cool, clammy skin

56. An object impaled in the eye should be:
    A. stabilized with gauze and protected with a disposable cup.
    B. removed carefully and a pressure dressing applied.
    C. shielded with a cup taped over the orbit.
    D. removed and a dressing applied with minimum pressure.

57. A lacerated eyelid or injury to the eyeball should be:
    A. flushed with water.
    B. covered with a cold pack.
    C. covered with folded 4 × 4s.
    D. covered with dark patches.

58. All open wounds to the chest should be considered:
    A. life-threatening.
    B. potentially infectious.
    C. a low priority.
    D. an indication for PASG.

59. Before moving a supine patient with possible spinal injuries onto a long spine board, you should always:
    A. align the teeth and tape the jaw in place.
    B. apply a short spine board.
    C. apply a rigid collar.
    D. secure a KED to the patient.

60. The initial effort to control bleeding from a severed neck artery should be:
    A. direct pressure or pinching.
    B. applying tape.
    C. pressure points.
    D. occlusive dressing.

61. The most reliable sign of spinal-cord injury in conscious patients is:
    A. pain without movement.
    B. paralysis of extremities.
    C. pain with movement.
    D. tenderness along the spine.

62. When caring for an open abdominal wound with evisceration:
    A. replace the organ but cover with occlusive material.
    B. replace the organ but cover with a bulky dressing.
    C. do not replace the organ but cover with occlusive material.
    D. do not replace the organ but cover with a moistened dressing.

63. A patient in acute abdominal distress without vomiting should be transported:
    A. in the Trendelenburg position with legs straight.
    B. in the coma position.
    C. face up with the knees bent.
    D. in the recumbent position with one knee bent.

64. When a joint is locked into position, the EMT should:
    A. pull traction on the extremity.
    B. straighten it.
    C. splint it in the position found.
    D. skip splinting and transport immediately.

65. A splint properly applied to an extremity should prevent all of the following except:
    A. circulation to the extremity.
    B. an open bone injury.
    C. motion of bone fragments.
    D. damage to muscles and blood vessels.

66. A fracture to the humerus shaft is best cared for by immobilizing with a(n):
    A. wrist sling.
    B. rigid splint or sling and swathe.
    C. air-inflated splint.
    D. sling and swathe.

©2009 Pearson Education, Inc.
Emergency Care, 11th Ed.

67. A fracture to the proximal end of the humerus is best cared for by immobilizing with a(n):
  A. wrist sling and swathe.
  B. padded board, sling, and swathe.
  C. air-inflated splint.
  D. sling and swathe.

68. The best way to immobilize a fractured elbow when the arm is found in the bent position and there is a distal pulse is to:
  A. straighten the arm and apply an air-inflated splint.
  B. keep the arm in its found position and apply a short padded board splint.
  C. keep the arm in its found position and apply an air-inflated splint.
  D. straighten the arm and apply a wire-ladder splint.

69. When splinting, if a severe deformity exists or distal circulation is compromised, you should:
  A. push protruding bones back into place.
  B. align to anatomical position under gentle traction.
  C. immediately move the patient to a stretcher.
  D. immobilize in the position found.

70. The first step in immobilizing a fractured wrist with distal pulse is to:
  A. correct angulation of the wrist.
  B. secure a padded board splint to the wrist.
  C. place the broken hand in its position of function.
  D. tape the wrist.

71. A patient with a fractured pelvis should be immobilized on an orthopedic stretcher or long spine board with:
  A. legs bound together with wide cravats.
  B. long padded boards secured down each side of the body.
  C. stabilizing sandbags placed between the legs.
  D. straps securing the torso and pelvis.

72. A fractured femur is best immobilized with a(n) _____ splint.
  A. long padded   **C.** rigid vacuum
  B. air-inflated   **D.** traction

73. Before immobilizing a fractured knee:
  A. assess distal PMS function.
  B. straighten the angulation.
  C. apply firm traction.
  D. flex the leg at the knee.

74. The best method for immobilizing a suspected ankle fracture is a(n) _____ splint.
  A. traction   **C.** padded board
  B. pillow splint   **D.** air-inflated

75. A sprain is an injury in which:
  A. tendons are torn.
  B. ligaments are torn.
  C. cartilage is crushed.
  D. muscles spasm.

76. Which of the following is <u>not</u> true of open extremity injuries?
  A. The skin has been broken or torn.
  B. There is increased likelihood of infection.
  C. Definitive care is provided in the prehospital setting.
  D. Such injuries require surgery at the hospital.

77. Muscle is attached to bone by:
  A. cartilage.
  B. ligaments.
  C. smooth muscles.
  D. tendons.

78. A partial thickness burn involves the:
  A. epidermis.
  B. epidermis and dermis.
  C. epidermis, dermis, and subcutaneous layers.
  D. epidermis, dermis, subcutaneous layers, and muscles.

79. The entire back of an adult patient's right arm and her entire chest have been burned. What percentage of surface burn would you report?
  A. 13.5%   **C.** 27%
  B. 18%   **D.** 36%

80. A moderate burn involves:
  A. partial and full thickness burns of the face and hands.
  B. full thickness burns over less than 2% of the body surface.
  C. superficial burns covering more than 50% of the body surface.
  D. superficial burns covering less than 20% of the body surface.

81. Partial thickness burns cause:
  A. swelling and blistering.
  B. nerve damage.
  C. slight swelling.
  D. scarring.

82. A patient is suffering from chemical burns to the skin caused by dry lime. After putting on PPE, your next step should be to:
  A. wash the area with running water.
  B. remove the lime with phenol.
  C. remove the lime with alcohol.
  D. brush away the lime.

83. Acid burns to the eyes should be flooded with water for at least _____ minute(s).
  A. 1   **C.** 10
  B. 5   **D.** 20

84. A method for estimating the extent of a burn is the:
  A. rule of nines.
  B. rule of percentages.
  C. rule of degree.
  D. burn assessment rule.

85. The number-one priority for all EMS personnel at a collision scene is:
  A. wearing the appropriate protective clothing.
  B. keeping the bystanders clear of the scene.
  C. assuring the patient's safety first.
  D. contacting medical direction for instructions.

86. When arriving at the scene of a collision, the first thing an EMT should do is:
  A. evaluate hazards and calculate the need for additional support.
  B. determine whether patients are low or high priority.
  C. check to see if the vehicles involved have deployed airbags.
  D. determine the extent of patient entrapment and the means of extrication.

87. The EMT is responsible for protecting the patient from all of the following except:
  A. broken glass from the wrecked car.
  B. sharp metal in the wrecked car.
  C. the environment.
  D. injuries sustained by not wearing a seatbelt.

88. At the scene of an auto collision, the EMT should try to do all of the following except:
  A. keep the patient's safety in mind.
  B. inform the patient of the unique aspects of the extrication.
  C. keep his or her own personal safety in mind.
  D. describe the extrication procedures to bystanders.

89. A vehicle involved in a collision that is determined to be a simple access will:
  A. not require towing.
  B. not require stopping traffic.
  C. not require equipment to get to the patient.
  D. require only basic air-powered tools.

90. Which of the following is not true of applying a short spine board?
  A. Secure the torso first, and then the head.
  B. Pad between the patient's head and the spine board if needed.
  C. Apply a single chin strap prior to moving the patient.
  D. Reassess the patient after the device is placed.

91. To assist with patient access, the EMT should initially do each of the following except:
  A. try opening each car door.
  B. roll down windows.
  C. ask the patient to unlock the doors.
  D. pull the patient out the side windows.

92. What dictates the specific technique used for spinal immobilization of a patient at a collision extrication?
  A. requirements for speed of removal
  B. how many rescuers are available for removal
  C. whether an airbag has deployed
  D. none of the above

93. Which step in the phases of the rescue process is out of order: (1) sizing up the situation, (2) gaining the access, (3) disentangling the patient, (4) stabilizing the vehicle?
  A. 1   C. 3
  B. 2   D. 4

94. Considerations for size-up of a collision include all of the following except:
  A. potential hazards.
  B. need for additional EMS units.
  C. number of patients involved.
  D. number of ambulances in the region.

95. To minimize injuries at a collision, the EMT should:
  A. use a limited number of tools.
  B. deactivate the safety guards on tools.
  C. wear highly visible clothing.
  D. wait until the police arrive on the scene.

96. The vehicle's catalytic converter can be a source of ignition at a collision because it:
  A. often emits sparks.
  B. is often over 1,200°F.
  C. may leak gasoline.
  D. pumps high-pressure fumes.

97. The three-step process of disentanglement described in the text includes all of the following except:
  A. open the trunk and cut the battery cable.
  B. create exitways by displacing doors and roof posts.
  C. disentangle occupants by displacing front end.
  D. gain access by disposing of the roof.

98. Which of the following is <u>true</u> about dealing with a collision vehicle's electrical system?
- **A.** It should be disabled by cutting a battery cable.
- **B.** If it must be disrupted, disconnect the ground cable from the battery.
- **C.** Cutting the battery cable can assist in rescue operations.
- **D.** Disconnecting the ground cable will produce a spark that can ignite battery gases.

99. When positioning flares, use a formula that includes the stopping distance for the posted speed plus the:
- **A.** angle of the road.
- **B.** radius of the danger zone.
- **C.** reaction distance.
- **D.** margin of safety.

100. Once the vehicle has been stabilized, the <u>next</u> part of an extrication procedure for patient rescue is to:
- **A.** dispose of the vehicle's roof.
- **B.** displace the front end of the vehicle.
- **C.** displace doors and roof posts.
- **D.** none of the above.

101. The Emergency Medical Dispatcher has told you the exact location of a collision, how many and what kinds of vehicles are involved, and any known hazards. What other information would you like the EMD to provide concerning this collision?
- **A.** how many persons are injured
- **B.** the direction designator
- **C.** how to contact the person who reported the collision
- **D.** the nature of the emergency

102. Which of the following is an <u>unnecessary</u> question for the Emergency Medical Dispatcher to ask when receiving a call for help?
- **A.** How old is the patient?
- **B.** What's the patient's sex?
- **C.** What's the patient's name?
- **D.** Is the patient conscious?

103. When operating a siren, be aware that:
- **A.** the continuous sound of a siren could worsen a patient's condition.
- **B.** all motorists will hear and honor your signal.
- **C.** the siren must be used continuously when carrying injured patients.
- **D.** it's necessary to pull up close to vehicles and sound the siren.

104. All of the following are factors that affect an ambulance's response to a scene <u>except</u>:
- **A.** day of the week.
- **B.** time of the day.
- **C.** detours.
- **D.** danger zones.

105. If a patient develops cardiac arrest during transport, have the operator of the ambulance:
- **A.** adjust the ambulance's speed.
- **B.** stop the ambulance.
- **C.** contact the hospital emergency department.
- **D.** assist you with CPR.

106. When transferring a nonemergency patient to the emergency department personnel, you should:
- **A.** wait for emergency staff to call for the patient.
- **B.** off-load, wheel to the designated area, and stay with the patient.
- **C.** check to see what is to be done with the patient.
- **D.** off-load, wheel to the designated area, and leave the patient.

107. The last step when transferring a patient is to:
- **A.** wait to help the emergency department staff.
- **B.** transfer the patient's valuables.
- **C.** obtain your release.
- **D.** transfer patient information.

108. At the hospital, as soon as you are free from patient-care activities, you should:
- **A.** notify dispatch you are back in service.
- **B.** quickly clean the vehicle's patient compartment.
- **C.** prepare the prehospital care report.
- **D.** check on patient status with the emergency department.

109. Which of the following is <u>not</u> a biohazard?
- **A.** suction catheters
- **B.** contaminated dressings
- **C.** blood-soaked linen
- **D.** unopened gauze bandages

110. Which of the following is <u>not</u> a benefit of an EMS/hospital equipment exchange program?
- **A.** Patients are not subjected to injury-aggravating movement.
- **B.** Delay of the crew at the hospital is prevented.
- **C.** Ambulances can return to quarters fully equipped.
- **D.** Completeness and operability of equipment is ensured.

111. Vigorous cleaning of the ambulance while parked at the hospital is prevented or restricted by all of the following limitations except:
    A. time.
    B. equipment.
    C. space.
    D. law.

112. When you return to quarters, do all of the following except:
    A. replenish oxygen cylinders.
    B. prepare for service.
    C. clean the interior of the ambulance.
    D. air the ambulance if necessary.

113. A poison-control kit should include all of the following except:
    A. paper cups.
    B. activated charcoal.
    C. drinking water.
    D. antivenin solution.

114. Which of the following is not a piece of equipment in the first-in kit?
    A. stethoscope
    B. penlight
    C. fixed suction system
    D. rigid cervical collar

115. The first thing to inspect on the ambulance when the engine is off is the:
    A. body of the vehicle.
    B. battery.
    C. siren.
    D. fuel level.

116. Rescue tools should always be examined for:
    A. electrolyte levels.
    B. rust and dirt.
    C. water pressure.
    D. dead batteries.

117. Along with physical and mental fitness, ambulance operators should be able to:
    A. move other vehicles off the roadway.
    B. perform under stress.
    C. always be up for a run.
    D. justify feelings of superiority.

118. When driving an ambulance, you should realize that there are no state laws that grant the:
    A. use of controlled additional speed.
    B. passage through traffic signals.
    C. privilege of special parking at the scene.
    D. absolute right of way.

119. The headlights of an ambulance should be turned on:
    A. only at night.
    B. whenever the vehicle is on the road.
    C. during the day, but only when raining.
    D. and off in a blinking fashion.

120. When a car collides with a utility pole, the EMT should assume all of the following except:
    A. obviously dead wires could be energized at any moment.
    B. severed conductors may be energizing every wire.
    C. wires may be charged at the highest voltage present.
    D. there is no electrical hazard.

121. The easiest way to break tempered window glass is with a:
    A. blunt object.
    B. spring-loaded center punch.
    C. Glas-Master® window saw.
    D. sledge hammer.

122. Which of the following signs is not an indication that a child has an airway disease?
    A. wheezing
    B. breathing effort on exhalation
    C. rapid breathing
    D. lack of airway passage swelling

123. The soft spot on top of an infant's head is called a:
    A. contusion.
    B. depression site.
    C. fontanelle.
    D. suture.

124. Small children are referred to as _____ breathers.
    A. neck
    B. abdominal
    C. head
    D. chest

125. A child's compensating mechanisms for shock fail at approximately _____ blood loss.
    A. 10%
    B. 20%
    C. 30%
    D. 40%

126. In cases of sudden infant death syndrome, the EMT should:
    A. hunt for evidence of child abuse.
    B. hold off on care and simply transport the body.
    C. declare the patient dead.
    D. provide resuscitation and transport to the hospital.

127. Which of the following might lead you to consider child abuse?
    A. multiple skinned knees
    B. a burn from chewing an electric cord
    C. injuries to the center of the back and upper arms
    D. both ankles are sprained

©2009 Pearson Education, Inc.
Emergency Care, 11th Ed.

128. A child who is hypoxic will:
A. have a slowed heart rate.
B. have an increased heart rate.
C. forget to breathe.
D. complain of neck pain.

129. Artificial ventilations for an infant or child under 8 years of age should be provided at a rate of _____ per minute.
A. 8   C. 16
B. 12   D. 20

130. If you suspect respiratory distress in a conscious toddler, you should <u>not</u>:
A. administer high-concentration oxygen.
B. insert anything into the patient's mouth.
C. open the airway.
D. allow the child to sit up.

131. Common causes of shock in children include infections, trauma, blood loss, and:
A. meningitis.   C. dehydration.
B. heart failure   D. lack of insulin.

132. A sunken fontanelle may indicate:
A. elevated intracranial pressure.
B. hypertension.
C. dehydration.
D. fever.

133. Flowing oxygen over the face of a small child so it will be inhaled is referred to as the _____ technique.
A. blow-by   C. supplemental
B. rebreather   D. flow-by

134. A complication of a rapidly rising temperature in a child is often:
A. hyperactivity.
B. a seizure.
C. vomiting.
D. ringing in the ears.

135. A group of viral illnesses that results in inflammation of the larynx, trachea, and bronchi is called:
A. meningitis.   C. asthma.
B. anaphylaxis.   D. croup.

136. The strong, white, fibrous material covering the bones is called the:
A. shell.   C. marrow.
B. perineum.   D. periosteum.

137. The coming apart of a joint is referred to as a:
A. fracture.   C. dislocation.
B. sprain.   D. strain.

138. Overstretching or overexertion of a muscle is called a:
A. strain.   C. dislocation.
B. sprain.   D. fracture.

139. Proper splinting of a closed fracture is:
A. done with the PASG.
B. designed to prevent closed injuries from becoming open ones.
C. completed in the hospital by a surgeon.
D. done with an air splint.

140. Any force strong enough to fracture the pelvis also can cause injury to the:
A. clavicle.   C. rib cage.
B. spine.   D. tibia.

141. Examples of a bipolar traction splint include all of the following <u>except</u>:
A. Hare®.   C. half-ring.
B. Fernotrac®.   D. Sager®.

142. The indications for a traction splint are painful, swollen, deformed mid-thigh with
A. an open fracture of the lower leg.
B. extensive blood loss and shock.
C. no joint or lower leg injury.
D. either ankle or knee involvement.

143. The level of training established by OSHA for those who actually plug, patch, or stop the release of a hazardous material is called:
A. First Responder Awareness.
B. First Responder Operations.
C. Hazardous Materials Technician.
D. Paramedic.

144. At a hazardous materials accident site, the "safe zone" should be located:
A. downwind/downhill.
B. downwind/same level.
C. upwind/same level.
D. upwind/downhill.

145. A resource that must be maintained at the work site by the employer and that must be available to all employees working with hazardous materials is called:
A. NFPA 704.
B. Material Safety Data Sheet.
C. *North American Emergency Response Guidebook*.
D. shipping manifest.

146. The responsibilities of EMS personnel at a hazmat incident include caring for the injured and:
A. staging personnel and equipment in the warm zone.
B. monitoring and rehabilitating the hazmat team members.
C. decontaminating those exiting the hot zone.
D. notifying medical direction about the incident.

147. When a patient is categorized as Priority-1 at an MCI, this means the patient:
- **A.** is serious, but does not have life-threatening injuries or illness.
- **B.** has minor musculoskeletal or soft-tissue injuries.
- **C.** is dead or fatally injured.
- **D.** has treatable life-threatening illness or injuries.

148. The MCI supervisor responsible for communicating with each treatment area to determine the number and priority of the patients in that area is called the _____ supervisor.
- **A.** staging
- **B.** triage
- **C.** treatment
- **D.** transportation

149. When identifying a patient's treatment priority at an MCI, a Priority-2 patient would be color-coded as:
- **A.** black
- **B.** green
- **C.** yellow
- **D.** red

150. At an MCI, patients who are assessed to have minor injuries should be categorized as Priority-:
- **A.** 1.
- **B.** 2.
- **C.** 3.
- **D.** 4.

Now that you have completed the three interim exams in this student workbook, you are ready to prepare for your state and/or national EMT exam. Review all the exercises in this book and consider taking Brady's online EMT practice examinations at www.prenhall.com/emtachieve.

Interim Exam 3 Answer Sheet

Fill in the correct answer for each item. When scoring, note there are 150 questions valued at 0.666 points each.

1. [ ] A	[ ] B	[ ] C	[ ] D		**37.** [ ] A	[ ] B	[ ] C	[ ] D
2. [ ] A	[ ] B	[ ] C	[ ] D		**38.** [ ] A	[ ] B	[ ] C	[ ] D
3. [ ] A	[ ] B	[ ] C	[ ] D		**39.** [ ] A	[ ] B	[ ] C	[ ] D
4. [ ] A	[ ] B	[ ] C	[ ] D		**40.** [ ] A	[ ] B	[ ] C	[ ] D
5. [ ] A	[ ] B	[ ] C	[ ] D		**41.** [ ] A	[ ] B	[ ] C	[ ] D
6. [ ] A	[ ] B	[ ] C	[ ] D		**42.** [ ] A	[ ] B	[ ] C	[ ] D
7. [ ] A	[ ] B	[ ] C	[ ] D		**43.** [ ] A	[ ] B	[ ] C	[ ] D
8. [ ] A	[ ] B	[ ] C	[ ] D		**44.** [ ] A	[ ] B	[ ] C	[ ] D
9. [ ] A	[ ] B	[ ] C	[ ] D		**45.** [ ] A	[ ] B	[ ] C	[ ] D
10. [ ] A	[ ] B	[ ] C	[ ] D		**46.** [ ] A	[ ] B	[ ] C	[ ] D
11. [ ] A	[ ] B	[ ] C	[ ] D		**47.** [ ] A	[ ] B	[ ] C	[ ] D
12. [ ] A	[ ] B	[ ] C	[ ] D		**48.** [ ] A	[ ] B	[ ] C	[ ] D
13. [ ] A	[ ] B	[ ] C	[ ] D		**49.** [ ] A	[ ] B	[ ] C	[ ] D
14. [ ] A	[ ] B	[ ] C	[ ] D		**50.** [ ] A	[ ] B	[ ] C	[ ] D
15. [ ] A	[ ] B	[ ] C	[ ] D		**51.** [ ] A	[ ] B	[ ] C	[ ] D
16. [ ] A	[ ] B	[ ] C	[ ] D		**52.** [ ] A	[ ] B	[ ] C	[ ] D
17. [ ] A	[ ] B	[ ] C	[ ] D		**53.** [ ] A	[ ] B	[ ] C	[ ] D
18. [ ] A	[ ] B	[ ] C	[ ] D		**54.** [ ] A	[ ] B	[ ] C	[ ] D
19. [ ] A	[ ] B	[ ] C	[ ] D		**55.** [ ] A	[ ] B	[ ] C	[ ] D
20. [ ] A	[ ] B	[ ] C	[ ] D		**56.** [ ] A	[ ] B	[ ] C	[ ] D
21. [ ] A	[ ] B	[ ] C	[ ] D		**57.** [ ] A	[ ] B	[ ] C	[ ] D
22. [ ] A	[ ] B	[ ] C	[ ] D		**58.** [ ] A	[ ] B	[ ] C	[ ] D
23. [ ] A	[ ] B	[ ] C	[ ] D		**59.** [ ] A	[ ] B	[ ] C	[ ] D
24. [ ] A	[ ] B	[ ] C	[ ] D		**60.** [ ] A	[ ] B	[ ] C	[ ] D
25. [ ] A	[ ] B	[ ] C	[ ] D		**61.** [ ] A	[ ] B	[ ] C	[ ] D
26. [ ] A	[ ] B	[ ] C	[ ] D		**62.** [ ] A	[ ] B	[ ] C	[ ] D
27. [ ] A	[ ] B	[ ] C	[ ] D		**63.** [ ] A	[ ] B	[ ] C	[ ] D
28. [ ] A	[ ] B	[ ] C	[ ] D		**64.** [ ] A	[ ] B	[ ] C	[ ] D
29. [ ] A	[ ] B	[ ] C	[ ] D		**65.** [ ] A	[ ] B	[ ] C	[ ] D
30. [ ] A	[ ] B	[ ] C	[ ] D		**66.** [ ] A	[ ] B	[ ] C	[ ] D
31. [ ] A	[ ] B	[ ] C	[ ] D		**67.** [ ] A	[ ] B	[ ] C	[ ] D
32. [ ] A	[ ] B	[ ] C	[ ] D		**68.** [ ] A	[ ] B	[ ] C	[ ] D
33. [ ] A	[ ] B	[ ] C	[ ] D		**69.** [ ] A	[ ] B	[ ] C	[ ] D
34. [ ] A	[ ] B	[ ] C	[ ] D		**70.** [ ] A	[ ] B	[ ] C	[ ] D
35. [ ] A	[ ] B	[ ] C	[ ] D		**71.** [ ] A	[ ] B	[ ] C	[ ] D
36. [ ] A	[ ] B	[ ] C	[ ] D		**72.** [ ] A	[ ] B	[ ] C	[ ] D

73.	[ ] A	[ ] B	[ ] C	[ ] D
74.	[ ] A	[ ] B	[ ] C	[ ] D
75.	[ ] A	[ ] B	[ ] C	[ ] D
76.	[ ] A	[ ] B	[ ] C	[ ] D
77.	[ ] A	[ ] B	[ ] C	[ ] D
78.	[ ] A	[ ] B	[ ] C	[ ] D
79.	[ ] A	[ ] B	[ ] C	[ ] D
80.	[ ] A	[ ] B	[ ] C	[ ] D
81.	[ ] A	[ ] B	[ ] C	[ ] D
82.	[ ] A	[ ] B	[ ] C	[ ] D
83.	[ ] A	[ ] B	[ ] C	[ ] D
84.	[ ] A	[ ] B	[ ] C	[ ] D
85.	[ ] A	[ ] B	[ ] C	[ ] D
86.	[ ] A	[ ] B	[ ] C	[ ] D
87.	[ ] A	[ ] B	[ ] C	[ ] D
88.	[ ] A	[ ] B	[ ] C	[ ] D
89.	[ ] A	[ ] B	[ ] C	[ ] D
90.	[ ] A	[ ] B	[ ] C	[ ] D
91.	[ ] A	[ ] B	[ ] C	[ ] D
92.	[ ] A	[ ] B	[ ] C	[ ] D
93.	[ ] A	[ ] B	[ ] C	[ ] D
94.	[ ] A	[ ] B	[ ] C	[ ] D
95.	[ ] A	[ ] B	[ ] C	[ ] D
96.	[ ] A	[ ] B	[ ] C	[ ] D
97.	[ ] A	[ ] B	[ ] C	[ ] D
98.	[ ] A	[ ] B	[ ] C	[ ] D
99.	[ ] A	[ ] B	[ ] C	[ ] D
100.	[ ] A	[ ] B	[ ] C	[ ] D
101.	[ ] A	[ ] B	[ ] C	[ ] D
102.	[ ] A	[ ] B	[ ] C	[ ] D
103.	[ ] A	[ ] B	[ ] C	[ ] D
104.	[ ] A	[ ] B	[ ] C	[ ] D
105.	[ ] A	[ ] B	[ ] C	[ ] D
106.	[ ] A	[ ] B	[ ] C	[ ] D
107.	[ ] A	[ ] B	[ ] C	[ ] D
108.	[ ] A	[ ] B	[ ] C	[ ] D
109.	[ ] A	[ ] B	[ ] C	[ ] D
110.	[ ] A	[ ] B	[ ] C	[ ] D
111.	[ ] A	[ ] B	[ ] C	[ ] D

112.	[ ] A	[ ] B	[ ] C	[ ] D
113.	[ ] A	[ ] B	[ ] C	[ ] D
114.	[ ] A	[ ] B	[ ] C	[ ] D
115.	[ ] A	[ ] B	[ ] C	[ ] D
116.	[ ] A	[ ] B	[ ] C	[ ] D
117.	[ ] A	[ ] B	[ ] C	[ ] D
118.	[ ] A	[ ] B	[ ] C	[ ] D
119.	[ ] A	[ ] B	[ ] C	[ ] D
120.	[ ] A	[ ] B	[ ] C	[ ] D
121.	[ ] A	[ ] B	[ ] C	[ ] D
122.	[ ] A	[ ] B	[ ] C	[ ] D
123.	[ ] A	[ ] B	[ ] C	[ ] D
124.	[ ] A	[ ] B	[ ] C	[ ] D
125.	[ ] A	[ ] B	[ ] C	[ ] D
126.	[ ] A	[ ] B	[ ] C	[ ] D
127.	[ ] A	[ ] B	[ ] C	[ ] D
128.	[ ] A	[ ] B	[ ] C	[ ] D
129.	[ ] A	[ ] B	[ ] C	[ ] D
130.	[ ] A	[ ] B	[ ] C	[ ] D
131.	[ ] A	[ ] B	[ ] C	[ ] D
132.	[ ] A	[ ] B	[ ] C	[ ] D
133.	[ ] A	[ ] B	[ ] C	[ ] D
134.	[ ] A	[ ] B	[ ] C	[ ] D
135.	[ ] A	[ ] B	[ ] C	[ ] D
136.	[ ] A	[ ] B	[ ] C	[ ] D
137.	[ ] A	[ ] B	[ ] C	[ ] D
138.	[ ] A	[ ] B	[ ] C	[ ] D
139.	[ ] A	[ ] B	[ ] C	[ ] D
140.	[ ] A	[ ] B	[ ] C	[ ] D
141.	[ ] A	[ ] B	[ ] C	[ ] D
142.	[ ] A	[ ] B	[ ] C	[ ] D
143.	[ ] A	[ ] B	[ ] C	[ ] D
144.	[ ] A	[ ] B	[ ] C	[ ] D
145.	[ ] A	[ ] B	[ ] C	[ ] D
146.	[ ] A	[ ] B	[ ] C	[ ] D
147.	[ ] A	[ ] B	[ ] C	[ ] D
148.	[ ] A	[ ] B	[ ] C	[ ] D
149.	[ ] A	[ ] B	[ ] C	[ ] D
150.	[ ] A	[ ] B	[ ] C	[ ] D

ALS-ASSIST SKILLS

MATCH TERMINOLOGY/ DEFINITIONS

A. Drip chamber used when minimal flow of fluid is needed (with children, for example)

B. Stopcock located below the drip chamber that can be pushed up or down to start, stop, or control the flow rate

C. Chamber from which the drops of IV fluid flow

D. Drip chamber used when a higher flow of fluid is needed (for a multi-trauma victim in shock, for example)

E. Measurement of the electrical activity of the heart on a graph

F. When an IV needle has either punctured a vein and exited the other side or has pulled out of the vein and the fluid is flowing into the surrounding tissues instead of into the vein

G. Gently pressing the thumb and index finger just to either side of the medial throat and over the cricoid cartilage to bring the patient's vocal cords into view

H. Intravenous line inserted into a vein so that blood, fluids, or medications can be administered directly into a patient's circulation

I. Opening below the flow regulator on an IV set into which medication is injected

_____ **1.** Cricoid pressure

_____ **2.** Drip chamber

_____ **3.** ECG

_____ **4.** Flow regulator

_____ **5.** Infiltration

_____ **6.** IV

_____ **7.** Macro drip

_____ **8.** Mini drip

_____ **9.** Needle port

MULTIPLE-CHOICE REVIEW

_____ **1.** Traditionally, although currently in controversy, the "gold standard" of airway care is the:
   A. jaw-thrust maneuver.
   C. endotracheal tube.
   B. ATV.
   D. nasal airway.

_____ **2.** Typical patients who need an advanced airway inserted include all of the following except:
   A. pulmonary or cardiopulmonary arrest patients.
   B. trauma patients in need of airway control.
   C. patients with respiratory failure due to overdose.
   D. patients with full thickness burns to the extremities.

_____ **3.** Prior to an intubation attempt, you may be asked to:
   A. ventilate the patient.
   C. flex the neck.
   B. insert a gastric tube.
   D. press on the neck.

_____ 4. During the intubation attempt, you may be asked to do any of the following except:
  A. shock the patient.
  B. stand by and be prepared to begin ventilations.
  C. gently press on the sides of the cricoid cartilage.
  D. maintain neck stabilization.

_____ 5. Once the endotracheal tube is inserted in the trachea and the cuff is inflated, the paramedic should:
  A. extend the patient's neck.
  B. use an esophageal intubation detector.
  C. tape the endotracheal tube in place.
  D. insert an oral airway as a bite block.

_____ 6. After inserting the tube, the intubator should listen with a stethoscope in all of the following locations except the:
  A. left lung.
  B. right lung.
  C. epigastrium.
  D. lower abdomen.

_____ 7. If, during the movement of the patient, the advanced airway is moved, you should:
  A. notify the paramedic, who will immediately recheck placement.
  B. apply the pulse oximeter to the patient.
  C. increase the oxygen concentration.
  D. quickly pull out the tube and replace it.

_____ 8. If you are ventilating a breathing patient with a BVM, you should:
  A. increase the liter flow to at least 25 liters per minute.
  B. time your ventilations with the patient's respiratory efforts.
  C. decrease the oxygen concentration.
  D. ventilate at a faster rate than you normally would.

_____ 9. If, when ventilating, you feel a sudden change in the resistance, this could be caused by:
  A. shock.
  B. anaphylaxis.
  C. air escaping through a hole in the lungs.
  D. a sucking chest injury.

_____ 10. When ventilating a patient in cardiac arrest with a BVM, with each defibrillation attempt you should:
  A. drop the bag and move back.
  B. remove the bag from the tube.
  C. lower the ventilation rate.
  D. continue ventilations.

_____ 11. Why is it important to note the mental-status changes of patients who are intubated?
  A. They may not be getting enough oxygen.
  B. They may wake up and bite on the tube.
  C. They may need to be hypoventilated.
  D. They may need a larger tube.

_____ 12. After the paramedic injects some medication down the tube, if you are assigned to ventilations, you may be asked to:
  A. ventilate the patient.
  B. turn up the oxygen concentration.
  C. reassess the tube placement.
  D. hyperextend the neck.

©2009 Pearson Education, Inc.
Emergency Care, 11th Ed.

_____ 13. If the patient has a suspected cervical-spine injury, your role will be to:
A. hold the patient's chin forward during the intubation attempt.
B. hand the paramedic the equipment for intubation.
C. maintain in-line spinal stabilization throughout the procedure.
D. place your fingers on the patient's throat throughout the procedure.

_____ 14. A standard procedure used to alert EMS personnel to life-threatening heart rhythm disturbances is the:
A. myelogram.   C. ECG.
B. EEG.   D. AED.

_____ 15. The EMT should know how to turn on the ECG monitor and do all of the following except:
A. change the battery.
B. change the roll of paper.
C. record an ECG strip.
D. interpret the ECG.

_____ 16. When assisting with an ECG, you should try to get in the habit of applying the:
A. electrode to the patient right away.
B. leads to the electrode and then to the patient.
C. electrode to the patient and then the leads to the electrodes.
D. defibrillator to the patient to monitor the ECG.

_____ 17. Which of the following is not part of preparing the patient's skin for ECG electrodes?
A. drying the area
B. removing oil
C. shaving excessive hair
D. applying alcohol

_____ 18. In the most common electrode configuration, the red electrode is placed:
A. under the center of the left lower chest.
B. under the center of the left clavicle.
C. on the right lower chest.
D. on the left lower chest.

_____ 19. In the most common electrode configuration, the green or black electrode is placed:
A. under the center of the left lower chest.
B. under the center of the left clavicle.
C. on the right clavicle.
D. on the left lower chest.

_____ 20. A mini-drip IV administration set produces _____ drops for every cc.
A. 15   C. 45
B. 30   D. 60

_____ 21. A macro-drip IV administration set produces _____ drops for every cc.
A. 10 to 15   C. 30 to 40
B. 20 to 30   D. 40 to 50

_____ 22. When inspecting an IV fluid bag, always check for:
A. expiration date.
B. clarity of the fluid.
C. leaks in the bag.
D. all of the above.

_____ **23.** When removing the protective covering from the port of the IV fluid and the protective covering from the spiked end of the tubing:
  A. be very careful to maintain sterility.
  B. only touch the ends with gloves.
  C. hold the bag lower than the tubing.
  D. it is not necessary to protect the end of this tubing.

_____ **24.** Why is the IV line flushed prior to using it on a patient?
  A. It prevents the patient from developing a blood clot.
  B. It prevents introducing an air embolism.
  C. It helps to maintain sterility of the entire system.
  D. The fluid will run much faster without air in the line.

_____ **25.** Interruptions in the flow of an IV can be caused by each of the following <u>except</u>:
  A. a closed flow regulator.
  B. a constricting band left on the patient's arm.
  C. a rise in the patient's blood pressure.
  D. kinked tubing.

_____ **26.** A relatively new method of treating patients with certain respiratory diseases that is now found in the field is called:
  A. IPPV.   **C.** CPAP.
  B. FROPVD.   **D.** BVM.

_____ **27.** The effect of positive end expiratory pressure in managing a patient with a respiratory problem is:
  A. constriction of the bronchioles.
  B. expansion of collapsed alveoli.
  C. dilated bronchioles.
  D. collapsed alveoli.

_____ **28.** When administering CPAP in the field it is important that the mask fits _____ the face.
  A. tightly to
  B. loosely around
  C. over the head and
  D. none of the above; it does not have a mask

COMPLETE THE FOLLOWING

List four steps that you may be asked to perform in the process of applying electrodes.

A. _____

B. _____

C. _____

D. _____

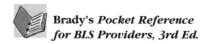
▶ **SETTING UP AND RUNNING AN IV LINE**

❑ Take Standard Precautions.

❑ Inspect IV fluid bag for clarity, expiration date, and leaks. Remove outer wrapper and gently squeeze bag.

❑ Select proper administration set, uncoil tubing, and keep ends sterile.

❑ Connect an extension set if using a mini drip. (Macro drips are not routinely used.)

❑ Make sure flow regulator is closed by rolling stopcock away from direction of fluid bag.

❑ Remove the protective coverings from the port of fluid bag and spiked end of tubing. Insert spiked end of tubing into fluid bag with a quick twist.

❑ Hold IV fluid bag higher than drip chamber. Squeeze drip chamber one or two times to start flow. Fill chamber to marker line (one-third full).

❑ Open flow regulator, and allow fluid to flush all the air from tubing. You may need to loosen the cap at the lower end to get fluid to flow. Be very careful to maintain sterility and to replace the cap.

BASIC CARDIAC LIFE SUPPORT REVIEW

Before beginning your EMT course, you are required to have completed a course in cardiopulmonary resuscitation. The elements of CPR are tested here as "extra value" for your review.

MATCH TERMINOLOGY/ DEFINITIONS

A. Providing artificial ventilations to a person who has stopped breathing or whose breathing is inadequate

B. Manual thrusts to the abdomen used to dislodge an airway obstruction

C. When breathing and heartbeat stop

D. Pulse felt between the groove of the Adam's apple and the muscles located along the side of the neck

E. Requirement that the amount of time you spend compressing the patient's chest should be the same as the time spent for release

F. Bulging of the stomach that may be caused by forcing air into the patient's stomach during rescue breathing

G. When brain cells die

H. Short triangular piece of cartilage (tough, elastic gristle) that extends from the bottom of the sternum

I. General term for the area of the lower border of the sternum

J. Maneuver that provides for maximum opening of the airway

K. Pulse measured by feeling the major artery of the arm; the absence of this pulse is used as a sign, in infants, that heartbeat has stopped and CPR should begin.

L. Actions you take to revive a person—or at least temporarily prevent biological death—by keeping the person's heart and lungs working

M. Maneuver used to open the airway of a patient with a suspected spine injury

N. Red or purple skin discoloration that occurs when gravity causes the blood to sink to the lowest parts of the body and collect there

O. Placing the patient on his side to allow for drainage from the mouth and to prevent the tongue from falling backward

_____ **1.** Biological death

_____ **2.** Brachial pulse

_____ **3.** Cardiopulmonary resuscitation

_____ **4.** Carotid pulse

_____ **5.** Clinical death

_____ **6.** 50:50 rule

_____ **7.** Gastric distention

_____ **8.** Head-tilt, chin-lift maneuver

_____ **9.** Abdominal thrust

_____ **10.** Jaw-thrust maneuver

_____ **11.** Line of lividity

_____ **12.** Recovery position

_____ **13.** Rescue breathing

_____ **14.** Substernal notch

_____ **15.** Xiphoid process

MULTIPLE-CHOICE REVIEW

_____ 1. When a patient's breathing and heartbeat stop, the _____ cells will begin to die after 4 to 6 minutes.
   A. heart
   B. brain
   C. liver
   D. kidney

_____ 2. Once clinical death occurs, how long does it usually take for biological death to occur?
   A. 4 minutes
   B. 6 minutes
   C. 8 minutes
   D. 10 minutes

_____ 3. In the ABC method of cardiopulmonary resuscitation, the "A" stands for:
   A. air flow.
   B. arterial pulse.
   C. airway.
   D. aorta.

_____ 4. In the ABC method of cardiopulmonary resuscitation, the "C" stands for:
   A. cardiac.
   B. compression.
   C. circulation.
   D. carotid.

_____ 5. To determine if an adult or a child is pulseless, the EMT should check for a pulse at the _____ artery.
   A. femoral
   B. brachial
   C. radial
   D. carotid

_____ 6. To determine pulselessness in an infant, the EMT should use the _____ artery.
   A. brachial
   B. carotid
   C. femoral
   D. apical

_____ 7. If you are alone, and do not have an AED, after determining unresponsiveness in the adult the next thing you should do before starting CPR is:
   A. reposition the patient.
   B. activate EMS.
   C. establish an open airway.
   D. check for breathing.

_____ 8. When an unconscious patient's head flexes forward, the _____ could cause an airway obstruction.
   A. hypopharynx
   B. uvula
   C. tongue
   D. larynx

_____ 9. One of the best methods to relieve an airway obstruction due to the positioning of the patient's tongue is the _____ maneuver.
   A. jaw-thrust
   B. abdominal-thrust
   C. head-tilt, chin-lift
   D. jaw-lift

_____ 10. The head-tilt, chin-lift maneuver should not be used on a:
   A. stroke victim.
   B. diabetic patient.
   C. diving accident victim.
   D. patient who had a seizure in bed.

_____ 11. The recommended maneuver for health care providers for opening the airway of a patient with possible cervical-spine injury is the _____ maneuver.
   A. jaw-thrust
   B. mouth-to-nose
   C. head-tilt, chin-lift
   D. jaw-lift

_____ 12. After opening the airway in a patient who requires rescue breathing, the EMT should inflate the patient's lung with:
   A. one quick, full breath.
   B. two breaths, 1 second each.
   C. one-half breath.
   D. four slow breaths.

©2009 Pearson Education, Inc.
Emergency Care, 11th Ed.

_____ **13.** Initial two ventilations did not result in chest rise. Your next step is to:
   A. continue standard mouth-to-mask ventilations.
   B. administer oxygen.
   C. continue the steps of CPR.
   D. deliver four quick breaths.

_____ **14.** A common problem in the resuscitation of infants and children caused by improper head position or too quick ventilations is:
   A. spinal injury.   **C.** pulmonary trauma.
   B. gastric distention.   **D.** airway injury.

_____ **15.** Adult rescue breathing should be provided at a rate of _____ breaths per minute.
   A. 5–7   **C.** 15–20
   B. 10–12   **D.** 21–25

_____ **16.** Infants should be ventilated at the rate of one breath every _____ seconds.
   A. 3   **C.** 8
   B. 5   **D.** 10

_____ **17.** When a patient has a distended abdomen due to air being forced into the stomach, the EMT should:
   A. manually press on the abdomen to relieve the distention.
   B. decrease the oxygen concentration being administered to the patient.
   C. be prepared to suction should the patient vomit.
   D. increase the force of the ventilation.

_____ **18.** Why is the recovery position used?
   A. It protects the airway and allows for drainage from the mouth.
   B. It forces the mouth to remain open at all times.
   C. It protects the patient's head during a seizure.
   D. It makes oxygen administration possible in the unconscious patient.

_____ **19.** When delivering chest compressions during CPR, which of the following is <u>not</u> correct?
   A. Keep your elbows straight.
   B. Keep your hands on the sternum.
   C. Deliver compressions with a stabbing motion.
   D. Move from your hips.

_____ **20.** The adult CPR compression point is located on the middle of the _____, centered between the nipples.
   A. clavicle   **C.** ribs
   B. substernal notch **D.** sternum

_____ **21.** Before beginning artificial ventilation, assess the patient's breathing for at least _____ seconds.
   A. 5   **C.** 15
   B. 25   **D.** 20

_____ **22.** For an adult, the one-rescuer compressions-to-ventilations ratio is:
   A. 5:1.   **C.** 15:2.
   B. 5:2.   **D.** 30:2.

_____ **23.** The adult CPR compression rate in one-rescuer CPR is _____ times a minute.
   A. 60   **C.** 100
   B. 80   **D.** 120

_____ **24.** The adult CPR compression rate in two-rescuer CPR is _____ times a minute when an advanced airway is in place.
   A. 60   **C.** 100
   B. 80   **D.** 120

_____ 25. The compression depth for an adult or older child should be:
    A. 1 to 1.5 inches.   **C.** $1/3$ to $1/2$ the depth of the chest.
    B. 1.5 to 2 inches.   **D.** $1/2$ to $3/4$ the depth of the chest.

_____ 26. The compression depth for a young child or infant should be:
    A. 1 to 1.5 inches.   **C.** $1/3$ to $1/2$ the depth of the chest.
    B. 1.5 to 2 inches.   **D.** $1/2$ to $3/4$ the depth of the chest.

_____ 27. The compression to ventilation ratio for a young child or infant when there are 2 rescuers should be:
    A. 15:1   **C.** 30:2
    B. 15:2   **D.** 5:1

_____ 28. The compression to ventilation ratio for a young child or infant when there is only one rescuer doing the CPR is:
    A. 15:1   **C.** 30:2
    B. 15:2   **D.** 5:1

_____ 29. The compression rate when performing CPR on an infant is at least _____ times a minute.
    A. 70   **C.** 90
    B. 80   **D.** 100

_____ 30. When opening the airway of an infant, use a:
    A. full head-tilt method.
    B. jaw-thrust method.
    C. slight head-tilt.
    D. neck hyperextension method.

_____ 31. With effective CPR, the patient's pupils may:
    A. dilate.
    B. constrict.
    C. assume a ground-glass appearance.
    D. begin to move.

_____ 32. CPR compressions are delivered to children:
    A. in the same manner as to adults.
    B. with the fingertips of index and middle fingers.
    C. with the palm of one hand.
    D. with the heel of one hand.

_____ 33. With the exceptions of advanced airway placement or defibrillation, CPR should not be interrupted for more than _____ seconds.
    A. a few   **C.** 15
    B. 10   **D.** 20

_____ 34. If you are treating a patient with a partial airway obstruction, poor air exchange, and gray skin, you should:
    A. wait for the patient to stop breathing, then ventilate.
    B. treat the patient for a complete airway obstruction.
    C. increase the delivered oxygen concentration.
    D. do none of the above.

_____ 35. Complete airway obstruction in a conscious patient is indicated by:
    A. crowing sounds.   **C.** gurgling sounds.
    B. an inability to speak.   **D.** snoring sounds.

_____ 36. When you recognize complete airway obstruction in a conscious adult patient, you should immediately:
    A. place the patient in the supine position.
    B. deliver four back blows in rapid succession.
    C. deliver abdominal thrusts five times.
    D. attempt to ventilate the patient.

_____ **37.** To deliver chest thrusts to an unconscious patient, place the patient in the _____ position.

    A. upright   **C.** coma

    B. prone   **D.** supine

_____ **38.** You are treating an unresponsive adult patient with a complete airway obstruction. You have been unsuccessful in your initial two attempts to ventilate the patient. Which is the correct sequence to continue your effort?

    A. finger sweeps, back blows, adominal thrusts

    B. adominal thrusts, finger sweeps, back blows

    C. ventilations, finger sweeps, adominal thrusts

    D. chest compressions, look in mouth, ventilations

_____ **39.** When treating an 8-month pregnant woman who has a complete airway obstruction, the EMT should:

    A. use abdominal thrusts.

    B. only use the back blows.

    C. use chest thrusts.

    D. start CPR immediately.

_____ **40.** If a patient has a partial airway (mild) obstruction and is able to speak and cough forcefully, you should:

    A. perform abdominal thrusts.

    B. carefully watch the patient.

    C. perform the chest thrust.

    D. position the patient on the floor.

_____ **41.** A major difference between the adult and infant obstructed airway procedure is:

    A. chest thrusts are used with children only.

    B. back slaps are administered to infants.

    C. blind finger sweeps are not used with infants.

    D. the number of abdominal thrusts is greater in the adult.

_____ **42.** While you are trying to clear an adult's obstructed airway, the patient loses consciousness. You open the airway, look in the mouth, and attempt to ventilate. If this fails:

    A. deliver chest thrusts/compressions.

    B. retilt the head and again attempt to ventilate.

    C. deliver four back blows.

    D. attempt another finger sweep.

_____ **43.** You have been unsuccessful in initially ventilating an unconscious infant. You reposition the infant's head and attempt to ventilate again but are unsuccessful. Your next step is to perform:

    A. a series of chest thrusts.

    B. back blows and chest thrusts.

    C. abdominal thrusts.

    D. a tongue-jaw lift.

_____ **44.** Which of the following is <u>not</u> a sign of choking in an infant?

    A. ineffective cough

    B. agitation

    C. wheezing

    D. strong cry

_____ **45.** In health care provider training, in respect to the procedure of CPR, children are treated as adult patients once they have reached:

    A. 8 years of age.   **C.** 10 years of age.

    B. puberty.   **D.** greater than 1 year of age.

COMPLETE THE FOLLOWING

1. List the special circumstances in which the EMT should not initiate CPR even though the patient is pulseless.

   _____

   _____

   _____

2. List situations in which the EMT may stop CPR.

   _____

   _____

   _____

3. List the following information missing from the chart below:

   A. _____

   B. _____

   C. _____

   D. _____

   E. _____

   F. _____

   G. _____

Age	Adult Puberty and older	Child 1 to puberty	Infant Birth to 1 year
Compression depth	**(A)**	1/3 to 1/2 depth of the chest	1/3 to 1/2 depth of the chest
Compression rate	100/min	**(B)**	At least 100/min (newly born 120/min)
Each ventilation	1 second duration	**(C)**	1 second duration
Pulse check location	Carotid artery	**(D)**	Brachial artery
One-rescuer compression-to-ventilation ratio	**(E)**	30:2	30:2
Two-rescuer compression-to-ventilation ratio	**(F)**	**(G)**	15:2

Answer Key

Note: Page numbers in parentheses ( ) refer to page numbers in the textbook where answers can be found or supported.

Chapter 1: Introduction to Emergency Medical Care

MATCH TERMINOLOGY/ DEFINITIONS

1. **(I)** Designated agent—an EMT or other person authorized by a Medical Director to give medications and provide emergency care (p. 17)

2. **(D)** EMS System—a system designed to get trained personnel to the patient as quickly as possible and to provide emergency care on the scene, en route to the hospital, and in the hospital (p. 7)

3. **(A)** Enabling legislation—state laws that allow an EMS system to exist (p. 6)

4. **(G)** Enhanced 911—a communications system that has the capability of automatically identifying the caller's phone number and location (p. 8)

5. **(C)** Medical direction—the provision for physician input and direction of patient care, training, and quality assurance of an emergency medical service or system (p. 16)

6. **(J)** Medical Director—a physician who assumes the ultimate responsibility for the patient-care aspects of the EMS system (p. 16)

7. **(H)** 911 system—a system for telephone access to report emergencies in which a dispatcher answers the call, takes the information, and alerts EMS or the fire or police departments as needed (p. 8)

8. **(F)** Protocols—lists of steps, such as assessment and interventions, that are developed by the Medical Director of an EMS system (p. 17)

9. **(B)** Quality improvement—a process of continuous self-review with the purpose of identifying and correcting aspects of the system that require improvement (p. 14)

10. **(E)** Standing order—policy or protocol issued by a Medical Director that authorizes EMTs or others to perform particular skills in certain situations (p. 17)

MULTIPLE-CHOICE REVIEW

1. **(B)** In the 1790s, France began to transport wounded soldiers so they could be cared for by physicians away from the scene of the battle. (p. 5)

2. **(C)** In 1966, the National Highway Safety Act charged the United States Department of Transportation with developing EMS standards. (p. 6)

3. **(B)** Computerization is helpful, but is not considered a major NHTSA EMS system assessment standard. (pp. 6–7)

4. **(C)** Specialty hospitals include poison control centers, trauma centers, burn centers, and pediatric centers. Most hospitals have an Emergency Department. Correctional facilities and primary care centers are not considered EMS specialty care units. (p. 8)

5. **(A)** The U.S. Department of Transportation publishes curricula for the First Responder, EMT-Basic, EMT-Intermediate, and EMT-Paramedic levels. (pp. 9–10)

6. **(C)** The EMT curriculum deals with basic assessment and care of the patient. The EMT course is not limited to immediate life-threatening care. Electrocardiograms are beyond the scope of the EMT curriculum, and advanced airway techniques are optional, not a major emphasis, in the EMT curriculum. (pp. 9–10)

7. **(B)** The care provided by the EMT is based upon assessment findings. It is not delayed until transportation, nor should it be guided by attorneys. EMTs do not make a diagnosis; rather treatment is based upon patient complaints. (pp. 9–10)

8. **(A)** During the transfer of care, continuity of care can be improved by providing pertinent patient information to the hospital staff. This includes information on the patient's condition and observation of the scene. (p. 11)

9. **(D)** While patient advocacy—speaking up for your patient—is one of the important roles of the EMT, it is not your primary responsibility. Your first responsibility is keeping yourself safe. (p. 11)

10. **(A)** Good personality traits of the EMT include: pleasant, cooperative, resourceful, a self-starter, emotionally stable, able to lead, neat and clean, of good moral character, having respect for others, in control of personal habits, and controlled in conversation. (p. 12)

11. **(D)** An EMT should be in control of personal habits such as smoking, drinking, and using inappropriate language in order to avoid contaminating the patient's wounds, making inappropriate decisions, and rendering improper care. (p. 12)

12. **(C)** Avoiding inappropriate conversation is paramount in protecting a patient's confidentiality. (p. 12)

13. **(C)** Continuing education includes attending conferences and watching training videos that further your education. Since procedures often change, rereading your old textbook cannot keep you up-to-date on these changes. (p. 13)

14. **(C)** By definition, quality improvement is a process of continuous self-review with the purpose of identifying and correcting aspects of the EMS system that require improvement. (p. 14)

15. **(B)** Additional ways of providing quality improvement are listed in answer 16 below. (p. 15)

16. **(C)** Participating in continuing education and keeping careful written documentation are just two of the ways EMTs can work toward quality care. Others include becoming involved in the quality improvement process, maintaining your equipment, and obtaining feedback from patients and the hospital staff. (p. 15)

17. **(D)** Each EMS system should have a Medical Director to provide oversight of patient care procedures. (p. 16)

18. **(C)** As an EMT, you act as an extender, or designated agent, of the Medical Director. (p. 16)

19. **(D)** On-line medical direction involves talking to a physician over the telephone or radio. Off-line medical direction includes the physician developing protocols and policies, advising the EMS service, and reviewing quality assurance issues. (pp. 16–17)

20. **(B)** Activated charcoal is one of the medications for which EMTs need on-line medical approval in order to administer. (pp. 16–17)

21. **(B)** Injury prevention programs are examples of community health initiatives EMTs may be involved in. (p. 22)

22. **(C)** EMTs should treat all patients in a nonjudgmental and fair manner. (p. 12)

23. **(C)** When the EMT makes a decision on the hospital to transport to, this is an example of a critical decision. (p. 9)

24. **(D)** The First Responder will be known as the Emergency Medical Responder in the future. (p. 10)

COMPLETE THE FOLLOWING

1. The categories and standards of an EMS system established by the National Highway Traffic Safety Administration are: (any six) (pp. 6–7)
   - regulation and policy
   - resource management
   - human resources and training
   - trauma systems
   - public information and education
   - communications
   - transportation
   - facilities
   - evaluation
   - medical direction

2. Six types of specialty hospitals are: (p. 8)
   - trauma centers
   - burn centers
   - cardiac centers
   - pediatric centers
   - poison control centers
   - stroke centers

3. Four levels of EMS certification are: (pp. 9–10)
   - First Responder/Emergency Medical Responder
   - EMT-Basic/EMT
   - EMT-Intermediate/Advanced EMT
   - EMT-Paramedic/Paramedic

STREET SCENES DISCUSSION

Scene safety, patient assessment (first), (and then) patient care, lifting and moving patients, and patient transport.

Chapter 2: The Well-Being of the EMT

MATCH TERMINOLOGY/ DEFINITIONS

1. **(J)** Anger—when a patient gets upset and questions, "Why me?" (p. 38)

2. **(G)** Bargaining—when a patient mentally tries to postpone death for a short time (p. 38)

3. **(M)** Biohazard—a potentially infectious material (p. 29)

4. **(A)** Standard Precautions—infection control based on the presumption that all body fluids are infectious (p. 22)

5. **(B)** Critical incident stress debriefing (CISD) teams—mental health professionals and peer counselors who work as a team to provide emotional and psychological support to EMS personnel who are or have been involved in a highly stressful incident (p. 37)

6. **(C)** Decontamination—the removal or cleansing of dangerous chemicals or other dangerous or infectious materials (p. 40)

7. **(L)** Denial—when the patient puts off dealing with the inevitable end of the process of dying (p. 38)

8. **(I)** Stress—a state of physical and/or psychological arousal to a stimulus (p. 33)

9. **(H)** Hazardous-material incident—the release of a harmful substance into the environment (p. 39)

10. **(N)** HEPA—a High-Efficiency Particulate Air respirator or mask designed to reduce the spread of TB (p. 25)

11. **(K)** Immunizations—injections given to a rescuer that are designed to prevent him or her from getting a disease (p. 33)

12. **(F)** MCI—an emergency involving multiple patients (p. 35)

13. **(E)** Pathogens—the organisms that cause infection, such as viruses and bacteria (p. 21)

14. **(D)** Personal protective equipment—equipment that protects the EMS worker from infection and/or from hazardous materials and the dangers of rescue operations (p. 23)

15. **(O)** PPD test—purified protein derivative test that determines if a person has been exposed to TB (p. 33)

MULTIPLE-CHOICE REVIEW

1. **(A)** The best EMT can be of no help to the patient if he or she is injured during a rescue situation or becomes ill. (p. 21)

2. **(D)** By definition, a pathogen is an organism that causes infection, such as a virus or bacteria. (p. 21)

3. **(C)** Since the EMT cannot identify patients who carry infectious diseases just by looking at them, all body fluids must be considered infectious and Standard Precautions must be taken all the time. (p. 22)

4. **(C)** BSI (Standard Precautions) involves handwashing, disposable gloves, and eye protection. A HEPA mask is used to protect against airborne particles that may cause TB. Leather gloves are helpful in a rescue to protect the EMT from cutting his or her hands but are not useful for Standard Precautions. (pp. 22–23)

5. **(B)** Surgical masks are routinely used for treating patients with a potential for blood or fluid spatter. If TB is suspected, a HEPA mask should be used. (p. 25)

6. **(A)** Whenever a mask is placed on a patient, the EMT will need to monitor the patient to assure respirations are adequate and the airway is open. Check often to ensure the patient doesn't vomit into the mask. If you think the patient has TB, you should wear a HEPA mask, not a surgical mask. (p. 25)

7. **(B)** In some states, keeping lists of certain types of patients, such as AIDS patients, may be a violation of the law. All other responses listed are ways to plan safety precautions. Since you never know which of your patients may have a communicable disease, you need to treat them all as if they do and take Standard Precautions. (pp. 28–29)

8. **(C)** The purified protein derivative (PPD) is a test for tuberculosis and is not a vaccine. (p. 33)

9. **(C)** The employee safety regulations come under the Occupational Safety and Health Administration (OSHA). The FDA regulates drugs and foods; the FCC regulates radio equipment; and the Public Health Service provides regulations and educational efforts to assure children are immunized, water is clean, and so on. (p. 29)

10. **(C)** Employers of EMTs must make available the hepatitis B vaccination series as outlined in the OSHA standards on bloodborne pathogens, which took effect in March 1992. Employers must also provide training and personal protective equipment. (pp. 29–30)

11. **(B)** The Ryan White CARE Act provides two different systems for infectious disease exposure—airborne disease exposure and bloodborne disease exposure. Ensure that you understand these notification procedures since treatment must be timely in order to be effective. (pp. 30–31)

12. **(C)** The designated officer is responsible for gathering facts surrounding emergency responder airborne or bloodborne infectious disease exposures. Be sure you know who the designated officer is in your organization. (pp. 31–32)

13. **(B)** It is safest to assume that any person with a productive cough may be infected with TB. Since there are rising cases of multidrug-resistant TB, you should learn to recognize situations in which the potential of TB exposure exists, as well as the signs and symptoms of TB patients. (p. 27)

14. **(D)** An EMT should never treat a contaminated patient. If you treated the patient in an ambulance, it would be contaminated. If you took the contaminated patient to the hospital, you could effectively close it down. (p. 26)

15. **(D)** The well-being of the EMT involves dealing with job stress, ensuring scene safety, and taking Standard Precautions to avoid contracting diseases. (p. 26)

16. **(B)** An adult cardiac arrest is considered a routine EMS call. Calls involving a higher potential for causing excess stress on EMS providers include calls involving infants and children, elder abuse, death or injury of a coworker, plus severe injuries and MCIs. (pp. 35–36)

17. **(C)** The warning signs that an EMT is being affected by stress include irritability with family, friends, and coworkers; inability to concentrate; changes in daily activities; difficulty sleeping or nightmares; loss of appetite; loss of interest in sexual activity; anxiety; indecisiveness; guilt; isolation; and loss of interest in work. (p. 37)

18. **(D)** Talking about your feelings with your partners is healthy. (p. 36)

19. **(C)** By definition, a critical incident stress debriefing is a process in which a team of trained peer counselors and mental health professionals meet with rescuers and health care providers who have been involved in a major incident. (p. 37)

20. **(D)** All are true. Also the normal reactions to stress should be discussed and provisions for follow-up set up for those who may need it. (pp. 37–38)

21. **(D)** The CISD is effective in accelerating the recovery process for the participants because it is nonthreatening and avoids performance review. It should never be combined with an incident critique or investigation. (pp. 37–38)

22. **(C)** The emotional stages that patients go through when they find out they are dying include denial, anger, bargaining, depression, and acceptance. (p. 38)

23. **(B)** The emotional stages have differing duration and magnitude but generally occur in the following order: denial, anger, bargaining, depression, and acceptance. (p. 38)

24. **(B)** All responses are correct except lying to the patient by saying everything will be all right when it will not. (pp. 24–25)

25. **(B)** It is not an EMTs responsibility to respond to dangerous situations. Rather, you should retreat, radio to police

for assistance, and reevaluate the scene once it has been secured by the police. (pp. 43–44)

26. **(D)** All of the stressors listed may affect the EMT. (pp. 35–36)

27. **(C)** Hans Selye, MD, first coined the phrase general adaptation syndrome as the body's response to stress. (p. 34)

28. **(C)** The three phases of general adaptation syndrome are: alarm, resistance, and exhaustion. (p. 34)

29. **(B)** Stress reactions occurring days, weeks, or even months after an incident are called post-traumatic stress reactions. (p. 35)

30. **(D)** The CDC recommends the use of alcohol-based hand cleaners when soap and water are not available. (p. 24)

31. **(C)** The normal mode of transmission of the disease chickenpox (varicella) is by airborne droplets. (p. 28)

32. **(A)** Hepatitis is not thought to be spread by respiratory secretions or oral or nasal secretions as bacterial meningitis, pneumonia, or tuberculosis would be. (p. 27)

33. **(B)** Mothers are thought to be able to pass the disease AIDS to their unborn child. (p. 28)

COMPLETE THE FOLLOWING

1. Types of calls with high potential of stress for EMS personnel include: (pp. 35–36)
   - MCIs
   - infants and children
   - severe injuries
   - abuse and neglect
   - death of a coworker

2. Signs and symptoms of stress include: (any five) (pp. 36–37)
   - irritability with family and friends and coworkers
   - inability to concentrate
   - changes in daily activities
   - loss of interest in sexual activity
   - anxiety
   - isolation
   - loss of interest in work
   - loss of appetite
   - difficulty sleeping

3. The critical elements of the infection control plan required by Title 29 Code of Federal Regulation 1910.1030 are: (any five) (pp. 28–32)
   - infection exposure control plan
   - adequate education and training
   - hepatitis B vaccination
   - personal protective equipment
   - methods of control
   - housekeeping
   - labeling
   - postexposure evaluation and follow-up

STREET SCENES DISCUSSION

1. Hepatitis B, C, or D, or HIV

2. AZT, safe sex with a condom, and regular blood tests

3. Yes, by being inoculated for hepatitis B, he may have prevented contraction of the disease.

4. Hepatitis B is a very hardy virus that kills approximately 200 health care workers each year.

MATCH TERMINOLOGY/ DEFINITIONS

1. **(M)** Abandonment—leaving a patient after care has been initiated and before the patient has been transferred to someone with equal or greater medical training (p. 55)

2. **(B)** Advance directive—a written order given by the physician based upon a decision by a patient prior to his demise (p. 51)

3. **(O)** Battery—subjecting a patient to unwanted care and transport can be considered this in a court of law (p. 51)

4. **(I)** Breach of duty—not providing the standard of care (p. 54)

5. **(L)** Confidentiality—the obligation not to reveal information about a patient except to other health care professionals involved in the patient's care, or under subpoena, or in a court of law (p. 56)

6. **(F)** Consent—permission from the patient to treat him or her (p. 49)

7. **(K)** DNR order—a legal document, usually signed by the patient and his or her physician, which states that the patient has a terminal illness and does not wish to prolong life through resuscitative efforts (p. 51)

8. **(D)** Duty to act—an obligation to provide care to a patient (p. 55)

9. **(N)** Emancipated minor—child who is married or of a specific age who, in certain states, can make his or her own legal decisions (p. 50)

10. **(E)** Expressed consent—permission given by adults who are of legal age and mentally competent to make a rational decision in regard to their medical well-being (p. 50)

11. **(G)** Good Samaritan laws—a series of laws, varying in each state, designed to provide limited legal protection for citizens and some health care personnel who are administering care (p. 56)

12. **(A)** Implied consent—permission to treat an unconscious patient until he or she becomes conscious (p. 50)

13. **(C)** Liability—being held legally responsible (p. 50)

14. **(J)** Negligence—a finding of failure to act properly in a situation in which there was a duty to act (p. 54)

15. **(H)** Scope of practice—the collective medical, legal, and ethical guidelines that govern the EMT (p. 48)

16. **(P)** HIPAA—a federal law protecting the privacy of patient-specific health care information (p. 56)

MULTIPLE-CHOICE REVIEW

1. **(B)** The collective set of regulations and ethical considerations governing the EMT's responsibilities is called the scope of practice. Duty to act is an obligation to provide care to the patient. Advance directives are the written and signed wishes of the patient in advance of any event where resuscitation might be undertaken. The Good Samaritan laws vary by state and often do not cover the EMT. (p. 48)

2. **(B)** Legislation that governs the skills and medical interventions that an EMT may perform not only differ from state to state, but may even vary from region to region within the state. (p. 48)

3. **(C)** Making the physical/emotional needs of the patient a priority is considered an ethical responsibility of the EMT. A legal responsibility would be assuring consent was gained prior to treating a patient. Advance directives involve orders on how a patient wants to be treated in the event resuscitation is needed. Protocols are models of care that an EMT follows in treating patients. (p. 49)

4. **(C)** Applied consent is a meaningless term that is often put on exams to test the student's understanding of consent terminology. The types of consent include consent for a minor or child, consent for a mentally incompetent adult, expressed consent (see answer 5), and implied consent (see answer 6). (pp. 49–50)

5. **(A)** Expressed consent is obtained by informing an adult patient of a procedure you are about to perform and its associated risks, then gaining his or her permission to proceed. Negligence is a finding of failure to act properly in a situation where there was a duty to act. Implied consent is defined in answer 6, and applied consent is a meaningless term. (p. 50)

6. **(C)** Consent that is based on the assumption that an unconscious patient would approve the EMT's life-saving interventions is called implied consent. Expressed consent, negligence, and applied consent are explained in answer 5. (p. 50)

7. **(C)** A patient refusal of medical aid or transport does not require any physician's signature. Your official record of a patient's refusal to accept medical aid must carefully and completely document the attempts you made to get the patient to accept care. Include the names of any witnesses to your attempts, and include the patient's "release" form with the patient's witnessed signature. (p. 50)

8. **(B)** Forcing a competent adult patient to go to the hospital against his will may result in assault and battery charges against the EMT. You could also be charged with kidnapping the patient. Both implied consent and negligence are discussed in answers 5 and 6. (p. 51)

9. **(C)** All choices are correct except C. In all cases of refusal, you should advise patients to call back at any time if there is a problem or they wish to be cared for or transported. While there may be patients who legitimately refuse care, such as for minor wounds, patients with any significant medical condition should be transported to the hospital. (p. 51)

10. **(D)** A DNR order is a physician's order to "do not resuscitate" a patient. This is also referred to as an advance directive. (p. 51)

11. **(A)** There are varying degrees of DNR orders, expressed through a variety of detailed instructions that may be part of the order, such as allowing for CPR only if cardiac or respiratory arrest was observed. Comfort care measures such as intravenous feeding, administering pain medications, and the long-term use of a respirator are a part of a living will and are not part of a DNR order. These orders generally do not specify procedures that are improper, such as specifying that only 5 minutes of artificial respiration will be attempted. (pp. 53–54)

12. **(B)** In a hospital, long-term life-support and comfort care measures would consist of intravenous feeding and the use of a respirator. Once a patient is considered terminal, routine inoculations would not be needed. Infection control by the health care providers is a given. Documentation needs to be the same as it would be had the patient not had an advance directive. (p. 54)

13. **(B)** In order to prove negligence, an attorney must prove the EMT had a duty to the patient, failed to provide the

standard of care or breached his or her duty, and this failure caused harm to the patient. (pp. 54–55)

14. **(C)** Termination of care of the patient without assuring the continuation of care at the same level or higher is called abandonment. Liability is being held legally responsible. Battery is attacking someone physically; and a breach of duty is not acting when you have an obligation to act. (p. 55)

15. **(D)** Information considered confidential includes patient history gained through interview, assessment findings, and treatment rendered. The release of this information can cause embarrassment as well as potential harm to the patient. In the past, when the public was uninformed about the causes and consequences of AIDS, release of a patient's HIV positive status caused cross burnings and sick graffiti on the property of patients' homes. (pp. 55–56)

16. **(D)** The only times an EMT may release confidential patient information is to inform other health care professionals who need to know the information to continue care, to report incidents required by state law, such as rape or abuse, and to comply with a legal subpoena. It is not your responsibility to release confidential patient information in an effort to protect the other victims of a motor vehicle collision. (p. 56)

17. **(D)** Medical identification insignia that indicate serious patient medical conditions come in the form of bracelets, necklaces, and cards because patients wear/carry these all the time and they are easily located. Patches are not medical IDs. (p. 51)

18. **(B)** The patient is not dead yet, so treat the critical patient who has an organ donor card the same as any other patient and inform the ED physician. Withholding oxygen therapy from the critically ill patient will just speed up his or her demise. (p. 58)

19. **(A)** At a crime scene, the EMT should avoid disturbing any evidence unless emergency care requires. The patient himself provides valuable information. The position the patient is found in, condition of the clothing, and injuries are all pieces of evidence. Do not move obstacles from around the patient to make more room to work; this may destroy evidence. Leave the search of the house for clues to the police. It is not your responsibility. (pp. 58, 60)

20. **(B)** Commonly required reporting situations include sexual assault, domestic abuse, and child and elder abuse. A crime in a public place does not require the EMT to report the crime to the authorities. (p. 61)

21. **(C)** The extent (or limits) of the EMT's job is called the scope of practice (p. 48)

22. **(B)** The patient may not have a life-threatening injury but he was unconscious prior to your arrival and may not be mentally competent to refuse at this time based on all the alcohol he admits drinking within the last hour. (p. 50)

23. **(C)** The federal law designed to protect the patient's private medical information is the Health Insurance Portability and Accountability Act, or HIPAA. (p. 56)

24. **(A)** HIPAA requires an agency privacy officer. (p. 57)

25. **(B)** Dirt and carpet fibers are examples of microscopic evidence found at a crime scene. (p. 60)

COMPLETE THE FOLLOWING

1. In order for a patient to refuse care or transport, these four conditions must be fulfilled: (p. 50)
   - The patient must be mentally competent and oriented.
   - The patient must be fully informed.
   - The patient must sign a "release" form.
   - The patient must be of legal age or an emancipated minor.

2. Negligence, or failure to act properly, requires all of the following circumstances in order to be proven: (pp. 54–55)
   - The EMT had a duty to the patient.
   - The EMT did not provide the standard of care.
   - The actions of the EMT in not providing the standard of care caused harm to the patient.

3. Four examples of conditions that may be listed on a medical identification device (such as a necklace, bracelet, or card) include: (p. 57)
   - Heart conditions
   - Allergies
   - Diabetes
   - Epilepsy

STREET SCENES DISCUSSION

1. Not really. This is not a confidentiality issue. It is more of an ethical issue and a matter of professional behavior in any conversation you have about any patient's residence. If, however, there are hazards observed while treating the patient in his residence (e.g., fire hazards, uncaged dangerous animals, explosives, dangerous conditions to future responders as well as to the patient), you should seriously consider notifying the appropriate authorities in your community.

2. Yes, it is medical documentation. You can always write things that the patient says in quotes in the narrative section of the PCR, too.

3. The appropriate BSI (Standard Precautions) equipment would be gloves, and because the patient was vomiting, a mask and eye shield.

CASE STUDY—A WITNESSED COLLISION: FIRST ON THE SCENE

1. No, unless your state law requires you to stop. You should, however, understand that once you do stop, you should not leave the patient except in the hands of another EMT or advanced EMT. Leaving a patient is considered abandonment, an example of "gross negligence."

2. Yes and no! Anyone can be sued. Most states do have some form of Good Samaritan laws or laws dealing specifically with EMS personnel that protect you in this situation provided you do not render treatment that is grossly negligent.

3. Yes, in most states.

4. Nine-One-One (911).

5. **A)** What is the exact location of the sick or injured person?
   B) What is your call back number?
   C) How old is the patient?
   D) What's the problem?
   E) What's the patient's sex?
   F) Is the patient breathing?

6. The police, the fire department, and the ambulance service.

7. Assign them to perform manual stabilization of the head and neck and to help with lifting the patient once the ambulance arrives.

8. The patient could have additional broken bones, internal bleeding, a head or neck injury to name a few.

9. No permission is needed as consent is implied because the patient is unconscious.

Chapter 3 (continued)

10. He could have a ruptured spleen, fractured ribs, back and neck injuries, as well as the obvious fractured leg.

11. Assign someone to lift the patient's injured leg and hold it as still as possible.

12. Yes, he is conscious and must give expressed consent.

13. No, not until you check with the EMT or paramedic in charge to be sure your assistance is no longer needed.

14. Gross negligence due to abandonment.

Chapter 4: The Human Body

MATCH TERMINOLOGY/ DEFINITIONS

▶ PART A

1. **(O)** Arteries—vessels that carry blood away from the heart (p. 80)

2. **(B)** Atria—upper chambers of the heart (p. 77)

3. **(I)** Brachial pulse—pulse in the arm used to take a blood pressure (p. 80)

4. **(A)** Bronchi—main branch of the respiratory system that enters each of the lungs (p. 76)

5. **(E)** Capillaries—tiny blood vessels (p. 81)

6. **(G)** Cardiovascular system—body system that transports blood throughout the body (p. 77)

7. **(F)** Carotid pulse—pulse in the neck at the side of the larynx (p. 80)

8. **(K)** Cricoid cartilage—ring-shaped structure that forms the lower larynx (p. 76)

9. **(C)** Diaphragm—muscle that divides the chest cavity from the abdominal cavity (p. 76)

10. **(N)** Dorsalis pedis pulse—pulse on the top of the foot lateral to the large tendon of the big toe (p. 80)

11. **(M)** Epiglottis—leaf-shaped structure that closes to prevent food from going into the trachea (p. 76)

12. **(D)** Femoral pulse—the carotid and this pulse are considered central pulses (p. 80)

13. **(L)** Larynx—structure that contains the vocal cords (p. 76)

14. **(J)** Nasopharynx—area directly posterior to the nose (p. 75)

15. **(H)** Oropharynx—area directly posterior to the mouth (p. 75)

▶ PART B

1. **(I)** Acetabulum—socket that holds the ball of the proximal femur to form the hip (p. 72)

2. **(M)** Femur—long bone of the thigh (p. 73)

3. **(O)** Fibula—the smaller bone of the lower leg (p. 73)

4. **(K)** Involuntary muscle—muscle type that responds automatically without the patient thinking about its operation (p. 74)

5. **(A)** Pharynx—area posterior to the mouth and nose that includes the oropharynx and nasopharynx (p. 75)

6. **(B)** Platelets—parts of the blood needed to form blood clots (p. 82)

7. **(C)** Plasma—watery, salty fluid that makes up over one-half of the blood's volume (p. 82)

8. **(D)** Posterior tibial pulse—pulse that may be palpated on the posterior aspect of the medial malleolus (p. 80)

9. **(N)** Radial pulse—pulse on the thumb side of the wrist (p. 80)

10. **(H)** Respiratory system—body system that takes in oxygen and eliminates carbon dioxide (p. 75)

11. **(G)** Systolic—blood pressure created in the arteries when the left ventricle contracts and forces blood out into circulation (p. 83)

12. **(E)** Trachea—structure that carries inhaled air from the larynx to the lungs; also called the windpipe (p. 76)

13. **(F)** Veins—vessels that carry blood from the capillaries back to the heart (p. 81)

14. **(L)** Venae cavae—two large veins that return blood to the heart (p. 77)

15. **(J)** Ventricles—the two lower chambers of the heart (p. 77)

▶ PART C

1. **(C)** Anatomical position—standing face forward with palms forward (p. 66)

2. **(M)** Cervical spine—seven vertebrae in the neck (p. 72)

3. **(D)** Coccyx—inferior-most division of the spine that is referred to as the tailbone (p. 72)

4. **(H)** Iliac crest—wide bony ring that can be felt near the waist (p. 72)

5. **(J)** Lateral malleolus—round ball of bone on the outside of the ankle (p. 73)

6. **(F)** Mandible—lower jaw bone (p. 70)

7. **(E)** Medial—toward or closer to the midline (p. 66)

8. **(G)** Medial malleolus—round ball of bone on the inside of the ankle (p. 73)

9. **(K)** Orbit—facial bone that surrounds each of the eyes (p. 71)

10. **(I)** Peripheral nervous system—system that consists of sensory and motor nerves (p. 83)

11. **(A)** Pubis—medial anterior portion of the pelvis (p. 72)

12. **(B)** Sacral spine—vertebrae that form the back of the pelvis (p. 72)

13. **(L)** Sternum—breastbone (p. 72)

14. **(N)** Tarsals—bones of the ankle (p. 73)

15. **(O)** Tibia—medial and larger of the two bones of the lower leg (p. 73)

▶ PART D

1. **(M)** Anterior—front side of the body or body part (p. 67)

2. **(N)** Calcaneus—heel bone (p. 73)

3. **(J)** Dermis—inner layer of the skin in which blood vessels and nerves are located (p. 87)

4. **(G)** Distal—when two points on the extremities are compared, the point further away from the torso (p. 67)

5. **(L)** Elbow—joint where three bones of the upper arm and forearm are connected (p. 73)

6. **(F)** Epidermis—outermost layer of the skin (p. 87)

7. **(B)** Humerus—upper arm bone (p. 74)

8. **(C)** Lateral—away from the midline (p. 66)

9. **(H)** Motor nerves—nerves that carry messages from the brain to the body (p. 83)

©2009 Pearson Education, Inc.
Emergency Care, 11th Ed.

10. **(K)** Phalanges—bones in the fingers and toes (p. 73)

11. **(O)** Posterior—back side of the body or body part (p. 67)

12. **(E)** Proximal—when two points on the extremities are compared, the point closer to the torso (p. 67)

13. **(D)** Sensory nerves—nerves that transmit information from the body to the spinal cord and brain (p. 83)

14. **(I)** Superior—above or toward the head end of the torso (p. 67)

15. **(A)** Xiphoid process—inferior tip of the sternum (p. 72)

▶ **PART E**

1. **(E)** Acromion process—highest portion of the shoulder (p. 74)

2. **(N)** Bilaterally—similar on both sides of the body (p. 67)

3. **(G)** Carpals—bones that make up the wrist (p. 74)

4. **(I)** Clavicle—bone in the front of the shoulder or collarbone (p. 73)

5. **(A)** Endocrine system—body system that regulates metabolic functions such as sugar absorption by the cells (p. 88)

6. **(M)** Fowler's—the sitting position (p. 69)

7. **(D)** Metacarpals—bones that make up the hand (p. 74)

8. **(L)** Mid-clavicular—an imaginary line drawn vertically from the center of the clavicle to the nipple below (p. 68)

9. **(B)** Nervous system—body system that governs sensations, movement, and thought (p. 83)

10. **(C)** Radius—lateral bone of the forearm aligned with the thumb (p. 74)

11. **(H)** Scapula—shoulder blade (p. 73)

12. **(K)** Supine—lying on the back (p. 68)

13. **(J)** Torso—the body less the extremities and the head (p. 67)

14. **(O)** Trendelenburg—lying supine (flat) with the legs elevated a few inches (p. 70)

15. **(F)** Ulna—medial bone of the forearm (p. 74)

▶ **PART F**

1. **(B)** Abdominal quadrants—four divisions of the abdomen used to pinpoint the location of pain (p. 68)

2. **(M)** Axilla—anatomical term for the armpit (p. 67)

3. **(D)** Coronary arteries—blood vessels that supply the muscle of the heart (p. 80)

4. **(H)** Diastolic—blood pressure in the arteries when the left ventricle is refilling (p. 83)

5. **(E)** Dorsal—referring to the back of the body (p. 67)

6. **(N)** Left side—patient's left side (p. 68)

7. **(J)** Lumbar spine—vertebrae of the lower back (p. 72)

8. **(F)** Maxillae—upper jaw bone (p. 70)

9. **(L)** Midline—imaginary line drawn vertically through the middle of the body (p. 66)

10. **(G)** Musculoskeletal system—body system that provides protection and movement (p. 70)

11. **(I)** Patella—kneecap (p. 73)

12. **(C)** Plantar—referring to the sole of the foot (p. 67)

13. **(O)** Prone—lying on the stomach or face down (p. 68)

14. **(K)** Thoracic spine—rib area of the spinal column (p. 72)

15. **(A)** Voluntary muscle—muscle under conscious control of the brain (p. 74)

©2009 Pearson Education, Inc.
Emergency Care, 11th Ed.

MULTIPLE-CHOICE REVIEW

1. **(C)** The abdomen is a cavity of the body containing hollow and solid organs. Body systems include: respiratory, cardiovascular, musculoskeletal, skin (integumentary), nervous, endocrine, and digestive. (p. 69)

2. **(B)** If a patient is lying on his left side, this position is called the recovery, or left lateral recumbent, position. Fowler's position is sitting on a stretcher, supine is lying on the back, and prone is lying on the stomach. (pp. 68–69)

3. **(C)** When a patient is placed in a sitting-up position on a stretcher, this position is called Fowler's. Lying on the stomach is prone; lying on the back is supine. Trendelenburg is defined in answer 4. (p. 69)

4. **(D)** When a patient is lying flat with head lower than legs, this position is called Trendelenburg. For an explanation of the other choices, see answer 3. (p. 70)

5. **(B)** The musculoskeletal system has three main functions: It gives the body shape, provides for body movements, and protects vital internal organs. Body sensation is a function of the nervous system. The skin, or integumentary, system is the body's outer covering. The cardiovascular system, working along with the respiratory system, transports oxygen into the cells. (p. 70)

6. **(C)** The upper jaw is also called the maxillae. The way to remember which of the two jaw bones is which, maxillae or mandible, is to use the rhyme "the mandible is moveable." The orbit is the area around the eyes, and the nasal bone protects the nose. (p. 70)

7. **(A)** The spinal column consists of the 7 cervical, 12 thoracic, 5 lumbar, 5 sacral, and 4 coccyx bones. (p. 72)

8. **(C)** An injury to the cervical spine may be fatal because control of the muscles of breathing arise from the spinal cord at this level. The lumbar region is also subject to injury because it is not supported by other parts of the skeleton. The thoracic spine, as well as the sacral spine and coccyx, are less easily injured. (p. 71)

9. **(A)** Bones in the lower extremities include the femur, fibula, patella, tarsals, metatarsals, calcaneus, and phalanges. The ischium is a pelvic bone. The ulna and radius are bones in the forearm. The orbit is the area around the eyes in the face. (p. 73)

10. **(A)** Bones in the upper extremities include the humerus, ulna, radius, carpals, metacarpals, and phalanges. The cervical bones are in the neck, and the tibia and calcaneus are in the lower extremities. (p. 73)

11. **(D)** The types of muscle tissue include voluntary, involuntary, and cardiac. Cardiac muscle has a specific quality called automaticity, or the ability to generate and conduct electrical impulses on its own. (p. 74)

12. **(A)** The type of muscle that allows body movement such as walking is called voluntary. Involuntary and cardiac muscles are described in answers 11 and 13. Smooth is the same as involuntary. (p. 74)

13. **(B)** Involuntary, or smooth, muscle is found in the blood vessels, gastrointestinal system, lungs, and urinary system and controls the flow of materials through these systems. The heart has a special type of muscle (cardiac), and the quadriceps and biceps have voluntary, or (skeletal) striated, muscle. (p. 74)

14. **(B)** The larynx is the structure in the throat that is commonly known as the voicebox. The pharynx is the area

directly posterior to the mouth and nose; the trachea is the windpipe; and the sternum is the breastbone. (p. 76)

15. **(B)** The epiglottis is a leaf-shaped valve that prevents food and foreign objects from entering the trachea. The bronchi are the two major tubes that allow air to enter each of the two lungs. The pharynx and larynx are defined above in answer 14. (p. 76)

16. **(C)** The normal order of passage of oxygen from the environment to the lungs is through mouth and nose to the pharynx, through the larynx, through the trachea, into the bronchi, then down into the bronchioles, and then into the alveoli. Normally air does not go into the esophagus, which is a tube that brings food into the stomach. (pp. 75–76)

17. **(C)** When the diaphragm and intercostal muscles relax, the size of the chest cavity decreases, causing exhalation. When the diaphragm contracts, it moves down, enlarging the chest cavity; the intercostal muscles pull the chest upward and outward to enlarge the cavity. This rapid pressure change accounts for air moving from the outside environment to fill the cavity. (p. 76)

18. **(D)** The difference between the adult airway and the pediatric airway is that all structures are smaller and more easily obstructed in a child. Actually, the adult's tongue takes up proportionately less space in the mouth than the child's. The trachea and cricoid cartilage is softer and more flexible in a child. (pp. 76–77)

19. **(B)** The body system that is responsible for the breakdown of food into absorbable forms is called the digestive system. The nervous system controls the body, the endocrine system manages intricate functions like insulin balance and growth hormone, and the integumentary system covers the surface of the body. (p. 85)

20. **(C)** An organ that contains acidic gastric juices that begin the breakdown of food into components that the body will be able to convert to energy is the stomach. The other organs are parts of the digestive system, which handle the food once it is already broken down. (p. 85)

21. **(B)** The major artery in the thigh is called the femoral artery. The carotid is in the neck, radial is in the wrist, and brachial is in the arm. (pp. 80–81)

22. **(C)** The vessel that carries oxygen-poor blood from the portion of the body below the heart and back to the right atrium is called the inferior vena cava. The posterior tibial is a pulse that can be palpated on the posterior aspect of the medial malleolus. The internal jugular is a vein that drains blood from the head. The aorta is the largest artery, which carries oxygen-rich blood away from the left ventricle. (pp. 78–79)

23. **(B)** The left atrium receives blood from the pulmonary veins (the only veins that contain oxygenated blood). The left atrium then pumps the blood into the left ventricle, where it is then pumped out to the rest of the body. (pp. 78–79)

24. **(C)** The fluid that carries the blood cells and nutrients is called plasma. Platelets are defined in answer 25. Urine is a waste product of the body excreted by the kidneys and held in the urinary bladder prior to being excreted from the body. (p. 82)

25. **(B)** The blood component that is essential to the formation of blood clots is called platelets. Plasma is the fluid part of the blood that carries blood cells and nutrients. The white blood cells fight infection, and the red cells carry oxygen to or carbon dioxide away from tissues. (p. 82)

26. **(A)** The pressure on the walls of an artery when the left ventricle contracts is called the systolic pressure. The pressure upon relaxation is the diastolic pressure. Residual and arterial pressures are utilized in critical care monitoring. (p. 83)

27. **(A)** The two main divisions of the nervous system are the central and peripheral nervous systems. The bones, muscles, and spinal column are parts of the musculoskeletal system. The spinal cord and brain are major components of the central nervous system. (p. 83)

28. **(D)** Nerves that carry information from throughout the body to the brain are sensory nerves. The motor nerves allow for movement. Spinal nerves, along with the brain, are actually a part of the central nervous system. There is no specific category called cardiac nerves. (p. 83)

29. **(C)** One of the functions of the skin is to protect the body from the environment, bacteria, and other organisms. Other functions of the skin include water balance, temperature regulation, excretion, and shock absorption. The respiratory system eliminates excess oxygen into the atmosphere. The nervous system regulates the diameter of the blood vessels in the circulation. The skin prevents environmental water from entering the body. (p. 86)

30. **(C)** The system that secretes hormones, such as insulin and adrenaline, and that is responsible for regulating body activities, is called the endocrine system. The skin provides covering, and the nervous system provides overall control. The gastrointestinal system digests food. (p. 88)

COMPLETE THE FOLLOWING

1. Arteries in the body include: (p. 80)
   - Coronary
   - Aorta
   - Pulmonary
   - Carotid
   - Femoral
   - Brachial
   - Radial
   - Posterior tibial
   - Dorsalis pedis

2. Functions of the skin include: (p. 86)
   - Protection
   - Water balance
   - Temperature regulation
   - Excretion
   - Shock absorption

LABEL THE DIAGRAMS

▶ **ANATOMICAL POSTURES (p. 69)**

1. Supine
2. Prone
3. Recovery

▶ **ANATOMICAL POSITION (p. 68)**

▶ **DIAGRAM 1**

1. Distal
2. Proximal
3. Midline
4. Mid-clavicular line
5. Medial
6. Lateral
7. Palmar
8. Left
9. Dorsal
10. Right

▶ **DIAGRAM 2**

11. Anterior (ventral)
12. Posterior (dorsal)
13. Superior
14. Mid-axillary line
15. Inferior

1. Scapular region
2. Lumbar region
3. Iliac crest
4. Pubis
5. Costal arch (margin)
6. Xiphoid process
7. Thorax region
8. Sternoclavicular joints
9. Suprasternal (jugular) notch
10. Clavicle
11. Sternum
12. Diaphragm
13. Umbilicus

STREET SCENES DISCUSSION

1. Manual stabilization is needed because the slightest movement of the neck could cause serious, permanent damage—or death—if in fact there is an actual injury to the spine.

2. As an EMT who was dispatched to the scene, you clearly have a duty to act. That means, yes, he is a patient in need of evaluation.

Chapter 5: Lifting and Moving Patients

MATCH TERMINOLOGY/ DEFINITIONS

1. **(A)** Basket stretcher—stretcher, made of steel wire mesh and tubular steel rim or plastic and steel rim, used to transport patients from one level to another or over rough terrain (p. 119)

2. **(H)** Body mechanics—proper use of the body to facilitate lifting and moving and prevent injury (p. 106)

3. **(D)** Direct carry—method of transferring a patient from bed to stretcher in which two or more rescuers curl the patient to their chests, then reverse the process to lower the patient to the stretcher (p. 123)

4. **(M)** Direct ground lift—method of lifting and carrying a patient from ground level to a stretcher during which two or more rescuers kneel, curl the patient to their chests, stand, then reverse the process to lower the patient to the stretcher (p. 123)

5. **(K)** Draw-sheet method—method of transferring a patient from bed to stretcher by grasping and pulling the loosened bottom sheet of the bed (p. 123)

6. **(N)** Emergency move—removal of a patient from a hazardous environment in which safety is the first priority and spinal integrity is second priority (pp. 108–109)

7. **(F)** Extremity lift—method of lifting and carrying a patient in which one rescuer slips hands under the patient's armpits and grasps the wrists, while another rescuer grasps the patient's knees (p. 123)

8. **(O)** Log roll—procedure done by three or four rescuers that is designed to move a patient onto a long backboard without compromising spinal integrity (p. 109)

9. **(L)** Long axis—line that runs down the center of the body from the top of the head and along the spine (p. 109)

10. **(E)** Non-urgent move—patient move that may be made if speed is not priority (p. 112)

11. **(I)** Power grip—gripping with as much hand surface as possible the object being lifted, with all fingers bent at the same angle (p. 107)

12. **(G)** Power lift—also called the squat-lift position; a lift is made from a squatting position with weight to be lifted close to the body, feet apart and flat on the ground, body weight on or just behind the balls of the feet, back locked in (p. 107)

13. **(C)** Scoop (orthopedic) stretcher—stretcher that splits in halves, which can be pushed together under the patient (p. 119)

14. **(B)** Stair chair—portable folding chair with wheels used to transport patient in a sitting position up or down stairs (p. 117)

15. **(J)** Urgent move—patient move that should be done quickly yet without any compromise of spinal integrity (p. 109)

MULTIPLE-CHOICE REVIEW

1. **(C)** To assure your own safety when lifting a patient, it is important to use your legs, not your back, to lift. Some EMTs use a soft back brace when they lift. These devices should only be used if your physician suggests you do so. When lifting, keep the weight as close to your body as possible. Consider the weight of the patient you are lifting: be realistic about your limitations and ask for help. (p. 106)

2. **(B)** Avoid twisting motions while you are lifting; such motions can lead to a back injury. When lifting a patient, you should communicate clearly and frequently with your partner and know your limitations. (p. 106)

3. **(A)** When lifting a cot or stretcher, use an even number of people so that balance of the device is maintained. Your feet should be a comfortable distance apart so you can maintain balance. If a third person is positioned on the heaviest side, he or she stands a greater chance of being injured. If you must use only one hand to carry a piece of equipment, never compensate by using your back. (p. 107)

4. **(A)** When placing all fingers and the palm in contact with the object being lifted, you are using a power grip. A power lift involves squatting and using the legs. The lock grip and grip lift are inventive distracters for this question. (p. 107)

5. **(A)** When you must push an object, keep the line of pull through the center of your body by bending your knees. Also keep the weight as close to your body as possible, avoid pushing or pulling overhead, and keep elbows bent with arms close to your sides. (p. 108)

6. **(D)** The fact that the dispatcher has another more serious call is not an appropriate reason to compromise the patient's spine. The situations in which an emergency move would be used include fire or danger of fire, explosives or other hazardous chemicals, and inability to protect the patient from other hazards at the scene. (pp. 108–109)

7. **(C)** If the patient is on the floor or ground and the EMT has decided that an emergency move is appropriate, the patient can be moved by pulling on his or her clothing in the neck and shoulder area, which maintains some spinal integrity and doesn't require additional equipment or other rescuers. (p. 109)

8. **(B)** If the patient has an altered mental status, the EMT should consider an urgent move. The emergency move is used in situations where there is a real danger to rescuer or patient, such as a fire. (p. 109)

9. **(C)** When doing a log roll, lean from your hips and use your shoulder muscles to help with the roll. Also try to keep your back straight and position yourself right next to the patient. Maintaining spinal integrity is more important than speed. (p. 109)

10. **(A)** The final step in packaging a patient on a wheeled stretcher is securing the patient to the stretcher. The particulars about using towels under the head and top sheets are specific to the standard operating procedures of your

service. Adjusting the back rest is optional depending on the patient's condition. (p. 114)

11. **(D)** If you are carrying a patient down stairs, when possible use a stair chair since it weighs less than a stretcher. Do not flex at the waist with or without bent knees. Both hands should be used to carry the stair chair. (p. 106)

12. **(B)** A scoop stretcher does not offer any support directly under the spine. It does work well for nonspinal-injured patients found in narrow places like bathrooms or hallways that will not accommodate the wheeled stretcher. (p. 119)

13. **(A)** You have a patient positioned on a scoop-style stretcher and wish to lower the patient from a roof top. You should place the stretcher and patient in a plastic basket stretcher. Make sure the basket is rated for the lift and you have the appropriate training in high-angle rescue techniques. It is not necessary to take the patient out of the scoop to place him into the wire basket. Never lower the patient in the scoop alone, as this could lead to serious injury or death. (p. 119)

14. **(A)** To avoid trauma to an injured spine, the best patient-carrying device would be the long spine board for immobilization. Then place the patient on the wheeled stretcher to move him. (p. 109)

15. **(D)** The direct ground lift is an example of a non-urgent move for a patient who has no spine injury. (p. 112)

16. **(B)** Power lifters or weight lifters use the squat-lift, and EMTs should also try to use this technique for their own safety. (pp. 106–107)

17. **(D)** Position your feet shoulder width and on firm, flat ground when lifting a patient. (p. 106)

18. **(B)** Do not compensate by leaning when lifting with one hand. (p. 106)

19. **(C)** A comfortable new device that can be used to transport a supine patient who has sustained a spinal injury is a vacuum mattress. The scoop, stairchair, and KED would *not* be used on a spinal-injured patient. (p. 119)

20. **(B)** When using an air vacuum mattress the patient is placed on the device and the air is withdrawn by the pump. The mattress will then form a rigid and conforming surface around the patient. These devices are new and rapidly expanding in their usage. (p. 119)

COMPLETE THE FOLLOWING

1. Seven patient-carrying devices include: (pp. 113–122)
   - wheeled ambulance stretcher
   - portable ambulance stretcher
   - stair chair
   - scoop stretcher
   - spine board
   - basket stretcher
   - flexible stretcher

2. Body mechanic principles include: (any four) (p. 106)
   - Position your feet properly.
   - When lifting, use your legs, not your back, to do the lifting.
   - When lifting, never twist or attempt to make any moves other than the lift.
   - When lifting with one hand, do not compensate by leaning.
   - Keep the weight as close to your body as possible.
   - When carrying a patient on stairs, use a stair chair instead of a stretcher when possible.

LABEL THE PHOTOGRAPHS (pp. 110–112)

1. Shoulder Drag
2. Incline Drag
3. Foot Drag
4. Clothes Drag
5. Firefighter's Drag
6. Blanket Drag
7. One-Rescuer Assist
8. Cradle Carry
9. Pack Strap Carry
10. Piggy-Back Carry
11. Firefighter's Carry
12. Two-Rescuer Assist

STREET SCENES DISCUSSION

1. You can try to use the vest-type immobilization device if she fits into it.

2. Just as long as the chest straps connect, the device should work to get her out of the car if you and your partners move her carefully. If the leg straps do not reach, you may need to omit them.

3. Obese people do not like to lie supine because it makes breathing difficult. Once she is on a long backboard, the vest can be loosened and 10-foot straps can be used around the long backboard to secure her chest, pelvis, and legs.

Chapter 6: Airway Management

MATCH TERMINOLOGY/ DEFINITIONS

▶ **PART A**

1. **(D)** Bronchi—the two large tubes that bring air to and from the lungs (pp. 76, 137)

2. **(F)** Cricoid cartilage—the ring-shaped structure that forms the lower portion of the larynx (pp. 76, 136)

3. **(H)** Diaphragm—the muscle of breathing that separates the abdomen from the thorax (pp. 76, 137)

4. **(A)** Epiglottis—the flap of tissue that caps the trachea as you swallow (pp. 76, 136)

5. **(I)** Exhalation—the process of breathing out (p. 76)

6. **(B)** Head-tilt, chin-lift maneuver—a means of correcting blockage of the airway by the tongue by tilting the head back and lifting the chin (p. 145)

7. **(G)** Inhalation—the process of breathing in (p. 76)

8. **(J)** Jaw-thrust maneuver—a means of correcting blockage of the airway by moving the jaw forward without tilting the head or neck (p. 145)

9. **(E)** Larynx—the voicebox, which contains the epiglottis and vocal cords (pp. 76, 136)

10. **(C)** Pharynx—the area inside the mouth joining the nasal passageways and the throat (pp. 75, 136)

▶ **PART B**

1. **(G)** Airway—the passageway by which air enters or leaves the body (p. 143)

2. **(H)** Artificial ventilation—forcing air or oxygen into the lungs when a patient has stopped breathing or has inadequate breathing (p. 146)

©2009 Pearson Education, Inc.
Emergency Care, 11th Ed.

3. **(B)** Bag-valve mask (BVM)—a handheld device with a face mask and self-refilling bag that can be squeezed to provide artificial ventilations to a patient (p. 150)

4. **(I)** Cyanosis—a blue or gray skin color resulting from lack of oxygen in the body (p. 142)

5. **(A)** Flow-restricted, oxygen-powered ventilation device—a device that uses oxygen under pressure to deliver artificial ventilation (p. 155)

6. **(C)** Gastric distention—expansion of the stomach caused by too forceful ventilation pressures, which cause excess air to enter the stomach instead of the lungs (p. 155)

7. **(F)** Humidifier—a device connected to the flowmeter to add moisture to the dry oxygen coming from an oxygen cylinder (p. 172)

8. **(D)** Respiration—another word for breathing (p. 136)

9. **(E)** Stoma—permanent surgical opening in the neck through which the patient breathes (p. 154)

10. **(J)** Ventilation—the breathing in of air or oxygen (p. 146)

▶ **PART C**

1. **(N)** Flowmeter—a valve that indicates the flow of oxygen in liters per minute (p. 171)

2. **(K)** Gag reflex—vomiting or retching that results when something is placed in the pharynx (p. 158)

3. **(G)** Ventilate—to provide ventilations at a higher rate than normal to compensate for oxygen not delivered during suctioning (p. 182)

4. **(M)** Hypoxia—an insufficiency of oxygen in the body's tissues (p. 167)

5. **(C)** Nasal cannula—a device that delivers low concentrations of oxygen through two prongs that rest in the patient's nostrils (p. 179)

6. **(A)** Nasopharyngeal airway—a flexible breathing tube inserted through the patient's nose into the pharynx to help maintain an open airway (p. 157)

7. **(B)** Nonrebreather mask—a face mask and reservoir bag device that delivers high concentrations of oxygen. The patient's exhaled air escapes through a valve. (p. 178)

8. **(J)** Oropharyngeal airway—a rigid curved device inserted through the patient's mouth into the pharynx to help maintain an open airway (p. 157)

9. **(H)** Oxygen cylinder—container filled with oxygen under pressure (p. 169)

10. **(E)** Pocket face mask—a device, usually with a one-way valve, to aid in artificial ventilation. A rescuer breathes through the valve when the device is placed over the patient's face. It also acts as a barrier to prevent contact with a patient's breath or body fluids and can be used with supplemental oxygen when fitted with an oxygen inlet. (p. 148)

11. **(O)** Pop-off valve—a valve on a BVM designed to blow off excessive pressure; this valve is no longer allowed per AHA standards on any BVM due to the danger of underinflation of the lungs. (p. 151)

12. **(D)** Pressure regulator—a device connected to an oxygen cylinder to reduce cylinder pressure to a safe pressure for delivery of oxygen to a patient (p. 171)

13. **(P)** Respiratory arrest—when breathing completely stops (p. 138)

14. **(L)** Respiratory failure—the reduction of breathing to the point where not enough oxygen is being taken in to sustain life (p. 137)

15. **(I)** Suctioning—use of vacuum device to remove blood, vomitus, and other secretions or foreign materials from the airway (p. 162)

16. **(F)** Patent airway—an open and clear passageway for air into the lungs (p. 143)

MULTIPLE-CHOICE REVIEW

1. **(A)** When we breathe in, or inspire, 21% oxygen enters the body (lungs); when we breathe out, or expire, carbon dioxide, the major waste product of respiration, and 16% oxygen exits the body. (pp. 76–77, Chapter 4)

2. **(B)** Respiratory failure is the reduction of breathing to a point where it is not sufficient to support life. Electrocution causes respiratory arrest, which is the cessation of breathing. (p. 137)

3. **(C)** Abdominal breathing, a sign of inadequate breathing, is the result of a patient using the abdomen to push up on the diaphragm in an effort to force air out of the lungs. Remember, however, that infants and children normally use their abdominal muscles more than adults do. Look, listen, and feel for air exchange to determine adequate breathing; if air is entering and leaving the nose, mouth, and chest without abnormal sounds, and at a regular rate, the patient has adequate breathing. (p. 142)

4. **(D)** All are signs of inadequate breathing. Cyanosis is common in both adults and children. Retractions (a pulling in of muscles) above the clavicles and between and below the ribs, as well as nasal flaring, occur especially in children. (pp. 142–143)

5. **(B)** In an adult, the normal respirations (in Table 6-2) are 12 to 20 a minute; therefore 14 to 18 is normal. (p. 142)

6. **(B)** When air can be felt at the mouth and nose, it may be a sign of adequate breathing. Remember, even if air can be felt at the mouth and nose, the respiratory rate must still be adequate for the breathing to be considered adequate. All other choices indicate signs of inadequate breathing. (pp. 137–139)

7. **(C)** When breathing is too slow or too fast, it can be inadequate. According to Table 6-2, for a child, that would be less than 15 per minute or greater than 30 per minute. (p. 142)

8. **(A)** According to Table 6-2, the normal adult breathing rate is 12 to 20 times a minute. (p. 142)

9. **(D)** All of the locations listed are correct, as well as the skin and lips. (p. 142)

10. **(C)** The short, choppy sentences are due to the patient being short of breath, therefore forcing him or her to take a breath between syllables. (p. 142)

11. **(D)** An open airway is paramount, since the patient who is not breathing deteriorates rapidly. This is a life-threatening situation. Open the airway, then clear the mouth and administer oxygen. (pp. 143–144)

12. **(B)** Trauma victims require the jaw-thrust maneuver to open the airway. (p. 145)

13. **(B)** The head-tilt, chin-lift maneuver provides for the maximum opening of the airway on a patient with no suspected head, neck, or spine injury. (p. 145)

14. (A) Do not allow the mouth to close when using a head-tilt, chin-lift or you will have difficulty ventilating the patient. (p. 145)

15. (D) Do not tilt or rotate the patient's head. All other choices are steps to perform the jaw-thrust maneuver. In addition, you will need to retract the patient's lower lip with your thumb to keep the mouth open. (p. 145)

16. (B) The jaw-thrust is used when you suspect possible neck, head, or spinal trauma. (p. 145)

17. (C) The American Heart Association recommends the order of preference as 4, 3, 2, 1. (p. 146)

18. (C) The patient's color would not improve if artificial ventilations were inadequate. (pp. 146–147)

19. (A) Each ventilation should be delivered over 1½ to 2 seconds for an adult. Remember that 1 to 1½ seconds is the rate for infants and children. (p. 150)

20. (B) The BVM should have a self-refilling bag, a standard 15/22-mm fitting, and a non-jam valve with an oxygen inlet. Studies show that pop-off valves prevent adequate ventilations. (p. 150)

21. (A) It is important for the BVM to perform in cold temperatures. High pressure in the chest and airway is not desirable as it increases gastric distention. As noted above, a pop-off (blow-off) valve is also undesirable. The oxygen inlet flow should be 15 liters per minute. (p. 150)

22. (D) When trauma is suspected, you should always use the jaw-thrust maneuver. All other answer choices are correct. Also make sure you use an airway and 100% oxygen reservoir system. (pp. 150–151)

23. (D) To be complete, all items listed must be used with the BVM when ventilating an unconscious patient. (pp. 150–151)

24. (D) Increasing the rate at which the bag is squeezed will *not* help. All other answer choices are correct. Also check for airway obstruction or obstruction in the BVM system. If all else fails, try a pocket mask. (pp. 153–154)

25. (C) Of the choices listed, the BVM is the best to use on a stoma, which is a surgical hole in the neck that creates an opening to the airway. (p. 154)

26. (D) All are correct. In addition, the FROPVD should have a peak flow of 100% oxygen at up to 40 liters per minute. (p. 155)

27. (C) The main function of oral or nasal airways is to keep the tongue from blocking the airway. These airways are not reusable. A patient with an amputated hand is critically injured yet probably does not need an airway. When an airway adjunct is in place, you must still remain ready to suction the patient's airway. (p. 157)

28. (C) A gag reflex causes vomiting or retching but not deep breaths or passing out. (p. 158)

29. (A) The oropharyngeal airway is measured from the corner of the patient's mouth to the tip of the earlobe on the same side of the face. (pp. 158–159)

30. (C) Both methods are acceptable, but the first method is preferred for adults. (p. 159)

31. (B) A nasopharyngeal airway should be measured from the patient's nostril to the earlobe (or angle of the jaw), which assures a proper diameter. Most nasopharyngeal airways are designed to be placed in the right nostril. The bevel should face toward the base of the nostril or toward the septum, which is in the medial portion of the nose. (p. 159)

32. (D) Always use a water-based lubricant. Petroleum and oil-based or silicone-based lubricants could cause aspiration pneumonia. (p. 159)

33. (C) The purpose of suctioning is to remove blood, vomitus, and other secretions. Teeth and large pieces need to be scooped out with a gloved hand. Try not to remove excess oxygen while suctioning. (p. 162)

34. (A) The suction unit is helpful in case the airway needs to be cleared. (p. 163)

35. (C) The Yankauer is most successfully used with an *unresponsive* patient, especially if the patient is not completely unresponsive or may be regaining consciousness. But caution must be used with rigid-tip suction; when the tip is placed into the pharynx, the gag reflex may be activated, producing additional vomiting. (p. 163)

36. (D) All choices are incorrect. The length of the catheter that should be inserted into the patient's mouth is equal to the distance between the corner of the patient's mouth and the earlobe. (p. 164)

37. (C) Never suction for longer than 15 seconds at a time, since supplemental oxygen or ventilations cease during suctioning. (p. 165)

38. (A) It is not necessary to measure when using a rigid-tip suction catheter. Rather, you should be sure not to lose sight of the tip when inserting it. (p. 164)

39. (C) The atmosphere provides 21% oxygen. Exhaled air has an oxygen concentration of 16%. (p. 167)

40. (C) Fully pressurized, a tank holds approximately 2,000 to 2,200 psi. (p. 169)

41. (B) An E cylinder is the largest portable cylinder of those listed, having 625 liters when full. The M cylinder is not a portable cylinder. (p. 169)

42. (B) Before connecting the regulator to the tank, the EMT should stand to the side and crack the valve slightly. This will clean the opening prior to attaching the regulator. Opening the valve before attaching the regulator will cause uncontrolled rushing of oxygen and is dangerous. Attach the nonrebreather mask to the regulator after it has been attached to the tank. (p. 171)

43. (C) In short term use, the dryness of the oxygen is not a problem; however, the patient is usually more comfortable when given humidified oxygen. This is true if the patient has COPD or is a child. (p. 172)

44. (A) It is now widely believed that more harm is done by withholding high-concentration oxygen from COPD patients than could be done by administering it. (p. 174)

45. (D) The nonrebreather mask provides oxygen concentrations from 80% to 100%. The nasal cannula and venturi are low concentration; the simple face mask is a medium concentration device. (p. 179)

46. (D) As noted above, the nonrebreather mask will provide concentrations of oxygen ranging from 80% to 100%. (p. 179)

47. (B) The maximum flow can range from 12 to 15 liters per minute. The reservoir bag must always contain enough oxygen so that it does not deflate by more than one-third when the patient takes his deepest inspiration. (p. 179)

48. (C) A nasal cannula provides low concentrations of oxygen between 24% and 44%. (p. 179)

49. (B) A rapid breathing rate that is shallow often means a diminished minute volume, which can be life-threatening. (p. 141)

50. (D) The areas of the lungs outside the alveoli are known as anatomic dead space. About 30% of inhaled air rests in this dead space. (p. 141)

COMPLETE THE FOLLOWING

1. The signs of inadequate breathing are: (any six) (p. 142)
   - Chest movements are absent, minimal, or uneven.
   - Movements associated with breathing are limited to the abdomen (abdominal breathing).
   - No air can be felt or heard at the nose or mouth, or the amount of air exchanged is below normal.
   - Breath sounds are diminished or absent.
   - Noises such as wheezing, crowing, stridor, snoring, gurgling, or gasping are heard during breathing.
   - The rate of breathing is too rapid or slow—above or below normal rates.
   - Breathing is very shallow, very deep, or appears labored.
   - The patient's skin, lips, tongue, earlobes, or nail beds are blue or gray.
   - Inspirations are prolonged or expirations are prolonged.
   - The patient is unable to speak, or the patient cannot speak in full sentences because of shortness of breath.
   - In children, there may be retractions above the clavicles and between and below the ribs.
   - Nasal flaring may be present, especially in infants and children.

2. In order of preference, the four techniques available to the EMT to provide artificial ventilations are: (p. 146)
   - Mouth-to-mask (preferably with high flow supplemental oxygen at 15 liters per minute).
   - Two-rescuer bag-valve mask (preferably with high-flow supplemental oxygen at 15 liters per minute).
   - Flow restricted, oxygen-powered ventilation device.
   - One-rescuer bag-valve mask.

3A. (p. 170)
   - Always use pressure gauges, regulators, and tubing that are intended for use with oxygen.
   - Always use nonferrous metal oxygen wrenches for changing gauges and regulators or for adjusting flow rates.
   - Always ensure that valve seat inserts and gaskets are in good condition.
   - Always use medical grade oxygen.
   - Always open the valve of an oxygen cylinder fully, then close it half a turn to prevent someone else from thinking the valve is closed and trying to force it open.
   - Always store reserve oxygen cylinders in a cool, ventilated room, properly secured in place.
   - Always have oxygen cylinders hydrostatically tested every 5 years.

3B. (pp. 170–171)
   - Never drop a cylinder or let it fall against any object.
   - Never leave an oxygen cylinder standing in an upright position without being secured.
   - Never allow smoking around oxygen equipment in use.
   - Never use oxygen equipment around an open flame.
   - Never use grease, oil, or fat-based soaps on devices that will be attached to an oxygen supply cylinder.
   - Never use adhesive tape to protect an oxygen tank outlet or to mark or label any oxygen cylinders or oxygen delivery apparatus.
   - Never try to move an oxygen cylinder by dragging it or rolling it on its side or bottom.

LABEL THE DIAGRAM (p. 137)

1. Pharynx
2. Nasopharynx
3. Oropharynx
4. Epiglottis
5. Larynx
6. Thyroid cartilage
7. Cricoid cartilage
8. Trachea
9. Bronchiole
10. Left main bronchus
11. Right main bronchus
12. Diaphragm
13. Lungs

STREET SCENES DISCUSSION

1. An oropharyngeal (oral) airway. Try inserting one of the appropriate size straight in with a tongue depressor.

2. Quickly turn the patient onto his side, remove the airway adjunct and BVM, and allow him to vomit. Make sure you clear out the airway so he does not aspirate vomitus into his lungs.

3. Yes, consider an ALS unit. If one is not on scene when you are ready to transport, arrange an intercept en route to the hospital. ALS providers can intubate the patient and administer medication as needed.

CASE STUDY—THE COMPLICATED AIRWAY:

▶ THE SELF-INFLICTED SHOOTING

1. Open the patient's airway by jutting the jaw, if possible, or pulling the tongue forward away from the back of the throat.

2. **A)** Yes! The patient needs to be suctioned.
   B) The maximum time is about 15 seconds per attempt. Keep in mind, however, that you must adequately clear his airway so he does not aspirate any blood. If in cardiac arrest, maximum 10 seconds.

3. Yes, an oral or nasal airway would be helpful to this patient.

4. A bag-valve mask should be used to assist this patient's ventilations.

5. **A)** Use 12 to 15 liters per minute.

5. **B)** Use it, but do not rely solely on it as the patient may have poor perfusion so the device may have an inaccurate reading.

6. **A)** A full D tank has about 350 liters in it.
   B) A pressure of 2,000 to 2,200 pounds per square inch (psi).
   C) It takes about 19 minutes to run the tank down to 200 psi. (This is figured out by dividing 350 liters by 15 liters per minute, which equals 23 minutes.) Then use the formula from text page 142 for cylinder D.
   $$\frac{(2{,}000 - 200)30.16}{15} = \frac{288}{15} = 19.2 \text{ minutes}$$

7. **A)** Don't exceed 15 seconds.
   B) You are removing oxygen when you suction the patient.
   C) A rigid Yankauer suction tip is most appropriate in this patient.

8. **A)** This patient is a high priority.
   B) His complicated airway is the major problem making him a priority patient.
   C) He should be transported right away.
   D) Take him to a trauma center if there is one in your region.

9. The ALS (advanced life support) treatment that might be most helpful to this patient, if you can arrange for an ALS intercept, is endotracheal intubation.

10. If you hear hissing or bubbling around the mask as you ventilate, you should check the seal on the mask and reposition the mask if necessary. Also check the jutting of the jaw since it is possible the airway is not fully opened due to the presence of partial airway obstruction noises.

Interim Exam 1

1. **(C)** Most EMT courses today are based on models developed by the United States Department of Transportation (DOT). The American Red Cross (ARC) is involved in disaster relief and basic first aid and CPR training. The American Heart Association (AHA) is involved in basic and advanced cardiac life support as well as cardiovascular research. The National Institutes of Health (NIH) provides grants for health research. (p. 6)

2. **(D)** Being pleasant, cooperative, sincere, and a good listener inspires confidence in patients and bystanders. Do not put patient safety above your own, and do not lie to the patient by telling him or her everything is all right. (p. 12)

3. **(C)** Negligence is a failure to act properly in a situation in which there was a duty to act, needed care as would reasonably be expected of the EMT was not provided, and harm was caused to the patient as a result. Abandonment means you left the patient in no one's care. Breach of promise is a distracter. (p. 54)

4. **(D)** In order for a patient to refuse care or transport, he or she must be mentally competent, oriented fully, and informed of potential consequences of refusing care. Document the refusal on a release form. (p. 50)

5. **(B)** In the case of an unconscious patient, consent may be assumed. This is known as implied consent. Triage is a French word that means "to sort." Immunity is a protection from liability. Applied is a distracter. (p. 50)

6. **(D)** Since the child's injury is not described as life-threatening, parental consent is still required. A minor cannot give expressed consent. Only life-threatening situations involve implied consent. (p. 50)

7. **(C)** Good Samaritan laws (in a number of states) grant immunity from liability to off-duty rescuers who act in good faith to provide care to the level of his training. (p. 56)

8. **(A)** Entering hazmat scenes with SCBA is not the responsibility of an EMT. Protecting yourself and others, recognizing potential problems, and notifying the hazardous-material response team are the responsibilities of an EMT at a hazardous-material incident. (p. 10–11)

9. **(B)** The form of infection control based on the presumption that all body fluids are infectious is called body substance isolation. Standard Precautions are taken only in certain circumstances. An infectious disease is a reason to take Standard Precautions. (p. 22)

10. **(D)** While the distance the object is to be carried is a consideration when planning to lift, it is not as important as the other factors. (p. 106)

11. **(C)** Use the leg muscles. Do not twist or use your back muscles while lifting; both may cause injury. (p. 106)

12. **(C)** Use the stair chair whenever possible. (p. 106)

13. **(C)** Keep your arms bent, *not* fully extended, when pushing or pulling objects. (p. 106)

14. **(D)** Unconsciousness is not a reason to use an emergency move. Use an urgent move for an unconscious patient. (pp. 108–109)

15. **(A)** The greatest danger of an emergency move is that a spinal injury may be aggravated. (p. 109)

16. **(B)** This is an extremity lift. The draw-sheet method involves a sheet. The direct ground lift requires lifting the patient from a supine position onto the rescuer's knees and then to the stretcher. The direct carry involves two rescuers lifting and curling the patient into their chests, then returning to a standing position, and then walking together with the patient. (pp. 123–124)

17. **(B)** When moving a patient from the ambulance stretcher to the hospital stretcher, you probably will use the modified draw sheet method. (p. 127)

18. **(A)** The EMTs should move to opposite sides of the stretcher to load it into the ambulance. (p. 116)

19. **(B)** Patients without spinal injury or fractures can be moved to a stretcher or stair chair, using the extremity lift. A slide transfer is from a bed to a bed. Chair lift and indirect carry are distracters. (p. 123)

20. **(A)** Drags are used only for emergencies because they do not protect the neck and spine. (p. 109)

21. **(B)** Use an even number of rescuers to lift patient-carrying devices. Odd numbers will create an imbalance. (p. 107)

22. **(B)** In order to control the patient's airway and bleeding, use an urgent move, the rapid extrication procedure. Taking time to apply a short backboard may cause a deadly delay in removing the patient. (p. 112)

23. **(D)** The piggyback carry requires that the patient be conscious so he can hold on to the rescuer. (p. 111)

24. **(C)** The firefighter's carry is generally done in one sweeping motion. (p. 111)

25. **(C)** A flexible stretcher is used in narrow hallways or restricted areas to remove a patient without spinal injuries. (p. 119)

26. **(B)** Carefully drag the patient's clothing, trying to minimize further spinal injury. The other moves would not be used on a patient with a spinal injury. (pp. 109–110)

27. **(C)** If the patient has no spinal injury and there are no space restrictions, then move the patient on the wheeled-ambulance stretcher. (pp. 114–117)

28. **(D)** Proper personal protective equipment can prevent injuries to you and your crew. (p. 23)

29. **(A)** When a threat presents itself, retreat to a safe area. (pp. 43–44)

30. **(B)** Eustress is positive stress. Distress is negative, can be cumulative, and may require a critical incident debriefing. (p. 36)

31. **(C)** When responding to a violent situation, observation begins when you enter the neighborhood or immediate area of the scene. (pp. 43–44)

32. **(B)** One crew member should always carry a portable radio to enable him to call for police assistance. (p. 41)

33. **(B)** Quickly control bleeding; then have the dog locked in another room so it doesn't try to protect its owner by attacking you. (pp. 42–43)

34. **(C)** Treat life-threatening problems and transport a patient who refuses care and then becomes unconscious. (pp. 50–51)

35. (B) An advance directive is the expressed wishes of the patient or family in writing. If one of these documents is signed and at the patient's side, it can simplify resuscitation situations. (p. 51)

36. (C) The oral wishes of the patient's family are not a reason to withhold medical care. (pp. 51, 53)

37. (D) Providing care within the scope of your practice, using proper documentation, and being courteous and respectful can prevent lawsuits. (pp. 55–56)

38. (D) If you are proven negligent, you may be required to pay for the patient's lost wages, medical expenses, and pain and suffering. Generally, insurance costs would not be your responsibility. (pp. 54–55)

39. (D) The skin, not the musculoskeletal system, regulates body temperature. The musculoskeletal system gives the body shape, protects internal organs, and provides for body movement. (p. 70)

40. (C) The superior portion of the sternum is called the manubrium. (p. 71)

41. (B) The protrusion on the inside of the ankle is called the medial malleolus. The lateral malleolus is on the outside of the ankle. (p. 73)

42. (B) Automaticity is the ability of the heart to generate and conduct electrical impulses on its own. (p. 75)

43. (A) The autonomic nervous system, a division of the peripheral nervous system, controls involuntary motor functions. (p. 83)

44. (B) The anatomical position is a standard reference position for the body in which the body is standing erect, facing the observer. The arms are down at the sides, and the palms of the hands are facing forward. (p. 66)

45. (A) See answer 44. (p. 66)

46. (D) Plantar refers to the sole of the foot. (p. 67)

47. (C) The zygomatic bones are the cheekbones. (p. 72)

48. (D) The heart is superior, or above, the stomach. (p. 67)

49. (B) Knees are proximal, or closer, to the torso as compared to the toes. The toes are distal, or farther away, from the torso than are the knees. (p. 67)

50. (C) Supine means lying on the back. Prone means lying face down. (p. 68)

51. (C) The abdomen is divided into four parts, or quadrants. (p. 68)

52. (A) The torso consists of the abdomen, pelvis, and thorax. (p. 67)

53. (A) The heart is located in the center of the thoracic cavity. There is no such thing as the cardiac cavity. (p. 72)

54. (C) The structure that divides the chest from the abdominal cavity is the diaphragm. (p. 76)

55. (C) The kneecap is the patella. The ilium is a pelvic bone; the malleolus is in the ankle; and the phalanges are fingers and toes. (p. 73)

56. (C) The cranium is the skull minus the facial bones. (p. 70)

57. (A) The acromion process of the scapula is the highest portion of the shoulder. (p. 74)

58. (C) Good Samaritan Laws provide some limited immunity to EMS personnel in some states. (p. 56)

59. (B) Unconsciousness in adults or children allows implied consent, thus allowing for care to begin. (p. 50)

60. (C) For negligence, three actions must be proved: the EMT had a duty to act; the EMT breached that duty; this breach of duty caused harm (physical or psychological) to the patient. (pp. 54–55)

61. (B) Lying on the stomach face down is a prone position; recovery is on the side; and supine is lying face up. Coma is a distracter. (p. 68)

62. (C) In a trauma center, surgery teams are available all the time. (p. 7)

63. (B) The National Registry of Emergency Medical Technicians has established professional standards for EMS since 1970. (pp. 13–14)

64. (D) Most patients are transported by ground ambulance. (p. 6)

65. (B) EMT-Intermediates are trained to start IVs, perform advanced airway procedures, and administer some medications beyond the EMT. (p. 10)

66. (B) Quality improvement is a continuous self-review of the EMS system or service. (p. 14)

67. (B) The Medical Director assumes the ultimate responsibility for the patient care aspects of the EMS system. (p. 16)

68. (A) A common cause of lawsuits against EMS agencies is patients who refuse care. (p. 50)

69. (D) The scope of practice defines the legal limits of the EMT's job. (p. 48)

70. (A) Decisiveness is *not* a sign of stress. (p. 37)

71. (D) Most motor vehicle collisions don't result in excessive stress reactions. (pp. 35–36)

72. (B) Increasing consumption of fatty foods is the wrong reaction to stress. (p. 37)

73. (A) If you want to reduce stress, request a change in shift or work location. Increasing your workload in any way will further increase your stress level. (p. 37)

74. (D) After a CISD, a member of the peer team offers support and referrals to assist in coping and recovering. (p. 38)

75. (C) After a major EMS incident, stress is normal and expected. (p. 35)

76. (B) The five stages of grief include a stage where the patient may retreat to a world of his own. This is called depression. (p. 38)

77. (D) PPD (purified protein derivative) is a test that will detect exposure to tuberculosis; it is not a disease. EMS providers should be concerned with hepatitis B, tuberculosis, and HIV/AIDS. (p. 33)

78. (C) A disease spread by exposure to an open wound or sore of an infected individual is caused by a bloodborne pathogen. (p. 21)

79. (D) Hepatitis is an infection that causes inflammation of the liver. (p. 27)

80. (C) Airborne diseases are spread by inhaling or absorbing droplets from the air through the eyes, nose, or mouth. (p. 22)

81. (D) Hepatitis B virus kills approximately 200 health workers every year in the United States. (p. 27)

82. (B) Assume that a patient with a productive cough has TB. (p. 27)

83. (D) HIV is not an airborne disease; it is a bloodborne disease. (p. 27)

84. **(C)** There is about a 30% chance of spreading hepatitis B with an infected needle. (p. 27)

85. **(A)** There is about a 0.5% chance of spreading HIV with an infected needle. (p. 27)

86. **(C)** To protect yourself from TB, wear BSI equipment, and take Standard Precautions, as well as a HEPA respirator. A surgeon's mask will not protect you from this airborne disease. (p. 32)

87. **(A)** Use a pocket mask with one-way valve when you are confronted with a nonbreathing patient and you are alone. The bag-valve mask needs two rescuers in order to be used effectively. You do not blow directly into the ET tube or the one-way valve. (pp. 148–150)

88. **(C)** Handwashing after each patient contact is an effective method of infection control and will reduce others' exposure risks. (p. 24)

89. **(B)** The Ryan White CARE Act establishes procedures for emergency response workers to find out if they have been exposed to life-threatening infectious diseases. OSHA does not require this. There is no such thing as an AIDS protection act. (pp. 30–32)

90. **(A)** OSHA 1910.1030 requires an exposure control plan and annual training. (p. 29)

91. **(D)** The OSHA regulation requires that every employer of EMT provide hepatitis B vaccination. Insurance or annual physicals are not required. (p. 29)

92. **(D)** Engineering controls to prevent spread of infectious diseases include all those listed. (p. 29)

93. **(C)** The bloodborne pathogen OSHA standard does not address the use of HEPA respirators since they are used for an airborne disease (e.g, TB). (pp. 28–32)

94. **(B)** High-risk locations for TB do not include day-care centers since children are not prone to TB. (p. 32)

95. **(D)** Avoid approaching a scene with your lights and sirens on, since this attracts a crowd, which you wish to avoid. (pp. 42–43)

96. **(A)** Notify police immediately if there may be any weapons at the scene. The police are responsible for weapons control; your responsibility is patient care. (pp. 42–43)

97. **(A)** Respiratory failure is the reduction of breathing to the point where oxygen intake is not sufficient to support life. Respiratory support is what you provide. Respiratory arrest is when breathing stops. Anoxic metabolism occurs in the absence of breathing. (p. 137)

98. **(C)** Cyanosis, or blue or gray skin, is *not* a sign of adequate breathing. (p. 142)

99. **(B)** Widening of the nostrils with respirations is called nasal flaring. Increased breathing rate is hyperventilation. Wheezes are a musical tone caused by spasms of the small airways. (p. 142)

100. **(B)** Blue or gray skin is called cyanosis. Anemia is a disease in which the patient has too few red blood cells. (p. 142)

101. **(C)** Inability to speak in full sentences is a sign of shortness of breath. Snoring is a noise made from a partial airway obstruction caused by the tongue. (p. 142)

102. **(B)** EMTs do not routinely insert ET tubes. All other answers listed are principle procedures used by the EMT to treat life-threatening respiratory problems. (pp. 9–10)

103. **(A)** The tongue causes most airway problems. (p. 144)

104. **(D)** If the unconscious patient is found at the bottom of a stairwell, you will need to assume a neck or spine injury and use the jaw-thrust maneuver. (p. 145)

105. **(B)** Since the one-rescuer bag-valve mask is the least effective in creating a seal, it would be the last choice. (p. 146)

106. **(C)** A ventilation rate that is too fast or too slow may result in inadequate artificial ventilation. (p. 147)

107. **(A)** The standard respiratory fitting on a bag-valve mask is 15/22 mm. (p. 150)

108. **(D)** A bag-valve mask should not have a pop-off valve. (p. 151)

109. **(C)** The proper bag-valve mask oxygen flow rate is 15 liters per minute. (p. 150)

110. **(B)** The American Heart Association's 2005 Guidelines now state that ventilation (i.e., mouth-to-mask, bag mask, or other forms of ventilation with or without supplementary oxygen) should involve sufficient ventilation volume to achieve visible chest rise. (p. 150)

111. **(C)** The first step in artificial ventilation of a stoma breather is to clear any mucus or secretions that may be obstructing the stoma. (p. 154)

112. **(A)** The audible alarm on the flow-restricted, oxygen-powered ventilation device should go off when the relief valve is activated but not when ventilation is activated. (p. 155)

113. **(B)** The oropharangeal and nasopharyngeal airways are the most common airway adjuncts. (p. 157)

114. **(D)** Use an oropharangeal airway on all unconscious patients with no gag reflex. Airway usage is not restricted to only medical or only trauma patients. (p. 158)

115. **(C)** When suctioning a patient, never suction for longer that 15 seconds. You do not *hypo*ventilate, but do *hyper*ventilate the patient prior to and after suctioning. Always wear eye protection and a mask when suctioning. Suction on the way out. (p. 165)

116. **(C)** The emergency situation in which there is a failure of the cardiovascular system to provide sufficient blood to all the vital tissues is called shock. (p. 83)

117. **(C)** Insufficiency in the supply of oxygen to the body's tissues is called hypoxia. Anoxia means no oxygen is being supplied to the cells. No oxia is a distracter. Cyanosis is a result of hypoxia. (p. 167)

118. **(A)** Change the oxygen cylinder before the pressure gauge reads 200 psi at the lowest, otherwise you may damage the inside of the tank. (p. 170)

119. **(C)** Store cylinders in a cool, dry area, *not* in a warm, humid room. (p. 170)

120. **(A)** Use a nonrebreather mask for high-concentration oxygen delivery to the breathing patient. We do not use partial rebreather masks in the field. A nasal cannula is a low-concentration device. (p. 178)

121. **(B)** The concentration of oxygen administered by a nasal cannula is between 24% and 44%. (p. 179)

122. **(B)** Do not remove the dentures unless they are loose. Dentures allow for an improved seal between the patient's face and mask. (p. 181)

123. **(A)** A child's mouth and nose are smaller and more easily obstructed than an adult's. The child's chest wall is softer. The trachea is narrower, so it is more easily obstructed. (p. 181)

©2009 Pearson Education, Inc.
Emergency Care, 11th Ed.

124. (A) Respiratory arrest is complete breathing stoppage. (p. 138)

125. (C) The flow-restricted, oxygen-powered ventilation device is usually not used in children. Other devices listed are. (p. 155)

126. (A) A flowmeter allows the control of oxygen in liters per minute. A humidifier helps prevent the oxygen from being so dry. A reservoir is used on the BVM to increase the oxygen concentration. (p. 171)

127. (B) The constant flow selector valve flowmeter allows for the control of the flow of oxygen in liters per minute in stepped increments. The Bourdon gauge and pressure compensated flowmeters are adjustable without stepped increments. (p. 172)

128. (A) Some systems use oxygen humidification to prevent drying out the patient's mucous membranes. Humidifiers are usually not used in systems with short transports and, unless they are disposable,may actually increase the potential for infection spread. (p. 172)

129. (C) Patients in the end stage of a respiratory disease are often on hypoxic drive. Carbon dioxide drive is the normal drive mechanism for healthy people. (p. 174)

130. (D) COPD is chronic obstructive pulmonary disease. (p. 174)

131. (D) When using an air mattress the patient is placed on the device and the air is withdrawn by the pump. The mattress will then form a rigid and conforming surface around the patient. These devices are new and rapidly expanding in their usage. (p. 119)

132. (C) The body system that is responsible for the breakdown of food into absorbable forms is called the digestive system. The nervous system controls the body, the urinary system eliminates the liquid wastes from the bladder, and the integumentary system covers the surface of the body. (p. 85)

133. (C) A stress reaction that involves either physical or psychological behavior manifested days or weeks after an incident is called a post-traumatic stress disorder. Acute is based on a specific incident and occurs right after that incident. Burnout is an expression for a rescue worker who has become uncaring and completely disinterested, and cumulative stress is based on many incidents over a long period of time (pp. 34–35)

134. (B) An agency privacy officer is required by the HIPAA or Health Insurance Portability and Accountability Act. NFPA sets firefighting standards and electrical codes, the Ryan White Law deals with communicable diseases and notification of emergency services personnel. The Privacy Control Act of 2002 does not pertain. (pp. 56–57)

135. (D) 12 breaths per minute times 500 mL of air per breath = 6,000 ml per minute in the adult patient. (p. 138)

Chapter 7: Scene Size-Up

MATCH TERMINOLOGY/ DEFINITIONS

1. (H) Blunt-force trauma—injury caused by a blow that does not penetrate through the skin or body tissue (p. 203)

2. (G) CHEMTREC—agency that provides advice on hazardous materials via a hotline (pp. 192, 194)

3. (D) Danger zone—area around the wreckage of a vehicle collision or other incident within which special safety precautions should be taken (p. 192)

4. (J) Domestic violence—violence in the home (pp. 194–196)

5. (F) High index of suspicion—keen awareness that a person may have injuries (p. 204)

6. (E) Law of inertia—principle that a body in motion will remain in motion unless acted on by an outside force (p. 198)

7. (A) Mechanism of injury—force or forces that may have caused injury (p. 197)

8. (I) *North American Emergency Response Guidebook*—material available for rescuers to obtain quick information about hazardous materials (p. 192)

9. (B) Penetrating trauma—injury caused by an object that passes through the skin and other body tissues (p. 202)

10. (C) Scene size-up—steps taken by an EMS crew when approaching, arriving, and attending at the scene of an emergency call to ensure the safety of the crew, the patient, and bystanders (p. 189)

MULTIPLE-CHOICE REVIEW

1. (B) Personal safety is your top priority. Determine dangers to yourself or other EMS providers from sources such as unstable vehicles, machinery, toxic exposure, or violence. If you and other crew members are not safe, you will be unable to continue with other steps in the scene size-up. (pp. 189–190)

2. (D) Scene size-up is an ongoing process throughout the call. Emergencies are dynamic; events may change without warning. For example, family members who were docile when you first arrived could turn hostile; structures that were stable could become unstable. Keep alert at all times! (p. 191)

3. (B) Always conduct your own scene size-up, no matter how many rescue vehicles or personnel are at the scene when you arrive. Never assume a scene is safe because others may have taken care of the hazards. (pp. 191–192)

4. (D) Always try to park your vehicle *uphill* from a collision scene. This way your ambulance will be out of the path of dense smoke if fuel ignites. The other actions listed are appropriate and necessary actions to take as you near a collision scene. (pp. 191–192)

5. (A) When you are in sight of the collision scene, you should watch for the signals of police officers and other emergency service personnel because they may have information about hazards or the location of injured persons. Who is in charge depends on the type of incident. The police are not the medical care experts in most communities. (pp. 191–192)

6. (B) When there are no apparent hazards, consider the danger zone to extend 50 feet in all directions from the wreckage. (p. 192)

7. (C) When a collision vehicle is on fire, consider the danger zone to extend at least 100 feet in all directions, even if the fire appears small and limited to the engine compartment. (p. 192)

8. (A) A good scene size-up should identify the potential for a violent situation. The name and amount of toxic substances would be difficult to determine during the scene size-up. The number of patients should be identified, but diagnosis is not the responsibility of the EMT. (pp. 194–195)

9. **(D)** An oxygen mask is not considered a piece of equipment used for Standard Precautions. The EMT's BSI equipment during the scene size-up may include eye protection, disposable gloves, and a mask. (p. 196)

10. **(B)** The key element of body substance isolation is to always have personal protective equipment readily available. You only need to take Standard Precautions when you might actually be exposed. Standard Precautions equipment is not placed on the patient. It is not practicable for the EMT to try to determine which body fluids are a danger. (p. 196)

11. **(B)** Injuries to bones and joints are usually associated with falls and vehicle collisions. Fights usually produce blunt injuries, and drug usage often results in overdoses. Fires and explosions produce burns. Bullet wounds can cause damage to anything in their paths. (p. 197)

12. **(C)** Knowing the mechanism of injury assists the EMT in predicting various injury patterns. While it does not assist you in immobilizing the spine, it can tell you *when* immobilization may be needed. An EMT should always take Standard Precautions. (p. 198)

13. **(C)** The law of inertia states that a body in motion will remain in motion unless acted on by an outside force. Centrifugal force is a force that explains why the faster you enter a turn the more your vehicle will be pulled straight. The formula for kinetic energy states that the mass or weight of an object is the least important contributor to the injury. (p. 198)

14. **(A)** An unrestrained driver involved in a head-on, up-and-over collision may injure his skull as well as the neck. Injuries to the fibula, knees, and femur are seen in the down-and-under pattern. (pp. 199–201)

15. **(C)** The brake pedal is least likely to be a mechanism of injury in up-and-over and down-and-under collisions. In the up-and-over pattern, the patient commonly strikes his head on the windshield and may additionally strike his chest and abdomen on the steering wheel. In the down-and-under pattern, the patient typically strikes his knees on the dash. (pp. 198–199)

16. **(C)** Knee, leg, and hip injuries are common in a head-on, down-and-under collision since the patient strikes the knees and the force is projected to the hips. The head-on, up-and-over collision produces head, neck, chest, and abdominal injuries. (p. 199)

17. **(D)** The rollover collision is potentially the most serious because of the potential for multiple impacts. Rollover collisions frequently cause ejection of anyone who is not wearing a seat belt. Expect any type of serious injury pattern. (pp. 199–201)

18. **(D)** A patient who fell three times his height, a spiderweb crack in the windshield, and a broken steering column are examples of mechanisms of injury. A flat tire is not a mechanism of injury. (p. 202)

19. **(A)** A severe fall for an adult is over 15 feet or three times the patient's height because a fall from this height will most likely involve a spinal injury. Falls from great heights are not always fatal because patients often strike objects that break their fall, such as a canopy. (p. 202)

20. **(A)** A penetrating injury that is usually limited to the penetrated area is called a low-velocity injury. The medium- and high-velocity injuries have larger zones of damage due to cavitation in the tract of the projectile. (pp. 202–203)

21. **(C)** The pressure wave around the bullet's tract through the body is called cavitation. Exsanguination is when a patient rapidly bleeds to death. Gas penetration can occur with air rifles. Pressure damage occurs only occasionally. (p. 203)

22. **(C)** An injury caused by a blow that strikes the body but does not penetrate the skin is called blunt-force trauma. There is no such term as inertia trauma. Cavitation is defined in answer 21. Rotational impact is a type of automobile collision. (p. 203)

23. **(B)** It would most likely be necessary for you and your partner to call for additional assistance lifting the 350-pound patient with the broken leg. Two patients with flu-like symptoms, especially if one is a child, could easily be handled in one ambulance. The patient with a deep laceration in his right forearm could be handled by you and your partner. The patient who loses consciousness while you are carrying her to the ambulance should be managed immediately by you and your partner. (p. 204)

24. **(A)** While in the living room of a private house treating a patient for nausea, headache, and general body weakness, your eyes begin to tear and three family members have the same symptoms. You should immediately evacuate all people from the building. Don't automatically call for three additional ambulances until you evaluate the situation. It may be a local protocol to notify the police department, but notifying the fire department is more appropriate in this situation. Any flushing of the eyes should be done after determining the nature of the substance. (p. 204)

25. **(B)** If the number of patients is more than the responding units can effectively handle, the EMT should call for additional EMS resources immediately. (p. 204)

COMPLETE THE FOLLOWING

1. The four parts of the scene size-up include: (pp. 189–190)
   - Scene safety
   - Mechanism of injury or nature of illness
   - Number of patients
   - Additional resources

2. The five signs of danger from violence that you may observe as you approach the scene are: (pp. 194–195)
   - Fighting or loud voices
   - Weapons visible or in use
   - Signs of alcohol or other drug use
   - Unusual silence
   - Knowledge of prior violence

3. Five types of motor vehicle collisions include: (pp. 198–201)
   - Head-on
   - Rear-end
   - Side-impact
   - Rollover
   - Rotational impact

4. Three sources of information about the nature of illness include: (p. 204)
   - Patient
   - Family and bystander
   - Scene

1. Try to find out what the chemical is from the driver. Let the dispatcher know right away that this is a hazardous-material incident. (You will learn more about such incidents when you read Chapter 34.)

2. You must follow your local protocols in such a situation. In general, if you are alone, you should retreat to a position of safety, call for help, and return only after the scene has been secured by the police.

Chapter 8: The Initial Assessment

MATCH TERMINOLOGY/ DEFINITIONS

1. **(H)** Alert—awake and oriented (pp. 213–214)

2. **(F)** AVPU—memory aid for classifying the levels of responsiveness or mental status (p. 213)

3. **(C)** Capillary refill—method of assessing circulation in a pediatric patient (pp. 214–215)

4. **(D)** Chief complaint—reason EMS was called (p. 210)

5. **(E)** General impression—part of the EMT's evaluation that includes assessment of the environment and the patient's chief complaint and appearance (p. 210)

6. **(A)** Initial assessment—steps taken by the EMT for the purpose of discovering and dealing with a patient's life-threatening problems (p. 210)

7. **(G)** Interventions—actions taken to correct a patient's problems (p. 210)

8. **(B)** Mental status—level of a patient's responsiveness (p. 213)

9. **(J)** Responsive—ability to respond to stimuli (pp. 213–214)

10. **(I)** Unresponsive—lack of response to any stimuli (pp. 213–214)

MULTIPLE-CHOICE REVIEW

1. **(D)** The assessment of blood pressure is not part of the initial assessment. It is part of taking vital signs, which is performed after the initial assessment and is discussed further in Chapter 9. (p. 210)

2. **(D)** The patient's past medical history is *not* part of the general impression. (p. 210)

3. **(C)** Drug-use paraphernalia may give clues about the cause of the patient's problem. The dark alley is not a helpful clue. The bruise is not an environmental indicator. You would not know the patient's medical history at this point. (p. 210)

4. **(B)** Clinical judgment is the development of that sixth sense that provides clues to the severity of the patient's condition. EMTs do not judge patients for mental status—we test it. EMTs never make a diagnosis. (pp. 210–212)

5. **(D)** When forming a general impression, always look, listen, and smell. Note the patient's age and sex and look at the patient's position. Listen for sounds such as moaning or gurgling. Smell for hazardous fumes, urine, feces, vomitus, or decay. (p. 210)

6. **(B)** Rubbing the patient's sternum briskly is the most common way to determine the patient's level of responsiveness. Ammonia inhalants can cause injury. Applying ice to the groin doesn't work. Pressing on the person's nail beds is a way of assessing capillary refill. (p. 213)

7. **(D)** AVPU stands for alert, verbal, painful stimuli, unresponsive. (p. 213)

8. **(C)** See answer 7. (p. 213)

9. **(B)** See answer 7. (p. 213)

10. **(B)** The unresponsive patient will be a higher priority and in need of quicker transport. The jaw-thrust maneuver is usually not used on responsive patients unless they have head, neck, or spinal injuries. (p. 215)

11. **(D)** If a patient is not alert and his breathing rate is slower than 8, provide positive-pressure ventilations with 100% oxygen. (pp. 214–215)

12. **(B)** An alert patient with a breathing rate faster than 24 warrants high-concentration oxygen via nonrebreather. (p. 216)

13. **(D)** The circulation assessment includes evaluating pulses, skin (condition, color, and temperature), and bleeding. The blood pressure is a vital sign taken moments after the initial assessment. (pp. 214–215)

14. **(D)** Good circulation exhibits as warm, dry, and normal in color provided the assessment is not complicated by the environment in which you find the patient (e.g., rain or cold). (pp. 214–215)

15. **(C)** Poor circulation exhibits as cool, pale, and moist skin. Increased perfusion and high blood pressure may show as flush colored skin. Cold exposure exhibits as red in early stages, and then pale to cyanotic in prolonged cases. (pp. 214–215)

16. **(A)** To evaluate skin color or the presence of jaundice or cyanosis on a dark-skinned patient, look at the lips or nail beds. (pp. 214–215)

17. **(C)** If even one large vessel or several smaller ones are bleeding, a patient can lose enough blood in a minute or two to die. Severe blood loss is life-threatening. (p. 215)

18. **(B)** Any life threats observed during the initial assessment should be treated immediately. (p. 215)

19. **(D)** High-priority conditions include poor general impression, unresponsive, responsive but not following commands, difficulty breathing, shock, complicated childbirth, chest pain with systolic blood pressure less than 100, uncontrolled bleeding, severe pain anywhere. (p. 215)

20. **(C)** Uncomplicated childbirth is not a priority. See answer 19. (p. 215)

21. **(C)** During the initial assessment of an adult medical patient you note the breathing rate is 28. You should consider administering oxygen by nonrebreather mask. The nasal cannula is too little, BVM is not needed, and the paper bag trick is dangerous and can lead to hypoxia. (p. 216)

22. **(B)** If the adult trauma patient you are assessing has inadequate breathing with a rate greater than 24 you should provide positive ventilations and high-concentration oxygen. (p. 216)

23. **(B)** The initial assessment is also often called the primary assessment or primary survey. (p. 210)

COMPLETE THE FOLLOWING

1. List the six steps of the initial assessment. (p. 210)
   - Form a general impression
   - Assess mental status
   - Assess airway
   - Assess breathing
   - Assess circulation
   - Determine priority

2. State what the letters in AVPU stand for. (p. 213)
   A = alert—awake and oriented (person, place, and day)
   V = verbal—responds to verbal stimuli
   P = painful—responds to painful stimuli
   U = unresponsive—does not respond to any stimuli

3. List five high-priority conditions. (any five) (p. 215)
   - Poor general impression
   - Unresponsive
   - Responsive, but not following commands
   - Difficulty breathing
   - Shock
   - Complicated childbirth
   - Chest pain with systolic pressure less than 100
   - Uncontrolled bleeding
   - Severe pain anywhere

STREET SCENES DISCUSSION

1. The airway is always the highest priority. Suction the patient's airway while maintaining spinal stabilization. Once the airway is clear, administer high-concentration oxygen.

2. This patient is a high priority. ALS would be helpful for intubation and another set of trained hands.

3. Even though the patient seems to be okay, it is always a good idea to be checked in the hospital due to the potential for aspiration or damage to the structures of the airway.

Chapter 9: Vital Signs and SAMPLE History

MATCH TERMINOLOGY/ DEFINITIONS

▶ PART A

1. (L) Auscultation—when a stethoscope is used to listen for characteristic sounds (p. 236)

2. (C) Blood pressure—force of blood against the walls of the blood vessels (p. 234)

3. (J) Brachial artery—major artery of the arm (p. 236)

4. (B) Bradycardia—slow pulse; any pulse rate below 60 beats per minute in an adult. (p. 228)

5. (D) Carotid pulse—pulse felt along the large artery on either side of the neck (p. 228)

6. (N) Constrict—to get smaller (p. 233)

7. (M) Dilate—to get larger (p. 233)

8. (A) Diastolic blood pressure—pressure remaining in the arteries when the left ventricle of the heart relaxes and refills (p. 234)

9. (E) Palpation—feeling with the fingertips (p. 236)

10. (H) Pulse—rhythmic beats felt as the heart pumps blood through the arteries (p. 227)

11. (I) Pulse quality—rhythm (regular or irregular) and force (strong or weak) of the pulse (p. 228)

12. (F) Pulse rate—number of pulse beats per minute (p. 227)

13. (K) Pupil—black center of the eye (p. 233)

14. (O) Radial pulse—pulse felt at the wrist on the lateral (thumb) side (p. 228)

15. (G) Reactivity—reacting to light by changing size such as occurs in the pupils of the eyes (p. 233)

▶ PART B

1. (A) Respiratory quality—normal or abnormal (shallow, labored, noisy) character of breathing (p. 229)

2. (B) Respiratory rate—number of breaths taken in one minute in an adult. (p. 229)

3. (E) Respiratory rhythm—regular or irregular spacing of breaths (p. 231)

4. (F) SAMPLE history—information about the present problems (signs and symptoms) and past medical history of a patient (p. 242)

5. (G) Sign—an indication of a patient's condition that is objective—something you see, hear, feel, or smell (p. 242)

6. (I) Sphygmomanometer—cuff and gauge used to measure blood pressure (p. 236)

7. (H) Symptom—an indication of a patient's condition that cannot be observed but rather is subjective—something felt and reported by the patient (p. 242)

8. (D) Systolic pressure—pressure created when the heart contracts and forces blood into the arteries (p. 234)

9. (C) Tachycardia—rapid pulse; any pulse rate above 100 beats per minute in an adult (p. 228)

10. (J) Vital signs—outward signs of what is going on inside the body, including respiration; pulse; skin color, temperature, and condition; pupils; and blood pressure (p. 226)

MULTIPLE-CHOICE REVIEW

1. (D) Pulse oximetry is not officially considered a vital sign. The respiratory rate and quality, skin color and condition, and the pulse rate and quality are all vital signs. (p. 226)

2. (B) A sign that gives important information about the patient's condition but is *not* considered a vital sign is the mental status. All other signs listed are vital signs. (p. 236)

3. (B) Vital signs should be recorded as they are obtained to prevent you from forgetting them and to note the time they were taken. The vitals can change quickly as the patient's condition changes. They are taken at least twice to develop trends in vital signs. The first measurements you take are called baseline vital signs. (p. 236)

4. (D) When a patient's pulse rate exceeds 100 beats per minute, this is called tachycardia. See Table 9-1 for normal pulse rates and possible causes of change in pulse quality. (p. 228)

5. (D) Based upon the pulse alone, a sign that something may be seriously wrong with a patient could be a sustained rate below 50 beats per minute, a sustained rate above 120 beats per minute, and/or a rate above 150 beats per minute. (p. 227)

6. (B) In addition to answer 5, another serious indicator found in the pulse may be an irregular rhythm. An athlete with a pulse of 50 is not unusual because aerobic training will lower the at-rest pulse. Exercise normally increases the pulse rate. (p. 227)

7. **(C)** The quality of the pulse includes determining the rhythm and force. (p. 228)

8. **(C)** A patient described as having a "thready" pulse has a weak pulse. See Table 9-1. (p. 228)

9. **(C)** The normal pulse rate for a school-age child (6–10 years) is 70 to 110. See Table 9-1. (p. 228)

10. **(A)** The normal pulse rate for an adult is 60 to 100. See Table 9-1. (p. 228)

11. **(B)** The pulse at the thumb side of the wrist is referred to as the radial pulse. The femoral pulse is in the thigh. The carotid pulse is in the neck. The brachial pulse is in the arm. (p. 228)

12. **(C)** When assessing the carotid pulse, the EMT should be aware that excessive pressure can slow the heart, especially in older patients. Never assess the carotid pulses on both sides at the same time. (p. 229)

13. **(C)** The number of breaths a patient takes in one minute is called the respiratory rate. (p. 229)

14. **(A)** The respiratory rate is classified as normal, slow, or rapid. The respiratory *quality* is classified as normal, shallow, labored, or noisy. The pulse force is classified as weak, thready, or full. (p. 229)

15. **(C)** If the EMT is treating a patient with a sustained respiratory rate above 24 or below 8 breaths per minute, high-concentration oxygen must be administered. Also be prepared to assist ventilations. (pp. 230–231)

16. **(B)** The normal respiration rate for an adult at rest is 12 to 20. See Table 9-2. (p. 230)

17. **(C)** The normal respiration rate for a toddler (1–3 years) is 20 to 30. See Table 9-2. (p. 230)

18. **(A)** Shallow breathing occurs when there is only slight movement of the chest or abdomen. If there is stridor or grunting on expiration, this indicates an airway obstruction. The chest muscles normally expand fully with each breath. (pp. 230–231)

19. **(B)** Many resting people breathe more with their diaphragm than with their chest muscles. (p. 231)

20. **(D)** Delayed capillary refill is *not* a sign of labored breathing. When a patient has labored breathing, he/she may have an increase in the work of breathing, use of accessory muscles, nasal flaring, and retractions above the collarbones. (p. 231)

21. **(C)** A harsh, high-pitched sound heard on inspiration when a patient has labored breathing is called stridor. Nasal flaring, grunting, and gurgling are signs of upper airway problems. (p. 231)

22. **(C)** When the quality of a patient's respirations is abnormal due to something blocking the flow of air, this is referred to as noisy breathing. Sounds to be concerned with are snoring, wheezing, gurgling, and crowing. (p. 231)

23. **(A)** A sound made by the patient that usually indicates the need to suction the airway is called gurgling. Crowing and stridor are upper airway noises. Wheezing is usually an indication of a lower airway problem. (p. 231)

24. **(B)** The best places to assess skin color in adults are the inside of the cheek and the nail beds as well as the inside of the lower eyelids. (p. 231)

25. **(C)** Blood loss, shock, hypotension, or emotional distress may result in pale skin. Jaundiced skin is due to liver abnormalities. See Table 9-3. (p. 231)

26. **(D)** A patient with a lack of oxygen in the red blood cells resulting from inadequate breathing or heart function will exhibit cyanotic skin. Pink skin is normal; pale skin is due

to shock; and flushed skin is a result of hypertension. See Table 9-3. (p. 231)

27. **(D)** The skin of a patient who has liver abnormalities may appear jaundiced, or yellow tinged. See Table 9-3. (pp. 231–232)

28. **(B)** Cold, dry skin is frequently associated with exposure to cold. Shock and anxiety would result in skin that is cool and clammy. See Table 9-4. (p. 232)

29. **(A)** Hot, dry skin is frequently associated with high fever or heat exposure. See Table 9-4. (p. 232)

30. **(C)** If you notice that the patient's right arm is much cooler than the rest of the patient's body, this should lead you to consider a circulatory system problem. (pp. 232–233)

31. **(B)** If you press on a child's nail bed and watch how long it takes for the normal pink color to return, you are testing for capillary refill. Normally, this action takes no more than 2 seconds. If it takes longer, the patient's blood is probably not circulating well. (p. 233)

32. **(B)** If a patient is in direct sunlight or very bright conditions, the EMT should test the pupils by covering the patient's eyes for a few moments, then uncovering one eye at a time. (p. 233)

33. **(D)** A patient in shock does not normally have unequal pupils. The pupils may be unequal due to stroke, head injury, or eye injury. See Table 9-5. (p. 234)

34. **(B)** Fright, blood loss, drugs, and treatment with eyedrops may cause the patient's pupils to become dilated. Constricted pupils are often due to narcotics. Unequal pupils are addressed in answer 33. (p. 234)

35. **(A)** When the left ventricle of the heart relaxes and refills, the pressure in the arteries is called the diastolic pressure. (p. 234)

36. **(B)** The pulse oximeter should be used with patients complaining of respiratory problems. It is inaccurate with hypothermic or shock patients, and may produce falsely high readings in patients with carbon monoxide poisoning. (pp. 239–240)

37. **(A)** The pulse oximeter is helpful because it encourages you to be more aggressive about providing oxygen therapy. (pp. 239–240)

38. **(C)** The oximeter will produce falsely high readings in patients with carbon monoxide poisoning. (p. 241)

39. **(B)** Chronic smokers may have a pulse oximeter reading that is higher than normal. (p. 241)

40. **(C)** The normal pulse oximeter reading for a healthy person should be between 95% and 100% (p. 241)

41. **(C)** Feel the patient's skin with the back of the hand to determine the patient's skin temperature. (p. 232)

42. **(B)** Goose pimples or pilo erection is associated with the chills. (p. 232)

43. **(A)** The systolic blood pressure is created when the heart contracts. (p. 234)

44. **(C)** When it is noisy a BP can be taken by palpation without a stethoscope. This reveals only the systolic reading. (p. 236)

45. **(C)** 90 mmHg is the limit below which hypotension is considered serious in an adult patient. (p. 235)

46. **(D)** The "M" in SAMPLE can include prescribed medications, over the counter medications, vitamins, herbal supplements, and recreational drugs. (p. 226)

COMPLETE THE FOLLOWING

1. The five vital signs are: (p. 226)
   - pulse
   - pupils
   - respiration
   - blood pressure
   - skin (temperature, color, condition)

2. The components of the SAMPLE history include: (p. 242)

   <u>S</u>igns & symptoms

   <u>A</u>llergies

   <u>M</u>edications

   <u>P</u>ertinent past history

   <u>L</u>ast oral intake

   <u>E</u>vents leading to the injury or illness

LABEL THE DIAGRAM (p. 84)

1. carotid   **4.** femoral
2. brachial   **5.** pedal
3. radial

STREET SCENES DISCUSSION

1. No. The patient had a chief complaint of abdominal pain, which cannot be diagnosed and treated in the field, especially in an elderly patient.

2. Normal ranges for an adult are respirations between 12 and 20, pulse between 60 and 100, systolic blood pressure between 90 and 150, and diastolic blood pressure between 60 and 90. Pulse ox readings between 100 and 95 are considered normal.

3. Yes, as you would any information pertinent to the patient's current condition. (Black, tarry stools often indicate bleeding into the intestines or lower gastrointestinal tract.)

Chapter 10: Assessment of the Trauma Patient

MATCH TERMINOLOGY/ DEFINITIONS

1. **(E)** Colostomy—surgical opening in the wall of the abdomen with a bag in place to collect excretions from the digestive system (p. 267)

2. **(N)** Contusion—a bruise (p. 251)

3. **(O)** Crepitation—grating sensation or sound made when fractured bones rub against each other (p. 265)

4. **(F)** DCAP-BTLS—memory aid, the initials of which stand for deformities, contusions, abrasions, punctures/penetrations, burns, tenderness, lacerations, and swelling (p. 251)

5. **(L)** Detailed physical exam—an assessment of the head (including face, ears, eyes, nose, and mouth), neck, chest, abdomen, pelvis, extremities, and posterior of the body to detect signs and symptoms of injury. (p. 273)

6. **(K)** Distention—condition of being stretched, inflated, or larger than normal (p. 266)

7. **(I)** Focused history and physical exam—step of patient assessment that follows the initial assessment (p. 249)

8. **(H)** Jugular vein distention—bulging of the neck veins (p. 265)

9. **(J)** Laceration—a cut (p. 251)

10. **(B)** Paradoxical motion—movement of part of the chest in the opposite direction from the rest of the chest during respiration (p. 266)

11. **(C)** Priapism—persistent erection of the penis that can result from spinal cord injury or certain medical problems (p. 268)

12. **(D)** Rapid trauma assessment—quick assessment of the head, neck, chest, abdomen, pelvis, extremities, and posterior body to detect signs of injury (p. 265)

13. **(M)** Stoma—permanent surgical opening in the neck through which the patient breathes (p. 265)

14. **(A)** Tenderness—found upon palpation of a body part (p. 251)

15. **(G)** Tracheostomy—surgical incision in the neck held open by a metal or plastic tube (p. 265)

MULTIPLE-CHOICE REVIEW

1. **(C)** The EMT inspects and palpates each body part during the focused physical exam. He does not auscultate, or listen, to every body part; nor does he percuss, or tap, to elicit a tone from each body part. (pp. 249–250)

2. **(D)** The memory aid for the physical exam is DCAP-BTLS. D = deformities, C = contusions, A = abrasions, P = punctures/perforations, B = burns, T = tenderness, L = lacerations, S = swelling. (p. 251)

3. **(B)** contusions. See answer 2. (p. 251)

4. **(D)** abrasions. See answer 2. (p. 251)

5. **(A)** punctures/penetrations. See answer 2. (p. 251)

6. **(C)** swelling. See answer 2. (p. 251)

7. **(B)** A deformity is an abnormal shaped body part. A hematoma is a collection of blood under the skin. A fracture is a broken bone. Crepitation is the sound or feel of broken bones rubbing against each other. (p. 251)

8. **(B)** Burns involve reddened, blistered, or charred-looking areas. An abrasion is a scrape. A laceration is a cut, and a contusion is a bruise. (p. 251)

9. **(C)** Tenderness is usually not evident until you palpate the patient. Pain is usually present even without applying pressure, or palpation, at least until another stronger pain source overrides it. (p. 251)

10. **(A)** When capillaries bleed under the skin, this is called swelling. Punctures, lacerations, and abrasions are types of soft tissue injuries. (p. 251)

11. **(A)** If the mechanism of injury exerts great force on the upper body, a cervical collar would be appropriate. In addition, apply a cervical collar if there is any soft tissue damage to the head, face, or neck from trauma, if there has been a blow above the clavicles (collarbone), if the trauma patient has an altered mental status, or if injury cannot be ruled out—even if the mechanism of injury is not known. (p. 252)

12. **(A)** Any blow above the clavicles may damage the cervical spine. (p. 253)

13. **(B)** Experienced EMTs refer to soft collars as "neck warmers" because that is about all they are good for. Soft collars are inappropriate for field use because of their inability to provide rigid support. (p. 241)

14. **(B)** A cervical collar that is the wrong size may make breathing more difficult or obstruct the airway. The collar does not cause the spine injury although mishandling it may do so. (p. 254)

15. **(D)** Cervical immobilization is based upon the trauma patient's level of responsiveness, mechanism of injury, and location of injuries. (pp. 254–255)

16. **(C)** If you are applying a collar on the patient's neck, be sure to assess the neck before you cover it with the collar. (p. 245)

17. **(C)** A rollover collision, a motorcycle collision, a pedestrian struck by a vehicle, and an adult who fell more than *three times* his height (which often involves a spine injury) are significant mechanisms of injury. (p. 250)

18. **(B)** When a patient is unrestrained in the front seat of an auto involved in a collision, the tell-tale sign is a spider-web crack in the windshield. This is also a sign that the patient went "up and over" to sustain the injury, rather than "down and under," which would present with leg injuries. (p. 263)

19. **(C)** Airbags minimize lacerations caused by the head striking the windshield. However, airbags can hide signs that could help you predict the severity of injuries caused by the collision. Be sure to move the collapsed bag and examine the steering wheel, which may give clues to the extent of the impact on the patient's chest. (pp. 263–264)

20. **(C)** When assessing the head, do DCAP-BTLS and listen for crepitation, the sound or feel of broken bones rubbing against each other. (p. 265)

21. **(A)** When assessing the neck, do DCAP-BTLS and observe for jugular vein distention (JVD). The other responses are all parts of DCAP-BTLS. (p. 265)

22. **(B)** Neck veins should be flat and not visible when a patient is sitting up. Flat neck veins in a patient who is lying down, however, may be a sign of blood loss. (p. 265)

23. **(B)** When assessing the chest, in addition to DCAP-BTLS, inspect/palpate for paradoxical motion, movement of part of the chest in the opposite direction from the rest of the chest. This is a sign of serious injury since it indicates a great deal of force was applied to the patient's chest. (p. 266)

24. **(B)** When assessing the abdomen, in addition to DCAP-BTLS, check to see if the patient has a colostomy and/or ileostomy, a surgical opening in the wall of the abdomen with a bag in place to collect excretions from the digestive system. (pp. 266–267)

25. **(C)** When assessing the pelvis, in addition to DCAP-BTLS, check for priapism (persistent erection of the penis), a sign of a potential spinal cord injury. (pp. 268–269)

26. **(A)** The rapid trauma assessment is similar to the detailed physical exam except the rapid trauma assessment is less detailed and done more quickly. (p. 273)

27. **(B)** Critical trauma patients do not always have a detailed physical exam, especially on the scene. Performing a detailed physical exam is always a lower priority than addressing life-threatening problems. (p. 273)

28. **(A)** The detailed physical exam is more specific than the rapid trauma assessment when it comes to assessing the head. You should assess the face, ears, eyes, nose, and mouth. (pp. 273–274)

29. **(B)** The final step of the detailed physical exam is to reassess the vital signs. (p. 280)

30. **(C)** A bruise behind the ear is called Battle's sign, which is indicative of a basilar skull fracture. (p. 279)

31. **(C)** Blood in the anterior chamber (front) of the eye tells you the eye is bleeding inside and that the patient's eye has sustained significant force. (p. 279)

32. **(B)** Clear fluid draining from the ears and nose is called cerebrospinal fluid. Mucous fluid lines the respiratory tract. Lymph bathes the cells and circulates throughout the body. Synovial fluid is in the joints. (p. 278)

33. **(D)** You do *not* look for crepitation. The other choices are specific to the mouth. (pp. 279–280)

34. **(C)** The detailed physical exam is not designed for a medical patient because there are usually few signs that an EMT can find in the physical exam of a medical patient that are significant or about which you can or should do anything. (p. 280)

35. **(C)** The safest and best thing to do for a patient who could be either medical or trauma is to generally treat him or her as a trauma patient who receives the rapid trauma assessment, and if there is time, a detailed physical exam. Whenever possible, also obtain a history from any witnesses you can find. (p. 281)

COMPLETE THE FOLLOWING

1. The components of the focused history and physical exam for the trauma patient who is found with significant mechanism of injury are as follows: (p. 250)
   - Reconsider the mechanism of injury.
   - Continue spine stabilization.
   - Consider a request for advanced life support personnel.
   - Reconsider your transport decision.
   - Reassess mental status.
   - Perform a rapid trauma assessment.
   - Assess baseline vital signs.
   - Obtain a SAMPLE history.

2. The components of the rapid trauma assessment include: (pp. 260–262)
   - Head
   - Neck (Apply cervical collar after the neck has been assessed.)
   - Chest
   - Abdomen
   - Pelvis
   - Extremities
   - Posterior

3. Examples of significant MOI include: (p. 250)

SIGNIFICANT MECHANISMS OF INJURY
   - Ejection from vehicle
   - Death in same passenger compartment
   - Falls of more than 15 feet or 3 times patient's height
   - Rollover of vehicle
   - High-speed vehicle collision
   - Vehicle-pedestrian collision
   - Motorcycle crash
   - Unresponsive or altered mental status
   - Penetrations of the head, chest, or abdomen; e.g., stab and gunshot wounds

ADDITIONAL SIGNIFICANT MECHANISMS OF INJURY FOR A CHILD
   - Falls from more than 10 feet
   - Bicycle collision
   - Vehicle in medium-speed collision

LABEL THE PHOTOGRAPHS (p. 252–253)

1. Deformities
2. Contusions
3. Abrasions
4. Punctures/Penetrations
5. Burns
6. Tenderness
7. Lacerations
8. Swelling

COMPLETE THE CHART (p. 253)

1. Crepitation
2. JVD
3. Crepitation
4. Paradoxical motion
5. Crepitation
6. Breath sounds
7. Firmness
8. Softness
9. Distention
10. Pain
11. Tenderness
12. Motion
13. Distal pulse
14. Motor function
15. Sensation

STREET SCENES DISCUSSION

1. If assessment reveals respirations less than 12, greater than 28, or very shallow, you should immediately use the BVM to assist ventilation.

2. Yes, call for ALS. A patient with an open chest wound needs advanced care. If possible, arrange for ALS to intercept you en route to the hospital.

3. Emergency care priorities would be to maintain the airway and adequate ventilation of the patient.

4. If the patient is injured on the left side of the chest at the mid-clavicular line at nipple level, a lung and the heart may be injured.

CASE STUDY—MOTORCYCLE MISHAP

1. Body substance isolation—protect yourself from the blood and other body fluids found on the patient.

2. Scene safety—most notably the traffic

3. Mechanism of injury—a two-vehicle collision

4. The number of patients

5. Forming a general impression helps you to determine how serious the patient's condition is, which helps you set priorities for care and transport. The general impression is based on an immediate assessment of the environment and the patient's chief complaint and appearance. It gives you an idea of the sex and age of the patient, what happened and why EMS was called, whether the patient is injured or ill, and the severity of the patient's condition.

6. One of your partners should be holding manual stabilization of the patient's head and neck.

7. The patient appears to be alert, or "A" on the AVPU scale.

8. His broken legs may not be the worst problem, and you must assess him for life-threatening injuries first.

9. The initial assessment for Tony should consist of forming a general impression, assessing mental status (both of which you have already done), assessing his ABCs (airway, breathing, and circulation), and determining priority.

10. Signs of developing shock make Tony a high-priority patient. (You'll learn more about shock in Chapter 26.)

11. Call for ALS right away. If they are not there by the time Tony is packaged, then try to arrange a quick meeting en route to the hospital; but do not delay transport waiting for an ALS unit to arrive.

12. Deformities, Contusions, Abrasions, Punctures/penetrations, Burns, Tenderness, Lacerations, Swelling

13. Signs and symptoms, Allergies, Medications, Pertinent past medical history, Last oral intake, Events leading up to incident

14. Assess respirations, pulse, blood pressure, skin (color, condition, temperature), and pupils

15. A detailed physical exam of Tony would include an assessment of everything examined in the rapid trauma assessment, plus the face, ears, eyes, nose, and mouth.

Chapter 11: Assessment of the Medical Patient

MATCH TERMINOLOGY/ DEFINITIONS

1. **(I)** Chief complaint—reason why EMS was called, usually in patient's own words (p. 292)

2. **(F)** Medical identification device—necklace, bracelet or other device designed to notify emergency personnel that a patient has a specific medical history or condition (p. 298)

3. **(H)** Onset of pain—description of how fast or slow the pain came on and what the patient was doing when the pain started (p. 293)

4. **(E)** OPQRST—memory jogger designed to remind the EMT of what questions to ask the patient about his chief complaint (p. 293)

5. **(J)** Prior history—history relating to the patient's chief complaint (p. 295)

6. **(C)** Provocation of pain—description of what makes the pain worse, such as sitting, standing, or eating certain foods (p. 293)

7. **(B)** Quality of pain—description of the pain, such as stabbing, crampy, dull, or sharp (p. 293)

8. **(A)** Radiation of pain—description of where pain is located and where it spreads to (p. 293)

9. **(D)** Severity of pain—description of how bad the pain is, often described on a scale of 1 to 10 (p. 293)

10. **(G)** Vial of Life®—medicine-like bottle kept in the patient's refrigerator that contains a listing of his past medical history (p. 299)

MULTIPLE-CHOICE REVIEW

1. **(D)** The rapid trauma exam is not used on a responsive medical patient. (pp. 291–292)

2. **(B)** OPQRST is a memory aid to help the EMT remember questions that expand on the history of the present illness. The letters stand for onset, provokes, quality, radiation, severity, and time. (p. 293)

3. (B) Something that triggers the pain is what provokes it. Onset is when the pain started. Quality is a description of the type of pain. Radiation is where the pain is located and where it spreads. (p. 293)

4. (B) "How bad is the pain?" is a severity question usually evaluated on a scale of 1 to 10. (p. 293)

5. (C) "T" stands for time (the time the pain started). (p. 293)

6. (A) Vomiting is a sign of various medical illnesses. (p. 294)

7. (B) "P" in SAMPLE is for pertinent past history. (p. 294)

8. (C) "How have you felt today?" is a questions about the events leading up to the illness. (p. 294)

9. (D) Patients may carry an inhaler, nitroglycerin, or an epinephrine kit with them. You may need to contact the Medical Director to gain permission to assist the patient with his or her medications. (p. 295)

10. (C) When a medical patient complains of difficulty breathing, but does not have a prescribed medication for this condition, you should generally transport the patient to the hospital. (p. 295)

11. (B) The main difference in approach to the focused history and physical exam for the responsive versus the unresponsive patient is that the unresponsive patient will be given a rapid physical exam first. The responsive patient would get the OPQRST questions first. Bystanders and family are more important if the patient is unresponsive, because they must supply information about the patient since the unresponsive patient is unable to do so. (p. 296)

12. (D) An unresponsive patient would be unable to answer the SAMPLE history questions. (p. 296)

13. (B) Check the medical patient's extremities for sensation and motor function as well as pulse. (p. 296)

14. (C) The bracelet or necklace could be a medical identification device that gives clues to the patient's medical history. (p. 298)

15. (B) A Vial of Life® is usually stored in the refrigerator and may be helpful when treating an unconscious patient. (p. 299)

COMPLETE THE FOLLOWING

1. The components of a focused history and physical exam for an unresponsive medical patient include: (pp. 296–299)
   - Conduct a rapid physical exam.
   - Obtain baseline vital signs.
   - Consider a request for ALS personnel.
   - Take a history of the present illness (OPQRST) and a SAMPLE history from the family or bystanders.

2. Questions to ask a bystander who witnessed a patient's medical emergency are: (any four) (p. 299)
   - What is the patient's name?
   - What happened?
   - Did the bystander see anything else?
   - Did the patient complain of anything before this happened?
   - Does the patient have any known illnesses or problems?
   - Is the patient taking any medications?

COMPLETE THE CHART
(p. 293–294)

1. Signs and symptoms	5. Last meal
2. Allergies	6. Events leading up to illness
3. Medications	7. Onset
4. Pertinent past history	8. Provokes

9. Quality
10. Radiation
11. Severity
12. Time

STREET SCENES DISCUSSION

1. A patient with breathing difficulty who speaks in short, choppy sentences may be breathing inadequately.

2. No. If there are no chest sounds during an asthma attack, the patient may not be moving enough air.

3. The term for lung sounds described as "noisy, like a whistling sound" is wheezing. A wheeze is a musical tone caused by air being forced through constricted air passageways. This is due to bronchoconstriction and the build-up of mucus.

4. Yes. If the patient has a prescribed inhaler, you may be able to assist the patient in taking the medication. This may be done only after consultation with medical direction, often during transportation to the hospital.

5. SpO_2 of 96% means the hemoglobin is saturated 96% with oxygen. This is an acceptable reading.

Chapter 12: Ongoing Assessment

MATCH TERMINOLOGY/ DEFINITIONS

1. (B) Interventions—actions taken to prevent a patient's problems (p. 310)

2. (C) Ongoing assessment—four-step procedure for detecting changes in a patient's condition (p. 308)

3. (A) Trending—changes in a patient's condition over time, which may show improvement or deterioration, and which can be shown by documenting repeated assessments (p. 310)

MULTIPLE-CHOICE REVIEW

1. (D) It is important to observe and reobserve the patient. Therefore, in the ongoing assessment, you need to repeat key elements of assessment procedures already performed in order to detect any changes in patient condition. (p. 307)

2. (C) The ongoing assessment must never be omitted or skipped unless life-saving interventions prevent the EMT from doing it. Frequently, one partner can perform the ongoing assessment while the other performs the interventions. (p. 307)

3. (D) Use a quiet, reassuring voice when talking to the infant or child. Also maintain eye contact. Try to stay on the same level as the infant or child or close to or at eye level. (p. 307)

4. (D) The ongoing assessment does not involve repeating all interventions since some interventions may be adequate or are ongoing. However, it does involve evaluating the adequacy of your interventions more objectively and to adjust them as necessary. The ongoing assessment does include repeating the initial assessment for life-threats, the focused assessment, and the vital signs. (p. 308)

5. (B) The sequence for performing the ongoing assessment is: repeat the initial assessment, reassess vital signs, repeat the focused assessment, and last, check interventions. (pp. 308–310)

6. **(D)** Applying a cervical collar is part of the rapid trauma assessment, not the initial assessment. When repeating the initial assessment, make sure that you reestablish patient priorities, monitor skin color and temperature, and maintain an open airway. (p. 309)

7. **(D)** The onset of shock is signaled by rapid pulse and cool and pale skin. This is a life-threat and should be watched for continually and treated immediately. (p. 309)

8. **(C)** The mental status of an unresponsive child or infant can be checked by shouting (verbal stimulus) or by flicking the feet (painful stimulus). The parent can also be helpful by explaining how the child normally behaves. A sternal rub or pin to the foot is too aggressive and may injure the child. (p. 309)

9. **(D)** An example of checking interventions during the ongoing assessment of a medical patient is assuring adequacy of oxygen delivery. Taking a blood pressure is obtaining a vital sign and is not an intervention. Bandaging and applying a tourniquet are treatments. (p. 310)

10. **(C)** Frequent reassessment establishes trends, or changes over time, that the EMT needs to pay attention to. You may need to institute new treatments or adjust treatments you have already started based on these trends. (pp. 310–311)

11. **(C)** The best way to determine if the patient is improving or deteriorating is to do frequent ongoing assessments. (p. 312)

12. **(C)** If the patient is stable, reassessment of vitals should be every 15 minutes. If the patient is not stable, the reassessment should be every 5 minutes. (p. 312)

13. **(A)** See answer 12. (p. 312)

14. **(C)** You should repeat the initial assessment whenever you believe there may have been a change in the patient's condition. This will help you determine if the patient needs to be reprioritized. (p. 312)

15. **(B)** Gurgling sounds in a patient's airway indicate the patient needs to be suctioned immediately. (p. 313)

COMPLETE THE FOLLOWING

1. The six steps involved in repeating the initial assessment involve: (p. 308)
   - Reassess mental status.
   - Maintain an open airway.
   - Monitor breathing for rate and quality.
   - Reassess the pulse for rate and quality.
   - Monitor skin color and temperature.
   - Reestablish patient priorities.

2. The three steps for checking interventions are: (p. 310)
   - Assure adequacy of oxygen delivery and artificial ventilation.
   - Assure management of bleeding.
   - Assure adequacy of other interventions.

STREET SCENES DISCUSSION

1. In a stroke patient, if there is any paralysis, the patient may not be able to clear and maintain her own airway.

2. The sense of hearing is one of the last ones to go. So be very careful what you say, because the patient often can hear and understand you.

MATCH TERMINOLOGY/ DEFINITIONS

1. **(E)** Base station—two-way radio at a fixed site such as a hospital or dispatch center (p. 320)

2. **(H)** Cellular phone—phone that transmits through the air instead of over wires so that the phone can be transported and used over a wide area (p. 320)

3. **(I)** Digital radio equipment—equipment that permits transmission of standard messages in condensed form by punching a key (p. 320)

4. **(A)** FCC—(Federal Communications Commission) federal agency that regulates radio communications (p. 321)

5. **(G)** Mobile radio—two-way radio that is used or affixed in a vehicle (p. 320)

6. **(D)** Portable radio—handheld two-way radio (p. 320)

7. **(J)** PTT—"press to talk" button on the EMS radio (p. 322)

8. **(B)** Repeater—device that picks up signals from lower-power radio units such as mobile and portable radios and retransmits them at a higher power (p. 320)

9. **(F)** Verbal report—update on the patient's condition given to hospital personnel either face-to-face or over the radio (p. 326)

10. **(C)** Watt—unit of measurement of the output power of a radio (p. 320)

MULTIPLE-CHOICE REVIEW

1. **(C)** As an EMT, your ability to communicate is very important because describing your assessment findings to the hospital may make a difference in the care the patient receives. (p. 319)

2. **(B)** EMS has progressed over the years due to the development of radio links among dispatcher, mobile units, and hospitals. (p. 319)

3. **(D)** The components of a communications system include the base station, mobile units, portable radios, repeaters, and cellular phones. (pp. 320–321)

4. **(C)** A device that picks up a lower power signal and then retransmits it at a higher power is called a repeater. (p. 320)

5. **(A)** The Federal Communications Commission (FCC) is responsible for approving communications and maintaining order on the airwaves. The FAA is the Federal Aviation Administration. FEMA is the Federal Emergency Management Agency. DOT is the Department of Transportation. (p. 321)

6. **(C)** The purposes of always following the general principles of radio transmission is to allow all persons to use the frequencies and to prevent delays. EMTs *should* request a repeat of orders from medical direction if they are unclear. The EMT should *not* use codes, but communicate in plain English. (pp. 324–325)

7. **(C)** Of the items listed, their correct sequence in a radio report is unit identification and level of provider, chief complaint, major past illness, and emergency medical care given. (p. 324)

8. (B) The reason why the ambulance was called is the chief complaint. EMTs do not make diagnoses. (pp. 323–324)

9. (D) The fact that a patient's abdomen does not feel rigid during palpation is referred to as a pertinent finding from the physical exam and is reported to the hospital. (p. 324)

10. (C) Updating the physician on the patient's mental status is a way of telling him or her how the patient is responding to the emergency medical care that was given. (p. 325)

11. (A) Whenever the EMT requests an order for medical direction over the radio, it is a good practice to repeat the physician's order back word for word, question inappropriate orders, and speak slowly and clearly. (p. 325)

12. (B) Always question the physician about an order over the radio that you think is inappropriate or that you do not understand. The physician may have misinterpreted or misunderstood your communication. (p. 325)

13. (B) Crossing your arms and looking down at the patient sends the message, "I am not really interested." Be aware of the nonverbal messages you may send by your body position and posture. (p. 326)

14. (D) If it is determined that a patient has a broken leg, tell the patient the truth in a calm voice and gentle manner. (p. 327)

15. (A) When treating a toddler, kneel down at the child's level to talk. Do not stare at the child. Never lie by saying you know his or her parents if you actually do not. The child will figure out that you are lying and will not trust you. (p. 328)

COMPLETE THE FOLLOWING

1. Five components of a communications system are: (p. 320)
   - Base station
   - Repeaters
   - Mobile radios
   - Cell phones
   - Portable radios

2. Interpersonal communication guidelines to use when dealing with patients, families, friends, and bystanders include: (pp. 326–327)
   - Use eye contact.
   - Be aware of your position and body language.
   - Use language the patient can understand.
   - Be honest.
   - Use the patient's proper name.
   - Listen.

STREET SCENES DISCUSSION

1. Calling ahead gives hospital personnel time to prepare for the patient's arrival. This may mean calling in a surgeon or a specialist or ordering a special medication.

2. Check with your instructor for your local protocols. Generally, it is the highest medically trained rescuer on scene.

3. Other types of communication were nonverbal and face-to-face, including EMT to patient and other rescue personnel such as law enforcement, the extrication crew, the incident commander, and the helicopter flight crew.

MATCH TERMINOLOGY/ DEFINITIONS

1. **(G)** Data element—each individual box on a prehospital care report (p. 336)

2. **(C)** Falsification—inaccurate entry or misrepresentation on a prehospital care report usually intended to cover up serious flaws in assessment or in care (p. 345)

3. **(H)** Minimum data set—minimum elements that are recommended by the U.S. Department of Transportation to be included in all prehospital care reports nationwide (p. 337)

4. **(D)** Objective statement—observable, measurable, and verifiable information (p. 339)

5. **(B)** PCR—report form used by EMS agencies to document prehospital assessment and care (p. 332)

6. **(I)** Electronic clipboard—clipboard-format device that is able to recognize handwriting and convert it to computer text (pp. 332, 335)

7. **(E)** Pertinent negative—exam finding that is not present or not true but is important to note (e.g., patient denies any shortness of breath) (p. 340)

8. **(F)** Special situation report—report on unusual, complex, or involved situations that is completed according to your service's standard operating procedures (p. 346)

9. **(A)** Subjective information—information from an individual point of view (p. 339)

10. **(J)** Triage tag—item affixed to a patient at a multiple-casualty incident used to record chief complaint and injuries, vital signs, and treatment given (p. 346)

MULTIPLE-CHOICE REVIEW

1. **(C)** The prehospital care report serves as a legal document as well as an aid for research, education, and administrative efforts. We do not routinely report all calls to the local police department. Because call information is confidential, it would never be used as a press release or as a receipt for the patient. (p. 335)

2. **(B)** The written PCR record provides a means for the emergency department staff to review the patient's prehospital care. (p. 336)

3. **(C)** The copy of the PCR left at the hospital should become part of the patient's permanent hospital record. (p. 336)

4. **(C)** A complete and accurate PCR will be your best recollection of the call. (p. 336)

5. **(D)** The person who completed a PCR may be called to court to testify about the call in a criminal proceeding, the care provided to the patient, and the call in a civil proceeding. (p. 336)

6. **(B)** The routine review of PCRs for conformity to current medical and organizational standards is a process called quality improvement. (p. 336)

7. **(B)** Each individual box on a PCR is called a data element. The narrative is a written description. A key punch is used to input data into a computer. (p. 336)

8. **(C)** The patient's Social Security number is not part of the minimum data set. It may be collected as a part of insurance information. According to the U.S. DOT, the minimum data set on a PCR should include respiratory rate and effort; skin color and temperature; times of incident, dispatch, and arrival at the patient; and capillary refill for patients less than 6 years old. (p. 336)

9. **(B)** Vehicle mileage is not important data. The minimum data set includes vital signs, chief complaint, and times of the call. (pp. 336–337)

10. **(B)** The time of dispatch is an example of run data on the PCR. (p. 337)

11. **(A)** Examples of patient data on a PCR would be date of birth and age. The other information is included elsewhere on the form. (pp. 338–339)

12. **(C)** Experienced EMTs consider a good PCR as one that paints a picture of the patient. Attempting to identify symptoms the patient may have overlooked is falsification. (p. 339–340)

13. **(B)** The statement "The patient has a swollen, deformed extremity" on the narrative portion of the PCR is an example of objective information. This means it is observable, measurable, or verifiable. Subjective information is information from an individual point of view. Pertinent negatives are examination findings that are negative (things that are *not* true), but are important to note. Nonstandard abbreviations should be avoided on PCRs. (pp. 339–340)

14. **(C)** Objective information is factual and need not be put in quotation marks. Subjective statements that are from an individual's point of view and that include opinions or actual statements made by bystanders, the patient, or a police officer should be in quotation marks. (pp. 339–340)

15. **(B)** In the narrative section of a PCR, the EMT should include pertinent negatives. Do not write your personal conclusions about the situation or use the radio codes for each treatment. The vital signs and times they are taken are recorded in a different section along with additional objective information. (pp. 340–341)

16. **(C)** Medical abbreviations should be used only if they are standardized to ensure that everyone who reads them will understand them. They are not used solely to save space in the narrative section of a PCR, to replace all words you cannot spell, or to ensure correct interpretation by physicians. (p. 340)

17. **(B)** The PCR form itself and the information on it should be considered confidential information. The form is a medical document. (p. 342)

18. **(D)** When a patient refuses transport, before the EMT leaves the scene, he or she should document assessment findings and care given, try again to persuade the patient to go to a hospital, and ensure the patient is able to make a rational, informed decision. (pp. 342–343)

19. **(D)** EMTs do not make a diagnosis. When completing a PCR on a patient refusal, the EMT should document that she was willing to return if the patient changed his mind, a complete patient assessment, and that alternative methods of care were offered. (pp. 342, 344)

20. **(A)** If the EMT forgot to administer a treatment that is required by a state protocol, he or she should document on the PCR only treatment actually given. Never fill the form out with excuses. Recording that the patient was given the forgotten treatment would be falsification. (pp. 344–345)

21. **(A)** Falsification of information on a prehospital care report may lead to suspension or revocation of your license or certification. (p. 345)

22. **(B)** To correct an error discovered while writing out a PCR, the EMT should draw a single horizontal line through the error, initial it, and write the correct information. Scribbling on the form is sloppy. You should be using a ballpoint pen to fill out the report; therefore, erasures may be looked upon by others as an attempt to cover up a mistake in patient care. (p. 345)

23. **(C)** If information was omitted on a PCR, the EMT should add a note with the correct information, the date, and initial it. It usually is not necessary to notify the Medical Director in this situation. (p. 346)

24. **(A)** An example of an instance in which it would *not* be unusual for the EMT to obtain only a limited amount of information is a multiple-casualty incident. An interhospital transfer and a child abuse call would probably be thoroughly documented with pertinent information. (p. 346)

25. **(A)** Special situation reports are used to document events that should be reported to local regulatory authorities. They must be accurate, neat, and submitted in a timely manner. They are reserved for special instances such as exposure to infectious disease, injury to EMTs, hazardous scenes, child or elder abuse, etc. (p. 346)

26. **(B)** Ambulance services are required by the Health Insurance Portability and Accountability Act (HIPAA) to take certain steps to safeguard patient confidentiality. The other Federal agencies listed: OSHA, NHTSA, and U.S. DOT do not regulate patient rights and confidentiality. (p. 340)

27. **(A)** An example of a method that an ambulance service would use to safeguard patient confidentiality would include requiring employees to place completed PCRs in a locked box. It would be inappropriate to use a patient's last name on the radio or review PCRs during QA meetings with a patient's name still on them. (p. 336)

28. **(D)** The policy an ambulance service develops concerning patient rights and confidentiality must take into consideration: state regulations, local regulations, and HIPAA. (p. 340)

COMPLETE THE FOLLOWING

1. Patient data on a PCR includes: (pp. 336–341)
   - the patient's name, address, date of birth, age, sex
   - billing and insurance information
   - nature of call
   - mechanism of injury (MOI)
   - location where the patient was found
   - treatment administered before arrival of EMTs
   - signs and symptoms, including baseline and subsequent vital signs
   - SAMPLE history
   - care administered to and effect on the patient
   - changes in condition throughout the call

2. Guidelines to help the EMT prepare the narrative portion of the PCR: (pp. 339–341)
   - Include both objective and pertinent subjective information.
   - Include pertinent negatives.

- Avoid radio codes and nonstandard abbreviations.
- Write legibly and use correct spelling.
- Use medical terminology correctly.
- If it's not written down, you didn't do it.

STREET SCENES DISCUSSION

1. If the call really does end up in court, it will be difficult to prove that the patient had distal function prior to and after immobilization. He therefore may be able to say that he lost sensation as part of the actual care you provided.

2. Sloppy documentation could lead a jury to believe the EMT's emergency care was sloppy, too.

3. Yes, but since it is not objective information, you should put the patient's statement in quotes.

4. The emergency department staff should place the PCR into the patient's official emergency department chart.

Chapter 15: General Pharmacology

MATCH TERMINOLOGY/ DEFINITION

1. **(H)** Activated charcoal—powder, usually premixed with water, that will adsorb some poisons and help prevent them from being absorbed by the body (p. 335)

2. **(F)** Epinephrine—drug that helps to constrict the blood vessels and relax airway passages; it may be used to counter a severe allergic reaction. (p. 359)

3. **(C)** Gel—semisolid paste form of a drug (p. 360)

4. **(A)** Indications—specific signs or circumstances under which it is appropriate to administer a drug to a patient (p. 360)

5. **(B)** Inhaler—spray device with a mouthpiece that contains an aerosol form of a medication that a patient can spray directly into his airway (p. 357)

6. **(D)** Oral glucose—medication given by mouth to treat a conscious patient (one who is able to swallow) with an altered mental status and a history of diabetes (p. 355)

7. **(I)** Oxygen—This gas, in its pure form, is used as a drug to treat any patient whose medical or traumatic condition causes them to be hypoxic, or low in oxygen. (p. 356)

8. **(J)** Suspension—liquid form of a drug in which a powder is mixed with a slurry or water (p. 360)

9. **(G)** Tablet—solid form of a drug; compressed powder (p. 360)

10. **(E)** Trade name—brand name of a medication (p. 360)

11. **(L)** Contraindications—specific signs or circumstances under which it is not appropriate and may be harmful to administer a drug to a patient. (p. 360)

12. **(K)** Side effect—any action of a drug other than the desired action. (p. 360)

MULTIPLE-CHOICE REVIEW

1. **(D)** The study of drugs and their effects is called pharmacology. Anatomy is the study of the structure of the body. Physiology is the study of the functions of the body. Medicinology is a distracter. (p. 355)

2. **(A)** Medications that are routinely carried on the EMS unit are activated charcoal, oral glucose, and oxygen. The patients may carry nitroglycerin, epinephrine, and prescribed inhalers. (pp. 355–356)

3. **(A)** Activated charcoal is an example of a powder, usually premixed with water. (p. 355)

4. **(B)** Activated charcoal is given to a patient because it will bind some poisons to its surface. It does not prevent vomiting. (p. 355)

5. **(B)** The brain is very sensitive to low levels of sugar in the blood, which may be caused by poorly managed diabetes; this can be a cause of a diabetic patient's altered mental status. (pp. 355–356)

6. **(A)** Oral glucose is given between the patient's cheek and gum because this area contains many blood vessels that allow absorption into the bloodstream. It does not cause the patient to regurgitate the stomach's contents. Oral glucose does not dilate the coronary vessels. (p. 356)

7. **(C)** Examples of medications that the patient may have in his possession that the EMT may assist the patient in taking under the appropriate circumstances are epinephrine (EpiPen®), a prescribed inhaler, and nitroglycerin. Patients do not generally carry home oxygen with them. EMTs do not assist patients in the administration of glucose injections, anticonvulsants, anti-inflammatories, insulin, or antihypertensives. (p. 357)

8. **(C)** Patients who have a medical history of asthma, emphysema, and chronic bronchitis may carry a bronchodilator. (p. 357)

9. **(C)** The drug nitroglycerin is used to dilate the coronary vessels. It is not used to constrict or dilate the peripheral vessels. (p. 358)

10. **(C)** The government publication listing all drugs in the United States is called the *U.S. Pharmacopoeia*. (p. 360)

11. **(B)** The name that the manufacturer uses in marketing a drug is called the trade name. The generic name is used more generally by all manufacturers. (p. 360)

12. **(D)** A circumstance in which a drug should not be used because it may cause harm to the patient or offer no effect in improving the patient's condition or illness is called a contraindication. An indication is a specific sign or circumstance under which it is appropriate to administer a drug. An adverse reaction is usually not known in advance. Side effects, although not desirable, are not a reason to withhold a medication (e.g., headache from nitroglycerin). (p. 360)

13. **(A)** An action of a drug that is other than the desired action is called a side effect. See answer 12. (p. 360)

14. **(D)** Prior to administering a medication to a patient, you must know the route of administration, proper dosage, and the actions the medication will take. You should know the generic name but are not expected to know the chemical name. (p. 360)

15. **(B)** Drugs prescribed for pain relief are called analgesics. See Table 15-1. (pp. 362–363)

16. **(D)** Drugs prescribed to reduce high blood pressure are called antihypertensives. See Table 15-1. (pp. 362–363)

17. **(C)** Drugs prescribed for heart rhythm disorders are called antiarrhythmics. See Table 15-1. (pp. 362–363)

18. **(B)** Drugs prescribed to relax the smooth muscles of the bronchial tubes are called bronchodilators. See Table 15-1. (pp. 362–363)

19. **(C)** Drugs prescribed for prevention and control of seizures are called anticonvulsants. See Table 15-1. (pp. 362–363)

20. **(A)** Drugs prescribed to help regulate the emotional activity of the patient to minimize the peaks and valleys in their psychological and emotional state are called antidepressants. See Table 15-1. (pp. 362–363)

COMPLETE THE FOLLOWING

1. The six medications an EMT can administer or assist a patient in taking are: (p. 355)
   - activated charcoal
   - prescribed inhalers
   - oral glucose
   - nitroglycerin
   - oxygen
   - epinephrine auto-injectors

2. The four "rights" to adhere to when administering a medication are: (p. 360)
   - The right patient.
   - The right dose.
   - The right medication.
   - The right route.

STREET SCENES DISCUSSION

1. A side effect of nitroglycerin is a drop in blood pressure. If this should occur, you may need to lay the patient down and raise the legs as you recontact medical direction for advice.

2. The patient expects the nitroglycerin to relieve his pain by dilating the coronary arteries, which supply the heart muscle with blood.

3. Yes. They are: "He denies any radiation down his arm or toward his jaw. He also denies any relief with the brief wait while sitting."

Chapter 16: Respiratory Emergencies

MATCH TERMINOLOGY/ DEFINITION

1. **(B)** Agonal respirations—sporadic, irregular breaths that are usually seen just before respiratory arrest (p. 370)

2. **(C)** Bronchoconstriction—blockage of the bronchi that lead from the trachea to the lungs (p. 380)

3. **(E)** Expiration—passive process in which the intercostal muscles and the diaphragm relax, causing the chest cavity to decrease in size and forcing air from the lungs; also called exhalation (p. 369)

4. **(A)** Inspiration—active process in which the intercostal muscles and the diaphragm contract, expanding the size of the chest cavity and causing air to flow into the lungs; also called inhalation (p. 369)

5. **(D)** Retractions—pulling in of the accessory muscles to breathe (p. 371)

6. **(F)** Inhalation—another term for inspiration (p. 369)

MULTIPLE-CHOICE REVIEW

1. **(C)** The diaphragm separates the chest from the abdomen. The intercostal muscles are between the ribs. The sternocleidomastoid muscle is in the neck. The inguinal muscle is at the base of the abdomen. (p. 368)

2. **(B)** Expiration is a passive process in which the intercostal (rib) muscles and the diaphragm relax, causing the chest cavity to decrease in size and forcing air from the lungs. (p. 369)

3. **(C)** Although rhythm must be observed, it is not included under the *quality* of breathing. Quality includes breath sounds (diminished, unequal, or absent?), chest expansion (inadequate or unequal?), and depth of respirations (labored, increased respiratory effort, use of accessory muscles?). (pp. 369–370)

4. **(C)** An unresponsive patient with shallow breaths and gasping with only a few breaths per minute (agonal respirations) is clearly breathing inadequately. You must provide artificial ventilation with supplemental oxygen preferably via pocket face mask. (p. 371)

5. **(B)** Accessory muscles, such as those in the neck and abdomen, assist in breathing, especially when a patient is having difficulty breathing. Subdiaphragmatic is a location below the diaphragm. Smooth muscles line blood vessels. Extra muscles are an inventive distracter. (p. 371)

6. **(D)** Blue-colored skin (cyanosis) that feels clammy and cool is usually a sign of inadequate breathing. (p. 371)

7. **(A)** Snoring and gurgling sounds usually indicate a partially obstructed airway. Wheezing can be a sign of anything from airway obstruction to bronchoconstriction. Sniffling is usually from a runny nose. Whistling or grunting is a distracter. (p. 371)

8. **(C)** Respiratory conditions account for a large percentage of deaths in infants and children. Motor vehicle collisions cause child deaths, but not as high a percentage as respiratory conditions. Heart attacks are more rare in children. Infections are high in infants, but decrease in children. (p. 371)

9. **(D)** The cricoid cartilage of infants and children is less developed and less rigid than is an adult's. (p. 371)

10. **(B)** Infants and children depend more heavily on the diaphragm for breathing because the chest wall is softer. They do not inhale twice the air, and they may grunt only when they are in respiratory distress. (p. 371)

11. **(D)** Signs of inadequate breathing in infants and children include nasal flaring (widening of the nostrils), grunting, seesaw breathing, and retractions. Lip quivering is a distracter. (p. 371)

12. **(C)** It is not enough to simply make sure the patient is breathing. The patient must be breathing *adequately*. (p. 371)

13. **(A)** In order of preference, the means of providing artificial ventilation are as follows: 1. Pocket face mask with supplemental oxygen, 2. Two-person BVM with supplemental oxygen, 3. Flow-restricted, oxygen-powered ventilator, 4. One-person BVM with supplemental oxygen. (p. 371)

14. **(D)** If you are unsure about whether a patient needs artificial ventilation, you should provide artificial ventilation. (p. 372)

15. **(B)** Artificially ventilate at a rate of 10–12 breaths per minute for an adult and 12–20 breaths per minute for infants and children, according to American Heart Association standards. (p. 370)

16. **(C)** See answer 15. (p. 370)

17. **(C)** A low pulse in infants and small children in the setting of a respiratory emergency usually means trouble. In infants and children with respiratory difficulties, you may observe a slight increase in pulse early, but soon the pulse will drop significantly. (p. 373)

18. **(B)** Increase the force of ventilations for any patient—adult, child, or infant—if the chest does not rise and fall with each artificial ventilation, or the pulse does not return to normal. If the chest still does not rise, check that you are maintaining an open airway. (p. 373)

19. **(A)** With certain lower airway respiratory diseases or infections in infants and children, it is dangerous to probe or place anything in the patient's mouth or pharynx because this may set off spasms along the airway. (p. 373)

20. **(D)** Patients with lower airway obstruction may be wheezing, have increased breathing effort upon exhalation, and have rapid breathing without stridor. Their skin may be pale or blue, but not yellow. Yellow skin is an indication of liver abnormalities. (p. 373)

21. **(C)** A patient with breathing difficulty frequently speaks in short, choppy sentences. The other choices are distracters. (p. 374)

22. **(B)** In a tripod position, the patient is leaning forward with hands resting on the knees or table. The recovery position is lying on the side, which allows fluid to drain from the mouth. Supine with knees flexed is helpful with abdominal pain. (pp. 374–375)

23. **(D)** Headache and vomiting are *not* commonly associated with breathing difficulties. Crowing, retractions, an increased pulse, and coughing are all common signs associated with breathing difficulty. Restlessness, shortness of breath, and chest tightness are common symptoms of patients with breathing difficulty. (p. 376)

24. **(B)** If a patient is suffering from breathing difficulty and is breathing adequately, administer oxygen via nonrebreather mask. The BVM and pocket mask are for patients in severe distress. (p. 376)

25. **(C)** If a patient is experiencing breathing difficulty and is breathing adequately, it is best to place him in a position of comfort. This is frequently the sitting-up position. Most patients with breathing difficulty feel they can breathe better this way. The tripod position is a position the patient with breathing difficulty assumes. A patient with inadequate breathing would need to be supine to receive assisted ventilations. (p. 376)

26. **(C)** An inhaler, also referred to as a puffer, is commonly used for patients with respiratory problems that cause bronchoconstriction. (p. 380)

27. **(C)** When giving a medication by an inhaler, a syringe is not needed. The patient must be alert and cooperative, and the right dose of unexpired medication must be given. (p. 380)

28. **(A)** Prior to coaching the patient in the use of an inhaler, first shake it vigorously. It is not necessary to test the unit by spraying it into the air. (p. 381)

29. **(B)** To ensure that the most medication is absorbed when using an inhaler, encourage the patient to hold the breath as long as possible so the medication can be absorbed by the lungs. Unless the medication is held in the lungs, it will have minimal or no value. (p. 380)

30. **(C)** When documenting a respiratory complaint, ask the patient to describe the difficulty in his own words. Answering history questions is also helpful. It is not necessary to count respirations for two minutes. (pp. 369–370)

31. **(C)** A physician realizes that his patient may become anxious and use the inhaler improperly. To help improve the volume of the medication that the patient is able to self-administer when in distress, the physician may prescribe a spacer device. (p. 380)

32. **(B)** Advair is not considered a medication that would be used in an emergency to reverse airway constriction as its use is aimed at prevention of attacks by reducing inflammation. The others—Ventolin, Proventil, and Albuterol—are used in emergency situations. (p. 380)

33. **(D)** When assessing the lungs of a patient in respiratory distress you hear a fine bubbling sound upon inspiration. This sound is caused by fluid in the alveoli and called crackles. (p. 377)

34. **(C)** A device that is commonly used in the hospital setting which is now frequently used by COPD patients in their home for respiratory treatments is called a small volume nebulizer. The other devices are inappropriate for the home setting for the COPD patient. (p. 385)

COMPLETE THE FOLLOWING

1. Conditions of inadequate breathing include: (pp. 370–372)
   - breathing rate that is out of normal range
   - agonal respirations
   - irregular rhythm (not an absolute indicator)
   - diminished or absent breath sounds
   - inadequate or shallow depth of respirations
   - inadequate or unequal chest expansion and increased respiratory effort
   - use of accessory muscles in breathing
   - pale or cyanotic, cool and clammy skin
   - snoring or gurgling (in patients with a diminished level of responsiveness or who are totally unresponsive)

2. Signs of inadequate breathing in infants and children are: (p. 371)
   - nasal flaring (widening of the nostrils)
   - grunting
   - seesaw breathing
   - retractions between the ribs

3. Signs of breathing difficulty include: (any eight) (pp. 374–378)
   - increased pulse rate
   - decreased pulse rate
   - changes in breathing rate
   - changes in breathing rhythm
   - pale, cyanotic, or flushed skin
   - noisy breathing that may be described as: audible wheezing, gurgling, snoring, crowing, stridor
   - inability to speak in full sentences
   - use of accessory muscles to breathe
   - altered mental status
   - coughing
   - flared nostrils
   - pursed lips
   - patient positioning
   - unusual anatomy (barrel chest)

4. Pulse Oximeter Readings (p. 375)

   Oxygen should be administered to all patients with respiratory distress regardless of their oxygen saturation readings. The oximeter reading in a normal, healthy person is typically *(A) 95% to 99%*. An oximeter reading below *(B) 95%* indicates hypoxia. A reading of *(C) 91% to 94%* indicates mild hypoxia, *(D) 86% to 90%* indicates moderate hypoxia, and *(E) 85% or less* indicates severe hypoxia.

LABEL THE DIAGRAMS (p. 369)

1. Relaxation
2. Contraction (inspiration begins)
3. Inspiration
4. Relaxation (passive expiration begins)

STREET SCENES DISCUSSION

1. Anything related to the patient's respiratory condition is pertinent to the current problem. Document it!

2. Yes.

3. As you learned in Chapter 6, the procedures for airway evaluation, opening the airway, and artificial ventilation are best carried out with the patient lying supine, or flat on the back. However, if the patient must sit, sit her up on the stretcher, lay her head back, and work with her breathing efforts. This takes patience and practice.

Chapter 17: Cardiac Emergencies

MATCH TERMINOLOGY/ DEFINITIONS

▶ PART A

1. **(I)** Acute myocardial infarction—condition in which a portion of the myocardium dies as a result of oxygen starvation; often called a heart attack by laypersons (p. 406)

2. **(B)** Aneurysm—dilation, or ballooning, of a weakened section of the wall of an artery (p. 405)

3. **(J)** Angina pectoris—pain in the chest that occurs when the blood supply to the heart is reduced and a portion of the heart muscle is not receiving enough oxygen (p. 405)

4. **(G)** Arrhythmia (Dysrhythmia)—irregular, or absent, heart rhythm (p. 405)

5. **(D)** Arteriosclerosis—condition in which artery walls become hard and stiff due to calcium deposits (p. 400)

6. **(E)** Asystole—when the heart has ceased generating electrical impulses (p. 410)

7. **(A)** Atherosclerosis—buildup of fatty deposits on the inner walls of arteries (p. 400)

8. **(F)** Cardiac compromise—blanket term for any kind of heart problem (p. 392)

9. **(C)** Congestive heart failure—condition of excessive fluid buildup in the lungs and/or other organs and body parts because of the inadequate pumping of the heart (p. 406)

10. **(H)** Coronary artery disease—diseases that affect the arteries of the heart (p. 405)

▶ PART B

1. **(J)** Edema—swelling resulting from a buildup of fluid in tissues (p. 406)

2. **(G)** Embolism—clot of blood and plaque that has broken loose from the wall of an artery and then moves to smaller arteries and blocks blood flow (p. 405)

3. **(B)** Occlusion—blockage (p. 405)

4. **(C)** Pedal edema—accumulation of fluid in the feet or ankles (p. 406)

5. **(E)** Pulmonary edema—accumulation of fluid in the lungs (p. 406)

6. **(I)** Pulseless electrical activity—condition in which the heart's electrical rhythm remains relatively normal, yet the mechanical pumping activity fails to follow the electrical activity, causing cardiac arrest (p. 410)

7. **(D)** Sudden death—cardiac arrest that occurs within two hours of the onset of symptoms (p. 406)

8. **(H)** Thrombus—clot formed of blood and plaque attached to the inner wall of an artery (p. 405)

9. **(A)** Ventricular fibrillation—condition in which the heart's electrical impulses are disorganized, preventing the heart muscle from contracting normally (p. 409)

10. **(F)** Ventricular tachycardia—condition in which the heartbeat is quite rapid; if rapid enough, it will not allow the heart's chambers to fill with enough blood between beats to produce blood flow sufficient to meet the body's needs (p. 409)

MULTIPLE-CHOICE REVIEW

1. **(C)** Cardiac compromise is a term that refers to any kind of problem with the heart. A period of time when the heart stops is cardiac arrest. (p. 392)

2. **(C)** Tearing pain is usually the result of a dissecting aortic aneurysm. Chest pain from the heart is normally described as dull, squeezing, or crushing. (p. 392)

3. **(A)** The pain or discomfort from a heart problem commonly radiates to the arms and jaw. It may also radiate down to the upper abdomen. (p. 392)

4. **(C)** In addition to chest pain or discomfort, the patient with cardiac compromise will also complain of dyspnea. The patient with gastrointestinal distress will complain of diarrhea. Cardiac compromise patients usually have a sudden onset of sweating, *not* shivering. A headache is a side effect of nitroglycerin. (p. 392)

5. **(C)** Patients with heart problems may complain of pain in the center of the chest, mild chest discomfort, and difficulty breathing. They do not have sudden onset of sharp abdominal pain. (p. 393)

6. **(B)** If the heart is beating too fast or too slow, the patient with cardiac compromise may also lose consciousness. This is due to an inadequate supply of oxygenated blood to the brain. (p. 393)

7. **(C)** The signs and symptoms of cardiac compromise do not include sharp pain in the lower abdomen combined with a fever. (p. 393)

8. **(C)** The patient with cardiac compromise should be administered high-concentration oxygen; the nasal cannula does not provide high-concentration oxygen. (p. 396)

9. **(A)** The "position of comfort" for a patient who is having chest pain is typically sitting up. Patients who are hypotensive (systolic blood pressure less than 90) will usually feel better lying down since this position allows more blood flow to the brain. (p. 396)

10. **(C)** A patient with prescribed nitroglycerin should be given or assisted in taking nitroglycerin (up to three doses). Vital signs and chest pain should be reassessed after each dose. If this patient's blood pressure falls below 100 systolic, then treat for shock and transport promptly. (p. 397)

11. (B) You should consider using nitroglycerin when the patient is carrying his own nitro and has crushing chest pain. A side effect of nitro is a headache. Nitro is *not* given to unconscious patients or to those who are hypotensive, below 100 systolic. (p. 397)

12. (C) The role of medical direction in the treatment of a cardiac compromise patient is authorizing the EMT to assist the patient in taking prescribed nitroglycerin. (p. 397)

13. (C) In order to give nitroglycerin, the patient's blood pressure must *not* be lower than 100 systolic. Medical direction should authorize the administration of nitroglycerin, and the patient's physician should have prescribed it. (p. 397)

14. (C) The maximum number of doses of nitro routinely given in the field is three. (p. 397)

15. (C) If after administering three doses of nitroglycerin, the patient's blood pressure falls below 100 systolic, you should treat for shock and transport promptly. (p. 397)

16. (A) Nitroglycerin is contraindicated for a patient who has a head injury. (p. 398)

17. (D) Palpitations are *not* a side effect of nitroglycerin. They are a symptom of cardiac compromise, however. The common side effects of nitro administration include hypotension, headache, and changes in the pulse rate. (p. 398)

18. (C) After administering nitro, it is important to reassess the vital signs. It is not necessary to lay the patient down unless his blood pressure drops. Continue the oxygen administration. (p. 398)

19. (D) The majority of cardiovascular emergencies are *not* a result of complications of cardiovascular surgery. Rather, they are a result of changes in the inner walls of arteries or problems with the heart's electrical and mechanical functions. (p. 400)

20. (A) When the body is subjected to exertion or stress, the heart rate will normally increase. It would be unusual for the heart to stop with normal exertion. (p. 400)

21. (C) Arteriosclerosis is a stiffening or hardening of the artery wall resulting from calcium deposits that cause a vessel to lose its elasticity, which restricts the amount of blood passing through the artery. Atherosclerosis is a buildup of fatty deposits on an artery's inner wall, which also restricts the amount of blood passing through it. (p. 400)

22. (D) Risk factors for coronary artery disease and acute coronary syndromes include lack of exercise, cigarette smoking, and obesity; other risk factors include heredity, age, hypertension, elevated blood levels of cholesterol and triglycerides. (p. 400)

23. (C) Hypertension as well as smoking and diet are risk factors that can be modified to reduce the risk of coronary artery disease. Unfortunately, a patient cannot change his or her age or heredity factors. (p. 400)

24. (A) The reason an emergency occurs in most cardiac-related medical emergencies is due to reduced blood flow to the myocardium. This may in turn cause cardiac arrest, loss of consciousness, or breathing difficulty. (p. 400)

25. (B) Angina pectoris means, literally, a pain in the chest. (p. 401)

26. (B) Nitroglycerin is administered to the patient with chest pain because it dilates the blood vessels and decreases the work of the heart. A drop in blood pressure is a side effect of nitro. Nitro should not be administered to unconscious patients. (p. 402)

27. (B) A condition in which a portion of the myocardium dies as a result of oxygen starvation is known as acute myocardial

infarction. A coronary occlusion occurs when the coronary artery is completely blocked. Myocardial starvation is a distracter. (p. 402)

28. (C) When a cardiac arrest occurs within 2 hours of the onset of cardiac symptoms, this is referred to as sudden death. (p. 402)

29. (B) Unfortunately, nearly 25% of the patients who experience a cardiac arrest within two hours of the onset of symptoms have no previous history of cardiac problems. (p. 402)

30. (C) Changes in the field care of the acute coronary syndromes have made fibrinolytics and defibrillation two of the most important treatment methods. Defibrillation of a patient with a shockable rhythm offers the best chance for survival. Fibrinolytics (clotbusters) break up the clot, saving heart muscle tissue. (p. 403)

31. (B) Congestive heart failure is a condition in which excessive fluids build up in the lungs and/or other organs. An infection in the heart is a distracter. A chronic lung condition that requires a low concentration of oxygen administration is COPD. (p. 403)

32. (B) When there is damage to the left ventricle and blood backs up into the lungs, this usually presents in the form of pulmonary edema. Pedal edema is the accumulation of fluid in the feet or ankles. Thrombolytics or fibrinolytics are medications that dissolve blood clots. Diaphoresis is profuse sweating. (p. 403)

33. (D) The chain of survival does not include early diagnosis. The elements of the chain of survival include early access, early CPR, early defibrillation, and early advanced care. (p. 405)

34. (D) Ways to decrease the EMS access time include installing a 911 system, placing 911 stickers on telephones, and providing public information workshops. (p. 405)

35. (B) CPR training by heart specialists is unnecessary in order to decrease the time it takes to start CPR on a cardiac arrest victim. (p. 405)

36. (A) The typical cardiac arrest victim is a male in his sixties. (p. 406)

37. (D) The most common witness to a cardiac arrest is a female in her sixties. (p. 406)

38. (D) Early defibrillation and high quality CPR are the most important factors in determining survival from cardiac arrest. If the time from the call is received to arrival of the defibrillator is longer than 8 minutes, virtually no one survives cardiac arrest. (p. 406)

39. (B) See answer 38. (p. 406)

40. (B) When treating a cardiac arrest patient and there is no ACLS unit in the community, the EMT should then package quickly and transport to the closest medical facility. To call for ACLS from another town and wait for their arrival would take too much time. Do not delay on the scene until the patient regains a pulse. Transport! (pp. 406–407)

41. (D) The EMT does not need to know how to administer epinephrine via IV or ET tube to manage a patient in cardiac arrest. Epinephrine administration is designed for allergic or anaphylactic patients. (p. 407)

42. (D) When using a fully automated defibrillator, it is unnecessary to press the button to deliver the shock. This is because a *fully* automated defibrillator delivers the shock automatically once enough energy has been accumulated. (p. 409)

43. (B) The primary electrical disturbance resulting in cardiac arrest is ventricular fibrillation. (p. 409)

44. (A) The shockable rhythms include ventricular fibrillation, ventricular tachycardia, and pulseless ventricular tachycardia. Asystole and PEA are not shockable. (p. 409)

45. (A) A nonshockable rhythm that can be the result of a terminally sick heart or severe blood loss is called pulseless electrical activity. (p. 410)

46. (C) A nonshockable rhythm that is commonly called "flatline" is named asystole. This condition is called "flatline" because the wavy line displayed on an ECG when there is electrical activity goes flat with asystole. (p. 410)

47. (B) When the AED is analyzing the patient's heart rhythm, the EMT must avoid touching the patient. If you are touching the patient, there can be interference from the electrical impulses of your heart and from movement of the patient's muscles. This can fool the AED's computer into believing there is a shockable rhythm when there really isn't one or vice versa. Also, it's possible a shock could be delivered to you if you are touching the patient, which could injure you. (p. 410)

48. (D) The AED should routinely be used on patients with shockable rhythms. If the patient is an adult or a child who is at least 1 year old and who has not sustained a trauma, before collapse, proceed with the AED. If the patient is less than 1 year old or the patient has sustained trauma before collapse, do not attached the AED unless you are ordered to do so by medical direction. Continue CPR and transport. (pp. 410–411)

49. (C) The AED pads are first attached to the cables. Then the pad attached to the red cable is placed over the left lower ribs. The pad attached to the white cable is placed in the angle between the sternum and the right clavicle. (p. 416)

50. (C) After the first shock, if the patient has a pulse and is breathing adequately, give high-concentration oxygen via nonrebreather mask and then transport. (pp. 416–417)

51. (B) After three shocks, the EMT should transport the patient unless local protocol says otherwise. Termination of an arrest can only be done with the approval of medical direction. (pp. 416–417)

52. (A) Defibrillation comes first! Don't hook up oxygen or do anything that delays analysis of the rhythm or defibrillation. (p. 417)

53. (D) A patient with an implanted defibrillator can be defibrillated immediately. Emergency care, CPR, and defibrillation for this patient are the same as for other cardiac patients. A trauma patient with severe blood loss should not be defibrillated. If a patient is soaking wet or is touching anything metallic that another person is touching, you could receive a shock. Move these patients before defibrillating. (pp. 419–420)

54. (A) If it is necessary to remove a nitro patch to defibrillate a patient, you should wear gloves to prevent the nitro from being absorbed into your skin. Do not use alcohol to cleanse the patient's skin; this could burn the patient's skin during defibrillation. (p. 420)

55. (C) If a patient has a cardiac pacemaker and needs to be defibrillated, the EMT should place the pad several inches away from the pacemaker battery. If you do not do this, you could damage the pacemaker with the AED shock. You cannot change the AED's power setting. EMTs do not remove pacemakers; this involves surgery. (p. 421)

COMPLETE THE FOLLOWING

1. The chain of survival includes: (pp. 405–407)
- early access
- early CPR
- early defibrillation
- early advanced care

LABEL THE DIAGRAM (Chapter 4, pp. 78–81)

1. Aorta
2. Pulmonary vein
3. Left lung
4. Left ventricle
5. Artery
6. Arterioles
7. Capillary bed
8. Venules
9. Vein
10. Right ventricle
11. Inferior vena cava
12. Superior vena cava
13. Pulmonary artery

STREET SCENES DISCUSSION

1. Cardiac patients can deteriorate very quickly. This is usually due to fluid in the lungs, intense chest pain, or dysrhythmia. Each of these problems can be monitored and managed by advanced life support (ALS) personnel, so call for them early.

2. Give the patient (or help the patient take) nitroglycerin if all of the following conditions are met: she complains of chest pain; she has a history of cardiac problems; her physician has prescribed nitroglycerin (NTG); she has the nitroglycerin with her; her systolic blood pressure is greater than 90 mmHg; medical direction authorizes administration of the medication.

3. If the AED does not shock a pulseless patient, it means the patient does not have a shockable rhythm.

4. This patient is in critical condition, so she is a high priority. Vital signs should be taken every 5 minutes on a critical patient.

Chapter 18: Acute Abdominal Emergencies

MATCH TERMINOLOGY/ DEFINITIONS

1. (D) Tearing pain—sharp pain that feels as if body tissues are being torn apart (p. 433)

2. (B) Peritoneum—the membrane that lines the abdominal cavity and covers the organs within it (p. 432)

3. (E) Visceral pain—a poorly localized, dull, or diffuse pain that arises from the abdominal organs or viscera (p. 433)

4. (A) Parietal pain—a localized pain that arises from the parietal peritoneum, the lining of the abdominal cavity (p. 433)

5. (C) Referred pain—pain that is felt in a location other than where the pain originates (p. 433)

MULTIPLE-CHOICE REVIEW

1. (B) The membrane that covers the abdominal organs is called the visceral peritoneum. (p. 432)

2. (C) The organs outside the peritoneum that are found between the abdomen and the back are in the retroperitoneal space. (p. 433)

3. (D) Pain originating from an organ in the abdomen is called visceral. (p. 433)

4. (D) Pain from an organ is often described as dull, achy, or diffuse. (p. 433)

5. (C) When a patient has colicky pain, this is often visceral pain from a hollow organ in the abdomen. (p. 433)

6. (B) It is common for the patient who has a gallbladder attack to complain of pain in his right shoulder blade because nerve pathways from the gallbladder return to the spinal cord by way of shared pathways with the shoulder. (p. 433)

7. (A) The last oral intake would be important to ask if the patient has a chief complaint of abdominal discomfort because the food may have been spoiled. (p. 437)

8. (B) An EMT who asks a young adult female patient, who is complaining of abdominal discomfort, where she is in her menstrual cycle is doing this to begin to focus in on the possibility of an ectopic pregnancy. (p. 437)

9. (A) Palpate the quadrant of the abdomen with the pain last. (p. 438)

10. (B) When managing a patient who has a complaint of abdominal pain and has no difficulty breathing, yet has signs consistent with shock or hypoperfusion, the EMT should administer 10–15 lpm oxygen by nonrebreather mask. (p. 440)

COMPLETE THE FOLLOWING

1. List four solid organs of the abdomen. (p. 432)
   A. Liver   **C.** Spleen
   B. Kidney   **D.** Pancreas

2. List six hollow organs of the abdomen. (p. 432)
   A. Appendix   **D.** Stomach
   B. Large intestine   **E.** Bladder
   C. Small intestine   **F.** Gallbladder

LABEL THE DIAGRAM (p. 431)

▶ **SOLID ORGANS**
   A. Diaphragm   **D.** Pancreas
   B. Spleen   **E.** Kidneys
   C. Liver

▶ **HOLLOW ORGANS**
   A. Stomach   **D.** Large intestine
   B. Gallbladder   **E.** Small intestine
   C. Duodenum   **F.** Bladder

STREET SCENES DISCUSSION

1. If the patient was 25 years old, instead of 72 years old, you should definitely consider a complication of early

pregnancy or an ectopic pregnancy which can both be life-threatening to the patient and fetus.

2. If when examining the patient's abdomen you noticed that she has a pulsating mass and she complains of a tearing sensation in her abdomen radiating into her back, there is a good chance she may have an abdominal aortic aneurysm or "AAA." This is a high priority since if it bursts the patient will die.

3. If the patient suddenly begins to complain of pain in the epigastric area and breaks out in a cold sweat, think acute myocardial infarction or AMI and treat for it!

Chapter 19: Diabetic Emergencies and Altered Mental Status

MATCH TERMINOLOGY/ DEFINITIONS

1. (D) Convulsions—uncontrolled muscular movements (p. 458)

2. (B) Diabetes mellitus—condition brought about by decreased insulin production; also called "sugar diabetes" or simply "diabetes" (p. 449)

3. (G) Epilepsy—medical condition that sometimes causes seizures (p. 459)

4. (A) Glucose—form of sugar that provides the body's basic source of energy (p. 448)

5. (H) Hyperglycemia—high blood sugar (p. 449)

6. (F) Hypoglycemia—low blood sugar (p. 449)

7. (C) Insulin—hormone produced by the pancreas or taken as a medication by many diabetics that helps cells use glucose (p. 448)

8. (I) Seizure—sudden change in sensation, behavior, or movement that can, in its most severe form, produce convulsions (p. 458)

9. (E) Status epilepticus—prolonged seizure, or when a person suffers two or more convulsive seizures without regaining full consciousness (p. 460)

10. (J) Stroke—blockage or bursting of a major blood vessel supplying the brain; also called a cerebrovascular accident (CVA) (p. 462)

MULTIPLE-CHOICE REVIEW

1. (C) The relationship of glucose to insulin is often described as a lock-and-key mechanism. In order for sugar to enter the body's cells, insulin must be present. The relationship is not oppositional, synergistic, or antagonistic. (p. 448)

2. (A) The condition brought about by decreased insulin production is known as diabetes mellitus. Hypotension is low blood pressure resulting from hypoperfusion, or shock, or other causes; hypoglycemia is low blood sugar. A cerebrovascular accident occurs when an artery in the brain is blocked or ruptured. (p. 449)

3. (C) The most common medical emergency for the diabetic patient is called hypoglycemia. See also answer 2. (p. 449)

4. (A) When a diabetic overexercises or overexerts, a medical condition called hypoglycemia can develop because sugars in the body are used faster than normal. Hyperglycemia (high blood sugar) occurs because the diabetic does not produce enough natural insulin, which is needed to pass sugar from the blood into the cells. Acute pulmonary edema is fluid in the lungs, which is usually the result of left heart failure. (p. 449)

5. **(B)** Potential causes of hypoglycemia: the patient may have taken too much insulin by mistake, the patient has been vomiting, or the patient has been fasting. A person does not lower sugar in the blood by eating a box of candy; this increases the blood sugar level. (p. 449)

6. **(A)** If sugar is not replenished quickly, the hypoglycemic patient may have permanent brain damage. (pp. 449–450)

7. **(C)** The clues that a patient is a diabetic include a medical identification bracelet, the presence of insulin in the refrigerator, and information provided by family members. The fact that the patient eats low-fat food would have no effect on the patient's condition. (p. 451)

8. **(B)** Sugunoil is a distracter and is not an oral medication used to treat diabetes. (p. 450)

9. **(D)** An intoxicated appearance and uncharacteristic behavior are typical of diabetic emergency. (p. 450)

10. **(B)** Diabetics often present the EMT with cold, clammy skin, anxiety, and combativeness. It is unusual for them to have a decreased heart rate. (p. 450)

11. **(A)** In order for the EMT to consider administering oral glucose, the patient must have altered mental status and have a history of diabetes and be awake enough to swallow. Oral glucose is not administered to the patient with an absent gag reflex or a patient with a seizure history who is not a diabetic. (p. 455)

12. **(C)** When reassessing a patient to whom you have administered oral glucose, and you note the patient's condition has not improved, you should consult medical direction about whether to administer more glucose. (p. 455)

13. **(C)** The recovery position prevents aspiration of fluids or stomach content into the lungs. The position is used for all non-spine-injured patients who are unresponsive or have an altered mental status. (p. 455)

14. **(C)** Children are less likely to eat correctly, are more active, and as a result are more likely to exhaust blood sugar levels. As a result, children are more at risk for developing hypoglycemia. (p. 450)

15. **(C)** A sudden change in mental status may indicate an alteration in the patient's blood sugar level. (p. 450)

16. **(B)** Before and after administering oral glucose, make sure you document the mental status of the patient. Increasing the oxygen flow rate is not necessary since it should remain at 15 liters per minute by nonrebreather mask. The glass of water is not needed. (p. 455)

17. **(D)** One trade name of oral glucose is Insta-glucose. D_5W is an intravenous solution of dextrose in water. Lactose is another form of sugar, and insulin is a hormone produced by the pancreas to help the body break down sugar. (p. 456)

18. **(D)** When a patient is very confused and disoriented, before deciding the patient has a behavioral problem, the EMT should consider a potential head injury, a brain tumor, and hypoxia. There is no such thing as an allergy to glucose. (p. 450)

19. **(B)** Diabetics routinely test the level of sugar in their blood using a glucose meter. (p. 451)

20. **(D)** Complications of diabetes include: kidney failure, heart disease, and blindness. (p. 457)

21. **(C)** The reading on the glucose meter is reported in milligrams of glucose per deciliter of blood. (p. 454)

22. **(D)** A diabetic with sugar level below 80 is considered hypoglycemic. (p. 454)

23. **(A)** A diabetic with a sugar level above 120 is considered hyperglycemic. (p. 454)

24. **(C)** The most common cause of seizures in adults is not taking anti-seizure medication. (p. 458)

25. **(A)** Seizures are commonly caused by high fever, brain tumor, and infection. They are not generally a result of cold exposure. (pp. 458–459)

26. **(A)** Idiopathic seizures occur spontaneously, have an unknown cause, and often start in childhood. Seizures in children who frequently have them are rarely life-threatening, but you should treat seizures in an infant or child as if they are life-threatening. (pp. 458–459)

27. **(A)** Convulsive seizures may be seen with epilepsy or hypoglycemia. They are not seen with asthma, AMI, pulmonary embolism, or anaphylaxis. (pp. 459–460)

28. **(B)** The best-known condition that results in seizures is epilepsy. (pp. 459–460)

29. **(A)** Not all seizures are alike. The type of seizure that most people associate with epilepsy and seizure disorders is called generalized tonic-clonic seizure. The patient falls to the floor and has severe convulsions. (p. 461)

30. **(D)** The family's reaction to the seizure (e.g., they called 911 or were frightened by the seizure) is not important to emergency care. When obtaining the medical history of a seizure patient, find out how long the seizure lasted, what the patient did after the seizure, and what the patient was doing prior to the seizure. (p. 460)

31. **(C)** If a seizure patient becomes cyanotic, provide artificial ventilations with supplemental oxygen. (p. 460)

32. **(B)** When you arrive on the scene of a seizure patient, and you notice that a bystander has placed a tongue blade in the corner of the patient's mouth, you should carefully remove the object from his mouth. Any object in the patient's mouth could cause an airway obstruction. Then begin oxygen administration. (p. 460)

33. **(A)** A seizure will normally last about 1 to 3 minutes. (p. 460)

34. **(B)** When a patient has two or more back-to-back seizures without regaining consciousness (or a seizure lasts over 5 to 10 minutes), this is called status epilepticus. Status asthmaticus is a continuous asthmatic attack. Convulsions are uncontrolled muscular movements. (p. 460)

35. **(D)** If you suspect a conscious patient has had a stroke, transport in the semisitting position. If a suspected stroke patient was *unconscious*, you should transport in the recovery position. (p. 462)

36. **(B)** When a stroke patient has difficulty saying what he is thinking even though he clearly understands you, this is called expressive aphasia. (p. 462)

37. **(C)** When the patient can speak clearly but cannot understand what you are saying, this is called receptive aphasia. (p. 462)

38. **(D)** A common sign of a stroke is headache. (pp. 463–464)

39. **(D)** Signs and symptoms of a stroke include: vomiting, seizures, and loss of bladder control. (pp. 463–464)

©2009 Pearson Education, Inc.
Emergency Care, 11th Ed.

40. (B) When a patient has many of the signs and symptoms of a stroke, which completely resolve in less than 24 hours, this is called a TIA. (p. 462)

41. (C) When a patient faints, the medical term used to describe this is usually a syncopal episode. A stroke and a CVA are a disruption to the blood supply to a portion of the brain causing cell damage. Hyperglycemia may cause a coma over a long period of time, but not suddenly. (p. 466)

42. (B) Lightheadedness or dizziness is often due to poor perfusion to the brain. This is corrected by placing the patient in the supine position, administering oxygen, and increasing the volume as needed. (p. 469)

COMPLETE THE FOLLOWING

1. The signs and symptoms of a diabetic emergency include: (any six) (p. 450)
   - Rapid onset of altered mental status
   - Intoxicated appearance, staggering, slurred speech, to unconsciousness
   - Elevated heart rate
   - Cold, clammy skin
   - Hunger
   - Seizures
   - Uncharacteristic behavior
   - Anxiety
   - Combativeness

2. *Hyper*glycemia occurs because the diabetic does not produce enough natural insulin, which is needed to pass sugar out of the blood and into the cells. It usually involves a situation in which the diabetic: (p. 449)
   - has not taken enough insulin to make up for the deficiency in natural insulin.
   - has forgotten to take his insulin.
   - has overeaten.
   - has an infection that has upset his insulin/glucose balance.

STREET SCENES DISCUSSION

1. They should be told how important it is that the patient eats, since the oral glucose will wear off. Tell them not to hesitate to call EMS again if there is any change in the patient's mental status.

2. Too much exercise for the amount of sugar taken in, too much insulin, or vomiting a meal also could cause hypoglycemia.

3. If medical direction permits it, you could have tried giving the patient some orange juice with a teaspoon of sugar in it.

Chapter 20: Allergic Reactions

MATCH TERMINOLOGY/ DEFINITIONS

1. **(C)** Allergen—something that causes an allergic reaction (p. 474)

2. **(B)** Anaphylaxis—severe or life-threatening allergic reaction in which the blood vessels dilate, causing a drop in blood pressure, and the tissues lining the respiratory system swell, interfering with the airway (p. 474)

3. **(E)** Auto-injector—syringe pre-loaded with medication that has a spring-loaded device that pushes the needle through the skin when the tip of the device is pressed firmly against the body (p. 478)

4. **(D)** Epinephrine—hormone produced by the body; as a medication, it constricts blood vessels and dilates respiratory passages and is used to relieve severe allergic reactions (p. 482)

5. **(A)** Hives—red, itchy, possibly raised blotches on the skin that often result from an allergic reaction (p. 477)

MULTIPLE-CHOICE REVIEW

1. **(C)** An exaggerated response of the body's immune system to any substance is called an allergic reaction. Vasoconstricting is the constriction of the vessels. A syncopal episode is when the patient passes out momentarily. (p. 474)

2. **(D)** Allergic reactions are sometimes treated as a high priority because they can cause airway obstruction. In anaphylaxis (a severe allergic reaction), exposure to the allergen will cause blood vessels to dilate rapidly and cause a drop in blood pressure. Many tissues swell, including those that line the respiratory system. This swelling can obstruct the airway, leading to respiratory failure. Vomiting and hives are not life-threatening. Most patients can tolerate a rapid pulse for a short while. (p. 474)

3. **(C)** The first time a patient is exposed to an allergen, the person's immune system forms antibodies, which are an attempt by the body to "attack" the foreign substances (allergens). (p. 475)

4. **(A)** The second time a patient is exposed to an allergen, the body reactions may include dilation of the blood vessels, massive swelling, and difficulty in breathing. (p. 475)

5. **(D)** Red fruits and vegetables are not common causes of allergic reactions. Causes include hornet stings, eggs and milk, poison ivy, and penicillin. (pp. 475–476)

6. **(A)** It is important to find out if a patient is allergic to latex so you do not wear gloves that could cause an allergic reaction. Latex allergy does not cause antitoxins, immediate cardiac arrest, or an allergy to other substances such as milk. (pp. 475–476)

7. **(B)** Hives are not a *respiratory* sign or symptom but are an effect of an allergic reaction on the skin. The respiratory signs and symptoms of anaphylactic shock include rapid breathing, cough, and stridor, as well as tightness in the throat or chest, labored or noisy breathing, hoarseness or loss of voice, and wheezing. (p. 477)

8. **(D)** The effects of an allergic reaction on the cardiac system could include increased heart rate and decreased blood pressure. (p. 477)

9. **(C)** To be considered a severe allergic reaction, a patient must have signs and symptoms of shock and/or respiratory distress. (p. 478)

10. **(B)** After administering epinephrine, the EMT should reassess the patient after 2 minutes. Do not decrease the oxygen and do not allow the patient to remain at home. (p. 478)

11. **(B)** If a patient has no history of allergies and is having her first allergic reaction, you should treat for shock and transport immediately. (p. 479)

12. **(A)** If a patient has an epinephrine auto-injector, besides helping administer the medication you should always ask if

the patient has any spare auto-injectors for the trip to the hospital just in case you need to recontact medical direction for permission to administer another dose of epinephrine to the patient. (p. 482)

13. **(B)** The location for injection with the auto-injector is the lateral mid-thigh. Injecting epinephrine in the back could cause a pneumothorax. Injection into the buttocks would require too much medication and take too long to act. (p. 483)

14. **(B)** The adult epinephrine auto-injector contains 0.3 mg and the child's contains 0.15 mg, or 1/2 the adult dose. The child dose is indicated for children weighing less than 66 pounds. (p. 483)

15. **(B)** Children commonly outgrow allergies as they mature. Infants rarely experience anaphylaxis; anaphylactic reactions are common in *older* children. Parents frequently can provide useful medical history. (p. 485)

COMPLETE THE FOLLOWING

1. The signs and symptoms of allergic reaction or anaphylactic shock can include: (any ten) (p. 477)
   - itching
   - hives
   - flushing
   - swelling of the face, especially the eyes and lips
   - warm, tingling feeling in the face, mouth, chest, feet, and hands
   - feeling of tightness in the throat or chest
   - cough
   - rapid breathing
   - labored breathing/tripod position
   - noisy breathing
   - hoarseness
   - muffled voice
   - loss of voice entirely
   - stridor
   - wheezing
   - increased heart rate
   - decreased blood pressure
   - itchy, watery eyes
   - headache
   - runny nose
   - sense of impending doom
   - altered mental status
   - flushed, dry skin or pale, cool, clammy skin
   - nausea or vomiting
   - vital sign changes to: increased pulse, increased respirations and decreased blood pressure

2. The important thing to recognize in any presentation is the presence of either respiratory distress or signs and symptoms of shock. (p. 478)

LABEL THE DIAGRAMS (p. 475)

1. Insect bites or stings
2. Food
3. Plants
4. Medications

STREET SCENES DISCUSSION

1. Yes, it would be appropriate but only with medical direction's permission. It should get injected into the thigh.

2. Yes, it would be appropriate. If ALS will not be on scene momentarily, then you could plan for an intercept en route.

3. Your priorities would be the patient's ABCs and defibrillation.

CASE STUDY—THE LAKEFRONT EMERGENCY

1. No, there is only one patient.

2. Yes, to the scene, or at least an intercept en route to the hospital due to the breathing difficulty.

3. Because she has breathing difficulty and cannot inhale deeply enough to speak for normal time periods.

4. She is alert and oriented.

5. The sound is most likely a wheeze, which can be caused by asthma, upper airway obstruction, anaphylaxis, or right heart failure (cor pulmonale).

6. The posture or position of the patient, like an upright tripod position, intercostal separation or retractions, accessory muscle use, cyanosis, and others.

7. This patient should be given oxygen by a nonrebreather mask at 15 liters per minute.

8. This is a high-priority patient due to her breathing difficulty, and she should be rapidly transported.

9. The position of comfort is generally best. But if she is able to breathe adequately, lay her down to improve her dizziness.

10. SAMPLE (signs and symptoms, allergies, medications, past medical history, last intake, and events leading up to illness).

11. **A)** Epinephrine.

    B) It would be appropriate to assist her with her epinephrine auto-injector.

12. **A)** You must call medical direction for permission to administer epinephrine to the patient.

    B) Make sure the epinephrine auto-injector is prescribed to the patient, is not expired, and is clear.

13. **A)** Chief complaint is breathing difficulty with chest pain.

    B) OPQRST findings, vital signs, SAMPLE findings.

    C) Treatment given thus far (e.g., oxygen, positioning, epinephrine auto-injector per medical direction).

14. The paramedic would establish an IV, administer saline or Ringer's lactate, evaluate the need for airway or breathing management, and assess the need for additional epinephrine or other medications such as Benadryl. Some EMS systems may use the PASG.

Chapter 21: Poisoning and Overdose Emergencies

MATCH TERMINOLOGY/ DEFINITIONS

1. **(D)** Absorbed poisons—poisons that are taken into the body through unbroken skin (p. 492)

©2009 Pearson Education, Inc.
Emergency Care, 11th Ed.

2. **(H)** Activated charcoal—substance that adsorbs many poisons and prevents them from being absorbed by the body (p. 494)

3. **(O)** Antidote—substance that will neutralize a poison or its effects (p. 498)

4. **(J)** Delirium tremens—severe reaction that can be part of alcohol withdrawal, characterized by sweating, trembling, anxiety, and hallucinations (p. 506)

5. **(I)** Dilution—thinning down or weakening by mixing with something else (p. 497)

6. **(E)** Downers—depressants, such as barbiturates, that depress the central nervous system (p. 508)

7. **(L)** Hallucinogens—mind-affecting or mind-altering drugs that act on the central nervous system to produce excitement and distortion of perceptions (p. 508)

8. **(F)** Ingested poisons—poisons that are swallowed (p. 491)

9. **(K)** Inhaled poisons—poisons that are breathed in (p. 491)

10. **(G)** Narcotics—class of drugs that affect the nervous system and change many normal body activities; their legal use is for relief of pain. (p. 508)

11. **(A)** Poison—any substance that can harm the body by altering cell structure or functions (p. 490)

12. **(M)** Toxin—poisonous substance secreted by bacteria, plants, or animals (p. 490)

13. **(B)** Uppers—stimulants, such as amphetamines, that affect the central nervous system to excite the user (p. 508)

14. **(N)** Volatile chemicals—vaporizing compounds, such as cleaning fluid, that are breathed in by an abuser to produce a "high" (p. 508)

15. **(C)** Withdrawal—state in which a patient's body reacts severely when deprived of an abused substance (p. 506)

MULTIPLE-CHOICE REVIEW

1. **(B)** Empty pill bottles or containers are a good environmental clue of poisoning. Just because a patient has vomited, has an altered level of responsiveness, or has a headache does not necessarily indicate poisoning. (p. 490)

2. **(A)** A poison is any substance that can harm the body, sometimes seriously enough to create a medical emergency. (p. 490)

3. **(C)** Although some of the over one million cases of poisoning in the United States each year result from murder or suicide attempts, most poisonings are accidental and involve young children. (p. 490)

4. **(B)** A substance secreted by plants, animals, or bacteria that is poisonous to humans is called a toxin. A narcotic is a drug that relieves pain; a drug is a chemical used to treat illness. (p. 490)

5. **(D)** Due to the poisons they produce, plants or fungi such as mistletoe, mushrooms, rubber plants, and holly can be dangerous to humans or pets. (p. 491)

6. **(B)** Botulism is a deadly disease caused by a toxin produced by bacteria. HIV is a virus. Steroids and penicillin are medications that, when used properly, are not deadly. (p. 491)

7. **(B)** Reactions to poisons are most serious in the ill and elderly. (p. 491)

8. **(B)** Poisons interfere with, but do *not* enhance, the normal biochemical processes in the body. Poisons damage the body by destroying skin and other tissues, overstimulating

(or depressing) the central nervous system, and displacing oxygen on the hemoglobin. (p. 491)

9. **(D)** Excretion is not a route of entry to the body but rather is a route of exit. Poisons enter the body through inhalation, ingestion, injection, and absorption. (p. 491)

10. **(C)** Carbon monoxide, chlorine, and ammonia are examples of inhaled poisons. (p. 491)

11. **(A)** Insecticides and agricultural chemicals can be absorbed through the skin. Carbon monoxide and ammonia are inhaled. Insect stings and snake bites are injected. Aspirin and LSD are ingested. (p. 492)

12. **(B)** The venom of a snakebite is an injected poison. (p. 492)

13. **(A)** It is important to determine the time a poison was ingested because different poisons act on the body at different rates. Other answer choices are incorrect statements. (p. 493)

14. **(B)** If you suspect poisoning by ingestion, after assuring a child has a patent airway, ask the parent for the child's weight because the effects of most chemicals are weight dependent. (p. 493)

15. **(B)** The most common results of poisoning by ingestion are nausea and vomiting. All the other answers are plausible but not the most common. (pp. 491, 493)

16. **(C)** Activated charcoal is used to prevent poisons from being absorbed by the body. It does not speed up the digestion of most chemicals, rather, it prevents digestion. It does not dilute the poison or act as an antidote. (p. 494)

17. **(A)** The difference between activated charcoal and regular charcoal is that activated charcoal is manufactured to have many cracks and crevices that increase the amount of surface for the poison to bind to. (p. 494)

18. **(C)** The decision on when to use activated charcoal is best made with medical direction or poison control center consultation. It is not necessary to wait until the patient gets to the emergency department. The patient's family physician need not be consulted. (pp. 494–495)

19. **(D)** Activated charcoal is not routinely used with ingestion of caustic substances, strong acids, or strong alkalis. (p. 496)

20. **(B)** Venom is an injected poison from a snakebite or other animal. Examples of caustic substances include lye, toilet bowl cleaner, and oven cleaner. (p. 492)

21. **(A)** A patient who continues to cough violently after a gasoline ingestion should not be given activated charcoal as he may aspirate the gasoline into his lungs. (p. 497)

22. **(C)** When a physician orders dilution of an ingested substance, you can use either water or milk. A cola drink will burn the stomach as well as produce gas from the carbonation. Coffee has caffeine in it, which will speed up the heart. (p. 497)

23. **(C)** The most common inhaled poison is carbon monoxide. Carbon dioxide is a colorless gas that we exhale. Nitrogen is a gas that makes up about 79% of the air. Phosgene is a nerve gas. (p. 499)

24. **(A)** As you approach a patient who has passed out while cleaning a large tank, if you smell an unusual odor, you should stand back and attempt to learn more about the chemical involved. This action will also prevent you or your crew from being overcome by the chemical. (p. 500)

25. **(B)** The principal prehospital treatment of a patient who has inhaled poison is administering high-concentration oxygen. (p. 499)

26. **(C)** Besides motor-vehicle exhaust, you might also find carbon monoxide around an improperly vented wood-burning stove. Malfunctioning oil, gas, and coal-burning furnaces and stoves can also be sources of carbon monoxide. (p. 499)

27. **(B)** Carbon monoxide affects the body by preventing the normal carrying of oxygen by the red blood cells. It does not cause severe respiratory burns or airway swelling, nor does it stimulate the central nervous system to decrease oxygen consumption. (pp. 499, 501)

28. **(D)** Cherry-red lips are *not* typically seen. A conscious patient who you suspect has carbon monoxide poisoning may exhibit cyanosis, altered mental status, and dizziness. (pp. 499, 501)

29. **(A)** If a patient has been contaminated by poisonous powder, you should brush off as much as possible, then irrigate after determining that the powder does not react with water. (p. 502)

30. **(B)** If you smell alcohol on the breath or clothes of a patient, you should not let this sidetrack you from doing a complete assessment. Calling the police is not necessary unless the patient is a threat to your safety. (pp. 503, 505)

31. **(A)** Acetone breath is not seen with alcohol abuse but is with diabetes. Do not confuse the odor of alcohol on the breath with acetone breath. (p. 505)

32. **(C)** Sweating, trembling, anxiety, and hallucinations found in the alcohol withdrawal patient are called delirium tremens. (p. 506)

33. **(B)** The patient who has mixed alcohol and other drugs will exhibit with depressed vital signs. (p. 507)

34. **(B)** When interviewing an intoxicated patient, do not begin by asking if he has taken any drugs because the patient may think you are accusing him of a crime. (p. 507)

35. **(A)** Drugs that stimulate the nervous system to excite the user are called uppers. (p. 508)

36. **(B)** Tranquilizers or sleeping pills are examples of downers. (p. 508)

37. **(B)** Drugs that have a depressant effect on the central nervous system are called downers. (p. 508)

38. **(C)** Drugs capable of producing stupor or sleep that are often used to relieve pain are called narcotics. Narcotics also depress the respiratory system. (p. 508)

39. **(D)** Mind-altering drugs that act on the nervous system to produce an intense state of excitement or distortion of the user's perceptions are called hallucinogens. (p. 508)

40. **(C)** A class of drugs that have few legal uses and are dissolved in the mouth are called hallucinogens. In illegal forms, they usually are found as a colored dot on a piece of paper or in sugar cubes. (p. 508)

41. **(B)** Cleaning fluid, glue, and model cement are examples of volatile chemicals. Diuretics are medications that tend to increase the flow of urine in order to eliminate excess body fluids. (p. 511)

42. **(A)** A patient who has overdosed on an upper may have signs and symptoms such as excitement, increased pulse and breathing rates, dilated pupils, and rapid speech. (p. 510)

43. **(B)** A patient who has overdosed on a downer may have signs and symptoms such as sluggishness, sleepiness, and lack of coordination of body and speech. (p. 510)

44. **(C)** A patient who has overdosed on a hallucinogen may have signs and symptoms such as fast pulse rate, dilated pupils, flushed face, and "see" or "hear" things. (p. 510)

45. **(D)** A patient who has overdosed on a narcotic may have signs and symptoms such as reduced pulse rate and rate and depth of breathing, constricted pupils, and sweating. (p. 510)

COMPLETE THE FOLLOWING

1. If you suspect poisoning, document the following information: (pp. 493, 498, 502)
   - Route of poisoning
   - Substance
   - Amount
   - Time
   - Interventions
   - Patient's weight
   - Effects of poisoning
   - Effects of treatment

2. The signs and symptoms of alcohol abuse include: (any six) (p. 506)
   - Odor of alcohol on a patient's breath or clothing.
   - Swaying and unsteadiness of movement.
   - Slurred speech
   - A flushed appearance to the face
   - Nausea or vomiting
   - Poor coordination
   - Slowed reaction time
   - Blurred vision
   - Confusion
   - Hallucinations
   - Lack of memory
   - Altered mental status

LABEL THE DIAGRAMS (p. 492)

1. Inhalation
2. Injection
3. Ingestion
4. Absorption

COMPLETE THE CHART (p. 511)

1. Upper
2. Narcotic
3. Mind-altering
4. Mind-altering
5. Volatile chemical
6. Downer
7. Downer
8. Upper
9. Upper
10. Downer
11. Mind-altering
12. Mind-altering
13. Mind-altering
14. Narcotic
15. Volatile chemical
16. Mind-altering
17. Upper
18. Narcotic
19. Downer
20. Narcotic
21. Downer
22. Mind-altering
23. Narcotic
24. Volatile chemical
25. Volatile chemical

STREET SCENES DISCUSSION

1. No. Do not give activated charcoal to any patient with an altered mental status.

2. Your highest priority should be to keep the patient's airway clear and patent.

3. It is necessary to take the oil to the hospital so that hospital chemists can identify the substance that was ingested.

Chapter 22: Environmental Emergencies

MATCH TERMINOLOGY/ DEFINITIONS

▶ **PART A**

1. **(C)** Active rewarming—application of an external heat source to rewarm the body of a hypothermic patient (p. 520)

2. **(B)** AGE—abbreviation that stands for arterial gas embolism (p. 534)

3. **(J)** Air embolism—gas bubble in the bloodstream; more accurately called an arterial gas embolism (p. 534)

4. **(H)** Central rewarming—application of heat to the lateral chest, neck, armpits, and groin of a hypothermic patient (p. 521)

5. **(F)** Conduction—direct transfer of heat from one material to another through direct contact (p. 517)

6. **(D)** Convection—carrying away of heat by currents of air or water or other gases or liquids (p. 518)

7. **(G)** Decompression sickness—condition resulting from nitrogen trapped in the body's tissues caused by coming up too quickly from a deep, prolonged dive (p. 534)

8. **(E)** Drowning—death caused by changes in the lungs resulting from immersion in water (p. 530)

9. **(A)** Evaporation—change from liquid to gas; as perspiration on the skin vaporizes, the body experiences a cooling effect (p. 518)

10. **(I)** Hyperthermia—increase in body temperature above normal; life-threatening in its extreme (p. 526)

▶ **PART B**

1. **(F)** Hypothermia—generalized cooling that reduces body temperature below normal; life-threatening in its extreme (p. 518)

2. **(E)** Local cooling—cooling or freezing of particular parts of the body (p. 523)

3. **(A)** Drowning—the process of experiencing impairment from submersion/immersion in liquid; the person may live or die (p. 530)

4. **(B)** Passive rewarming—covering a hypothermic patient and taking other steps to prevent further heat loss and help the body rewarm itself (p. 520)

5. **(C)** Radiation—sending out energy, such as heat, in waves into space (p. 518)

6. **(D)** Respiration—breathing; during this process, the body loses heat as warm air is exhaled from the body (p. 518)

7. **(G)** Toxins—substances produced by animals or plants that are poisonous to humans (p. 538)

8. **(I)** Venom—toxin produced by certain animals such as snakes, spiders, and some marine life-forms (p. 538)

9. **(H)** Water chill—chilling caused by conduction of heat from the body when the body or clothing is wet (p. 518)

10. **(J)** Wind chill—chilling caused by convection of heat from the body in the presence of air currents (p. 518)

MULTIPLE-CHOICE REVIEW

1. **(A)** Water conducts heat away from the body 25 times faster than still air. (p. 518)

2. **(C)** The body loses heat from respiration, radiation, conduction, convection, and evaporation. Excretion is the elimination of solid wastes, and induction is to place something into the body. Condensation is the accumulation of moisture on an object. (p. 518)

3. **(C)** When there is more wind, there is greater heat loss. (p. 518)

4. **(C)** Most radiant heat loss occurs from a person's head and neck. This is why one should always cover the head when going outside on a cold day. (p. 518)

5. **(D)** Having a headache does not predispose the patient to hypothermia. Predisposing factors to hypothermia include burns, diabetes, and spinal-cord injuries. Other predisposing factors include shock, head injuries, generalized infection, and hypoglycemia. Also the elderly and infants and young children are at risk. (p. 518)

6. **(D)** Infants and children do *not* have more body fat than adults. Infants and children are more prone to hypothermia because they have small muscle mass, they have large skin surface in relation to their total body mass, and they are unable to shiver effectively. (p. 518)

7. **(B)** You should consider hypothermia when a patient has been in a cold environment for a considerable length of time. (p. 518)

8. **(B)** When a patient's core body temperature drops below 90°F, the patient may no longer be shivering. (p. 519)

9. **(A)** Hypothermic patients do *not* have a high blood pressure and low pulse. Signs and symptoms of hypothermia include stiff or rigid posture, cool abdominal skin temperature, and loss of motor coordination. (pp. 519–520)

10. **(B)** Passive rewarming involves simply covering the patient. Administering heated oxygen and applying heat packs are part of active rewarming. Never massage the limbs of any hypothermic patient. (p. 520)

11. **(C)** Never give hot liquids to a hypothermic patient quickly. You can give warm liquids slowly. The treatment of the hypothermic patient includes removal of all of the patient's wet clothing, actively rewarming the patient during transport, providing care for shock, and providing oxygen. (pp. 519–520)

12. **(A)** When actively rewarming a patient, apply heat to the chest, neck, armpits, and groin. Never give the person stimulants to drink. (p. 520)

13. **(A)** The reason why you should rewarm the body's core first is to prevent blood from collecting in the extremities due to vasodilation, which could cause a fatal form of shock. (p. 521)

14. **(C)** When transporting an alert patient with mild hypothermia, it is recommended you keep the patient at rest. Since the blood is the coldest in the extremities, unnecessary movement could quickly circulate the cold blood and lower the core body temperature. The wet clothing must come off so the patient can be dried and warmed. (pp. 525–526)

15. **(B)** In a heat emergency, EMT care of a patient with moist, pale, normal-to-cool skin includes placing the patient in an air-conditioned ambulance, elevating the patient's legs

(if appropriate), and administering oxygen. It may also include cooling or fanning, but never so far as to cause the patient to shiver. (p. 526)

16. **(C)** If in a heat emergency a patient with moist, pale, normal-to-cool skin is responsive and not nauseated, the EMT should have him drink water. (p. 526)

17. **(C)** When treating an unresponsive patient with severe hypothermia, provide high-concentration oxygen that has been passed through a warm humidifier. If necessary, the oxygen that has been kept warm in the ambulance passenger compartment can be used. If there is no other choice, oxygen from a cold cylinder may be used. (p. 522)

18. **(B)** Because patients with extreme hypothermia may not reach biological death for over 30 minutes, the medical philosophy is "they are not dead until they're warm and dead." In other words, a patient is not considered dead until after he is rewarmed and resuscitative measures are applied. (p. 522)

19. **(A)** A cold injury usually occurring to exposed areas of the body that is brought about by direct contact with a cold object or exposure to cold air is called an early local cold injury. This injury is commonly called frostnip. (p. 523)

20. **(A)** The skin color of a patient with a superficial local cold injury will change from red to white. (p. 523)

21. **(C)** If a superficial local cold injury is on an extremity, the EMT should not re-expose the injury to cold. Immersion in hot water will burn the injury. The extremity should be splinted, but should be covered. (p. 523)

22. **(C)** When muscles, bones, deep blood vessels, and organ membranes become frozen, this type of injury is called a deep local cold injury. (p. 524)

23. **(B)** In frostbite, the affected area first appears white and waxy. When the condition progresses to actual freezing, the skin turns mottled or blotchy and the color turns from white to grayish yellow and finally grayish blue. (p. 524)

24. **(C)** Do not allow the frostbite patient to drink alcohol or smoke because constriction of blood vessels and decreased circulation to the injured tissues may result. (p. 524)

25. **(A)** Active rewarming of a frozen part is seldom recommended in the field. Very hot water may burn the part; the patient's face should be left uncovered. (pp. 524–525)

26. **(C)** When assessing a patient you suspect is in extreme hypothermia, check the carotid pulse for 30–45 seconds. (p. 522)

27. **(C)** The environment associated with hyperthermia includes heat and high humidity. (p. 526)

28. **(B)** The higher the humidity, the less your perspiration evaporates. (p. 526)

29. **(B)** The medical problems resulting from dry heat are often worse than those from moist heat because moist heat tires people before they can harm themselves through overexertion. Dry heat does not affect the respiratory system more quickly than humid heat. (pp. 527–528)

30. **(D)** Fluid buildup in the lungs is related to *too much* salt in the body, not too little. When salts are lost by the body through sweating, the patient may have muscle cramps, weakness or exhaustion, and dizziness or periods of faintness. (p. 527)

31. **(B)** A patient with heat exhaustion will present with moist, pale, normal-to-cool skin. A rapid strong pulse and lack of sweating are sometimes found with heat stroke. (pp. 527–528)

32. **(B)** The signs and symptoms of a heat emergency in patients who have hot, dry or moist skin include seizures. Muscle cramps usually only occur in early heat exposure from salt loss. (p. 528)

33. **(C)** Heat emergency patients with hot, dry or moist skin have little or no perspiration. The signs and symptoms of a heat emergency in patients who have hot, dry or moist skin include generalized weakness, loss of consciousness or altered mental status, and a full and rapid pulse. (p. 528)

34. **(B)** Substance abuse is a large contributor to adolescent and adult drownings. Car crash immersions are rare. (pp. 528–529)

35. **(C)** During a drowning incident, water flowing past the epiglottis causes a reflex spasm of the larynx. (p. 530)

36. **(B)** About 10% of the drowning victims die from lack of air (suffocation). (p. 530)

37. **(A)** If you are not an experienced swimmer, you should never attempt to go into the water to do a rescue. You should wear a personal floatation device on the shore and the appropriate exposure suit if you are going into the water. Get qualified help immediately. (p. 530)

38. **(B)** If you suspect that a patient still in the pool has a possible spine injury, you should immobilize and spineboard him while still in the water. Expediting the removal from the water could complicate the injury. Do not encourage the patient to swim, as this may further injure him. (p. 531)

39. **(C)** Two special medical problems seen in scuba-diving accidents are decompression sickness and air embolism. (p. 534)

40. **(A)** The risk of decompression sickness is increased by air travel within 12 hours of a dive. (p. 534)

41. **(C)** A toxin produced by some animals that is harmful to humans is called venom. (p. 538)

42. **(D)** Typical sources of injected poisons include spider, scorpion, and snakebites and stings. (p. 538)

43. **(B)** While cleaning out the crawl space below the house, you experience blotchy skin, redness in your arm, weakness, and nausea. It is possible that you were bitten by a poisonous spider. (p. 539)

44. **(A)** Lack of sensation on one side of the body is usually due to a head injury or cerebrovascular accident. Signs and symptoms of injected poisoning include puncture marks, muscle cramps, chest tightening, joint pain, excessive saliva formation, and profuse sweating. (p. 539)

45. **(D)** Never transport a live snake in the ambulance. Arrange for separate transport of a live specimen. If you suspect that your patient has been bitten by a snake, you should call for medical direction, clean the injection site with soap and water, and remove rings, bracelets, or other constricting items on the bitten limb. (p. 540)

COMPLETE THE FOLLOWING

1. The signs and symptoms of heat exhaustion include: (any six) (p. 527)
   - muscular cramps
   - weakness or exhaustion
   - rapid, shallow breathing
   - weak pulse
   - moist, pale skin that may feel normal to cool
   - heavy perspiration
   - possible loss of consciousness

2. The signs and symptoms of heat stroke include: (any six) (p. 528)
   - rapid, shallow breathing
   - full and rapid pulse
   - generalized weakness
   - hot, dry or possibly moist skin
   - little or no perspiration
   - loss of consciousness or altered mental status
   - dilated pupils
   - seizures may be seen; no muscle cramps

3. The signs and symptoms of an insect sting, spider bite, or scorpion sting include: (any ten) (p. 539)
   - altered state of awareness
   - noticeable stings or bites on the skin
   - puncture marks
   - blotchy skin
   - localized pain or itching
   - numbness in a limb or body part
   - burning sensations at the site
   - redness
   - swelling or blistering at the site
   - weakness or collapse
   - difficult breathing and abnormal pulse rate
   - headache and dizziness
   - chills
   - fever
   - nausea and vomiting
   - muscle cramps, chest tightening, joint pains
   - excessive saliva formation, profuse sweating
   - anaphylaxis

4. List five signs and/or symptoms of snake bite. (pp. 541–542)
   - Noticeable bite on the skin. This may appear as nothing more than a discoloration.
   - Pain and swelling in the area of the bite. This may be slow to develop, taking from 30 minutes to several hours.
   - Rapid pulse and labored breathing
   - Progressive general weakness
   - Vision problems (dim or blurred)
   - Nausea and vomiting
   - Seizures
   - Drowsiness or unconsciousness

STREET SCENES DISCUSSION

1. Active rewarming involves heat packs, hot air, blankets, and warmed humidified oxygen. In the hospital environment, active rewarming may include warm fluids, dialysis, warm enemas, and bypass.

2. Yes, of course, and prepare to apply the AED.

3. In the early stages of hypothermia, the heartbeat may be rapid. In a later stage, it slows. In this patient's situation, it may have been that he was in early-stage hypothermia or he may have had another problem, such as shock from internal bleeding.

CASE STUDY—TOO COLD FOR COMFORT

1. Mental status, ABCs, and ruling out trauma.

2. No. The parent is on the way, so you can begin to talk to the children and patient.

3. SAMPLE history and OPQRST of the chief complaint, which is altered mental status in this case.

4. Comfortable, lying supine, wrapped in blankets.

5. A mild case of hypothermia.

6. Yes, oxygen would be helpful via nonrebreather mask.

7. A slightly decreased temperature but not as low at 90°F, which is considered severe hypothermia.

8. She is a child, she is skinny with little fat insulation, and she has been playing in cold water and the wind all afternoon.

9. Children love to swim and will do so all day long. Suggest that they have frequent breaks to warm up out of the water and wind.

Chapter 23: Behavioral Emergencies

MATCH TERMINOLOGY/DEFINITIONS

1. **(E)** Behavior—manner in which a person acts (p. 548)

2. **(D)** Behavioral emergency—when a patient's behavior is not typical for the situation; when the patient's behavior is unacceptable or intolerable to the patient, his family, or the community; or when the patient may harm himself or others (p. 548)

3. **(C)** Positional asphyxia—death of a person due to a body position that restricts breathing for a prolonged time (p. 556)

4. **(A)** Soft restraint—humane device made of leather used to hold a patient still to prevent the patient from injuring himself or others (p. 555)

5. **(B)** Stress reaction—display of emotions, such as fear, grief, or anger, in response to an accident, serious illness, or death (p. 550)

MULTIPLE-CHOICE REVIEW

1. **(D)** Differing lifestyles are not a *physical* cause of altered behavior. The behaviors of persons from other cultures and with different lifestyles may seem unusual to you but might be quite normal to the person performing them. (pp. 548–549)

2. **(C)** Hypoactivity is a distracter and incorrect response. Altered behavior ranging from irritability to altered mental status can be due to lack of oxygen (hypoxia), head trauma, or hypoglycemia. (p. 549)

3. **(C)** To calm a patient who is experiencing a stress reaction, you should explain things to the patient honestly. Do not lie, since this will lead to mistrust of anything you say or do. Quick movements not only confuse, but will scare the patient, not calm him. You, not the patient, should control the situation. Quickly restraining the patient will not calm him and should only be used as a last resort. (p. 550)

4. **(B)** Rather than having a neat appearance, a patient experiencing a behavioral emergency is more likely to have an unusual appearance, disordered clothing, or poor hygiene. In addition, he may exhibit panic and anxiety; agitated or unusual activity, such as repetitive motions; and unusual speech patterns, such as pressured-sounding speech. (pp. 550–551)

5. **(B)** When you are called to care for a patient who has attempted suicide, or is to attempt suicide, your first concern must be your own safety. Once you ensure your safety, treat the patient as you would other patients. (p. 552)

6. **(A)** High suicide rates occur at ages 15–25 and over age 40. Also, suicides among the elderly are increasing. (p. 552)

7. **(C)** Most suicidal patients will not deny suicidal thoughts, but rather will express them and tell others they are considering suicide. Take all threats of suicide seriously. Examples of a self-destructive activity include a defined lethal plan of action that has been verbalized, giving away personal possessions, and previous suicide threats. (pp. 552–553)

8. **(C)** A patient who has made the decision to commit suicide may actually appear to be coming out of depression, or improving. The fact that the decision has been made and an end is in sight can cause this apparent improvement. (p. 553)

9. **(D)** Stay out of kitchens when dealing with an aggressive patient. Kitchens are filled with dangerous weapons. Stay in a safe area until the police can control the scene. When assessing an aggressive patient for a possible threat to you or your crew, determine the patient's history of aggressive behavior, pay attention to the patient's vocal activity (is he shouting at you?), and the patient's posture (watch body language). (p. 554)

10. **(A)** If a patient stands in a corner of the room with fists clenched and screaming obscenities, you should request police backup and keep the doorway in sight. Raising your voice or challenging him could force a confrontation. Explaining that you would respond to the situation in the same way is simply being dishonest. (p. 555)

11. **(B)** The family's ability to pay for services is not a consideration in evaluating whether or not to restrain a patient. Use of reasonable force to restrain a patient should involve an evaluation of the patient's size and strength, the mental state of the patient, and the available methods of restraint. (pp. 555–556)

12. **(A)** The use of force by an EMT is allowed in most states in order to defend against an attack by an emotionally disturbed patient. While the police do not need to be present, it is very desirable to involve them. The fact that a patient has been drinking or refuses care does not take away his decision-making rights. (pp. 555–556)

13. **(D)** Four rescuers, not two, should be used to secure a disturbed patient. This allows one rescuer to control each limb. Monitor all restrained patients carefully. (p. 556)

14. **(D)** Apply a surgical mask, but ensure that the patient is not likely to vomit or does not have breathing difficulties before applying. Placing the patient in a prone position may limit, but will not eliminate, the patient's ability to spit. Never place roller gauze or tape over a patient's mouth due to the risk of aspiration. (p. 556)

15. **(C)** When a patient is a danger to himself and others and needs to be transported against his will, the EMT should contact the police for assistance. Most states have a legal provision that will allow such a patient to be transported and gives this authority to law enforcement personnel. Know your laws on treating patients without consent. (p. 558)

COMPLETE THE FOLLOWING

1. Risk factors for suicide include the following: (pp. 552–553)
   - depression
   - high current or recent stress levels
   - recent emotional trauma
   - age
   - alcohol and drug abuse
   - threats of suicide

- suicide plans
- previous attempts or suicide threats; history of self-destructive behavior
- sudden improvement from depression

2. When a patient acts as if he may hurt himself or others, take the following precautions: (p. 555)
   - Do not isolate yourself from your partner or other sources of help.
   - Do not take any action that may be considered threatening by the patient.
   - Always be on the watch for weapons.
   - Be alert for sudden changes in the patient's behavior.

STREET SCENES DISCUSSION

1. Restraint is the responsibility of law enforcement. However, while they call and wait for backup, you may offer your assistance, but remember: never assist unless there are sufficient personnel to do the job; you must be able to ensure your own safety and the safety of the patient; and, if you do assist, make certain the restraints used are humane.

2. The most humane form of restraint is a roller bandage or a sheet and tape. Leather restraints are also helpful. Metal and plastic handcuffs cut and rip the skin and should not be carried by EMTs.

3. No. You may need to convince the patient that vital signs are a part your normal routine, but do not skip them. Remember, there could be more than just a behavioral problem.

Chapter 24: Obstetrics and Gynecological Emergencies

MATCH TERMINOLOGY/ DEFINITIONS

▶ **PART A**

1. **(I)** Abortion—spontaneous (miscarriage) or induced termination of pregnancy (p. 590)

2. **(F)** Abruptio placentae—condition in which the placenta separates from the uterine wall; a cause of prebirth bleeding (p. 558)

3. **(D)** Afterbirth—placenta, umbilical cord, and some tissues from the lining of the uterus that are delivered after the birth of the baby (p. 565)

4. **(K)** Amniotic sac—thin, membranous "bag of waters" that surrounds the developing fetus (p. 565)

5. **(M)** Breech presentation—when the buttocks or both legs of a baby deliver first during birth (p. 565)

6. **(A)** Cephalic presentation—normal head-first birth (p. 565)

7. **(B)** Cervix—neck of the uterus at the entrance to the birth canal (p. 564)

8. **(O)** Crowning—when the presenting part of the baby first appears through the vaginal opening (p. 565)

9. **(C)** Ectopic pregnancy—implantation of the fertilized egg in an oviduct, the cervix of the uterus, or in the abdominopelvic cavity (p. 588)

10. **(E)** Fetus—baby developing in the womb (p. 564)

11. **(G)** Induced abortion—deliberate actions to stop a pregnancy (p. 590)

12. (J) Labor—three stages of the delivery of a baby that begin with the contractions of the uterus and end with the expulsion of the placenta (p. 565)

13. (L) Meconium staining—amniotic fluid that is greenish or brownish-yellow rather than clear; an indication of possible maternal or fetal distress during labor (p. 566)

14. (H) Multiple birth—when more than one baby is born during a single delivery (p. 584)

15. (N) Perineum—the surface area between the vagina and the anus (p. 581)

16. (P) APGAR—a way to assign a number to a newborn's condition and is the total of five values, ranging from 0 to 10. (p. 575)

▶ **PART B**

1. (H) Placenta—organ of pregnancy where exchange of oxygen, foods, and wastes occurs between a mother and fetus (p. 564)

2. (I) Placenta previa—condition in which the placenta is formed in an abnormal location (usually low in the uterus and close to or over the cervical opening) that will not allow for a normal delivery of the fetus (p. 588)

3. (F) Premature infant—any newborn weighing less than 5½ pounds or one that is born before the 37th week of pregnancy (p. 586)

4. (A) Prolapsed umbilical cord—when the umbilical cord presents first and is squeezed between the vaginal wall and the baby's head (p. 583)

5. (C) Spontaneous abortion—when the fetus and placenta deliver before the 28th week of pregnancy, commonly called a miscarriage (p. 590)

6. (E) Stillborn—born dead (p. 592)

7. (B) Supine hypotensive syndrome—dizziness and a drop in blood pressure caused when the mother is in a supine position and the weight of the uterus, infant, placenta, and amniotic fluid compress the inferior vena cava, reducing return of blood to the heart and cardiac output (p. 570)

8. (G) Umbilical cord—fetal structure containing the blood vessels that carry blood to and from the placenta (p. 565)

9. (D) Uterus—muscular abdominal organ where the fetus develops; also called the womb (p. 564)

10. (J) Vagina—birth canal (p. 564)

MULTIPLE-CHOICE REVIEW

1. (B) The 9 months of pregnancy are divided into three-month trimesters. During the second trimester, the uterus grows very rapidly while the woman's blood volume, cardiac output, and heart rate increase. (p. 565)

2. (B) The normal birth position is head first and is called a cephalic birth. Breech is buttocks or feet first birth. (p. 565)

3. (C) The first stage of labor starts with regular contractions of the uterus. This can occur earlier or later than 9 months. It ends with full dilatation of the cervix. (p. 565)

4. (D) The second stage of labor starts with the entry of the baby into the birth canal. (p. 565)

5. (A) The third stage of labor begins after the birth of the baby. (p. 565)

6. (B) The third stage of labor is complete when the afterbirth is expelled. Expulsion should occur within 20 minutes from the birth of the baby. (p. 565)

7. (B) The process by which the cervix gradually widens and thins out is called dilation. (p. 565)

8. (A) As the fetus moves downward and the cervix dilates, normally the amniotic sac breaks and fluid leaks out. If this fluid is greenish or brownish-yellow in color, it may indicate fetal or maternal distress. (p. 566)

9. (C) The greenish or brownish-yellow fluid expelled from the amniotic sac is called meconium staining. There is no such thing as amniotic bile. Bile is a chemical that helps break down fats during digestion. (p. 566)

10. (C) When a mother in labor states she feels the need to move her bowels, this means the birth moment is nearing. This does not indicate that the baby is in distress. (p. 567)

11. (B) The contraction duration is timed from the beginning of contraction to when the uterus relaxes. The contraction interval is defined in answer 12. (p. 567)

12. (A) The contraction interval, or frequency, is timed from the start of one contraction to the start of the next. The contraction duration is defined in answer 11. (p. 567)

13. (B) Delivery is imminent when the contractions last 30 seconds and are 2 to 3 minutes apart. (p. 567)

14. (B) The EMT's primary roles at a normal childbirth scene are to determine whether the delivery will occur at the scene and, if so, to assist the mother as she delivers the child. If delivery is imminent, do not delay it. There is no need to immobilize the patient during emergency childbirth. (p. 567)

15. (C) The sterile obstetrical kit does *not* contain heavy flat twine to tie the cord. Occasionally, in an off-duty situation, you may be required to improvise using heavy flat twine or new shoelaces to tie the cord. (pp. 567–568)

16. (B) When evaluating the mother for a possible home delivery, the EMT should ask the frequency and duration of contractions. If the mother feels the need to urinate, this is a normal process, but if she has to move her bowels, this is a signal that the infant is moving down the birth canal. The father's blood type is not important to field care but would be important to hospital care if a transfusion is necessary. (p. 568)

17. (A) It is important to ask the mother if you can examine for crowning if the mother is straining during contractions. If she is, birth will probably occur too soon for transport. EMTs do not automatically examine every woman in her 9th month for crowning, and you would need the patient's permission to do so. (p. 568)

18. (C) You should ask the mother if her water broke and prepare for a quiet ride to the hospital. Since this is her first pregnancy and only an 8-month term, this may be false labor or just the beginning of labor. (p. 568)

19. (A) If you determine that the delivery is imminent based on the presence of crowning and other signs, you should contact medical direction, or follow your local protocol. Do not ask the mother to go to the bathroom first, as the infant may be expelled into the toilet. Do not attempt to hold back a delivery by asking the mother to hold her legs closed. (p. 568)

20. (B) When a full-term pregnant woman in a supine position complains of dizziness and you note a drop in blood pressure, this could be due to a condition called supine hypotension syndrome. This is a condition in which the heavy mass created by the weight of the uterus, coupled with the infant's weight, placenta, and amniotic fluid, compresses the inferior vena cava, reducing return of blood to the heart, reducing cardiac output and resulting in low blood pressure. Cushing's reflex occurs in head injuries. (p. 569)

21. (B) To counteract the pressure of the uterus on the inferior vena cava, you should transport the patient on her left side to lessen the pressure. See answer 20. (p. 570)

22. (D) During a delivery, the EMT will need infection control gear such as surgical gloves, a mask, and eye protection as well as a gown. A Tyvek suit is not needed for protection against blood spraying. (p. 571)

23. (D) During delivery, encourage the mother to breathe deeply through her mouth. She may feel better if she pants, although she should be discouraged from breathing rapidly and deeply enough to bring on hyperventilation. (p. 572)

24. (A) Do not pull on the baby's shoulders or any other part of the baby. When supporting the baby's head during a delivery, the EMT should apply gentle pressure to control the delivery, place one hand below the head, and spread fingers evenly around the baby's head. (p. 572)

25. (B) If the amniotic sac has not broken by the time the baby's head is delivered, use your finger to puncture the membrane. Then pull the membranes away from the baby's mouth and nose. (p. 572)

26. (C) If you cannot loosen or unwrap the umbilical cord from around the infant's neck, you should clamp the cord in two places and cut between the clamps. This way the child will not strangle, and the cord will not tear. (p. 572)

27. (A) Most babies are born face down and then rotate to either side. (p. 574)

28. (B) When suctioning a newborn, compress the syringe before placing it in the baby's mouth to avoid blowing fluids into the baby's airway. (p. 574)

29. (B) Once the baby's feet are delivered, lay the baby on her side with head slightly lower than its torso. This is done to allow blood, fluids, and mucus to drain from the mouth and nose. Remember, newborns are very slippery; never pick up a baby by the feet since you could drop the child. (p. 574)

30. (D) To assess the newborn, the EMT does not check the response to a sternal rub; this could injure the child. A general evaluation usually calls for noting ease of breathing, the heart rate, crying (vigorous crying is a good sign), movement (the more active, the better), skin color (blue coloration at the hands and feet may or may not disappear, but it should not spread to other parts of the body). (p. 575)

31. (C) It is necessary to suction the baby's mouth before the nose because suctioning the nose first may cause the baby to gasp or begin breathing and aspirate any meconium, blood, fluids, or mucus from the mouth into the lungs. (p. 575)

32. (C) If assessment of the infant's breathing reveals shallow, slow, or absent respirations, the EMT should provide artificial ventilations at 40 to 60 per minute. Do not use an oxygen mask. (pp. 576–577)

33. (A) In a normal birth, the infant must be breathing on his own before you clamp and cut the cord. (p. 577)

34. (D) The first umbilical cord clamp should be placed about 10 inches from the baby. (p. 578)

35. (C) The second umbilical cord clamp should be placed about 7 inches from the baby. (p. 578)

36. (D) If the placenta does not deliver within 20 minutes of the baby's birth, transport the mother and baby to a medical facility without delay. (p. 579)

37. (B) It is not uncommon for the mother to tear part of the perineum during a delivery. If this occurs, apply a sanitary napkin and apply gentle pressure. Let the mother know that torn tissue is normal and that the problem will be quickly cared for at the medical facility. (p. 581)

38. (D) Initiate rapid transport on recognition of a breech presentation. Never pull on the baby's legs. Provide high-concentration oxygen. Place the mother in a head-down position with the pelvis elevated. (p. 582)

39. (A) If you see the umbilical cord presenting first, gently push up on the baby's head or buttocks to take pressure off of the cord. This may be the only chance that the baby has for survival, so continue to push up on the baby until you are relieved by a physician. All patients with prolapsed cords require rapid transport! (pp. 582–583)

40. (D) When a baby's limb presents first, the EMT should begin rapid transport of the patient immediately. Do not try to replace the limb into the vagina. (p. 583)

41. (B) When assisting with the delivery of twins, clamp the cord of the first baby before the second baby is born. Labor contractions will continue after the first baby is born. (p. 585)

42. (C) Premature infants are at high risk for hypothermia because they lack fat deposits that would normally keep them warm. (p. 586)

43. (B) When oxygen is administered to an infant, it should be given by flowing it past the baby's face. Use humidified oxygen, if available, so it doesn't dry out the baby's respiratory tract. (p. 586)

44. (B) If you suspect meconium staining when the infant is born, avoid stimulating the infant before suctioning the oropharynx. This reduces the risk of aspiration. (p. 587)

45. (D) A condition in which the placenta is formed low in the uterus and close to the cervical opening, preventing the normal delivery of the fetus, is called placenta previa. (p. 588)

46. (D) Seizures in pregnancy are usually associated with extreme swelling of the extremities. In addition, the patient will have *elevated* blood pressure. Seizures tend to occur *late* in pregnancy and pose a threat to *both* the mother and unborn baby. (p. 589)

47. (C) Massive bleeding and shock are the gravest dangers associated with blunt trauma to the pregnant woman's abdomen or pelvis. Perform a patient assessment and treat her injuries as you would those of any trauma patient. (p. 590)

48. (A) Because of the physiology of a pregnant woman, the vital signs of a pregnant woman may be interpreted as suggestive of shock when they are actually normal. The pregnant woman has a pulse rate 10–15 beats per minutes *faster* than her nonpregnant counterpart and a blood volume as much as 48% *higher* than her nonpregnant state. Shock is *more* difficult to assess in the pregnant patient, and it is the most likely cause of prehospital death from injury to the uterus. (p. 591)

49. (B) Unless a back or neck injury is suspected, all pregnant women who have suffered blunt trauma injury should be transported in the left lateral recumbent position. If you suspect neck or back injury, first secure the mother to a spine board, then tip board and patient as a unit to the left, relieving pressure on the abdominal organs and vena cava. (pp. 591–592)

50. **(C)** If vaginal bleeding is associated with abdominal pain, treat the patient as if she has a potentially life-threatening condition. The most serious complication of vaginal bleeding is hypovolemic shock due to blood loss. (p. 593)

COMPLETE THE FOLLOWING

1. When evaluating the expectant mother, the EMT should: (pp. 568–569)
   - Ask her name and age and expected due date.
   - Ask if this is her first pregnancy.
   - Ask her how long she has been having labor pains and how often, and if the "bag of waters" has broken.
   - Ask if she is straining or feels the need to move her bowels.
   - With patient's permission, examine for crowning.
   - Feel for uterine contractions.
   - Take vital signs.

2. Take the following steps when providing care for the premature infant: (p. 586)
   - Keep the baby warm.
   - Keep the airway clear.
   - Provide ventilations and/or chest compressions.
   - Watch the umbilical cord for bleeding.
   - Provide oxygen.
   - Avoid contamination.
   - Transport the infant in a warm ambulance.
   - Call ahead to the emergency department.

3. Complete the following (p. 575):
   (A) Extremities blue, trunk pink
   (B) >100
   (C) No reaction
   (D) Only slight activity (flexing extremities)
   (E) Good breathing, strong cry

LABEL THE DIAGRAMS (p. 564)

1. Amniotic sac
2. Umbilical cord
3. Placenta
4. Uterus
5. Pubic bone
6. Cervix
7. Vagina

STREET SCENES DISCUSSION

1. If the amniotic sac has not broken by the time the baby's head is delivered, use your finger to puncture the membrane. Then pull the membranes away from the baby's mouth and nose.

2. This is called meconium staining. Meconium-stained amniotic fluid is caused by fetal feces (wastes) released during labor, usually because of maternal or fetal stress. If meconium is present, suction the infant immediately—first the mouth and then the nose. Maintain an open airway and be prepared to provide artificial ventilation or CPR if needed. Transport as soon as possible.

3. Be sure to put the mother on high-concentration oxygen via nonrebreather mask, keep her warm, elevate her legs, and massage her abdomen above the uterus. It also may be

helpful to encourage the mother to nurse the infant, since sucking stimulates the uterus to contract.

Chapter 25: Putting It All Together for the Medical Patient

MATCH TERMINOLOGY/ DEFINITIONS

1. **(E)** Intervention—Action taken to correct a patient's problem (p. 601)
2. **(C)** Circulation—Movement of blood throughout the body (p. 601)
3. **(A)** Airway—Passageway by which air enters and leaves the body (p. 601)
4. **(H)** Priority determination—Decision on the seriousness of the patient's condition (p. 601)
5. **(G)** On-line medical direction—Orders from the on-duty physician given directly to an EMT in the field by radio or telephone (p. 606)
6. **(B)** Breathing—Respiration, or the process by which a person inhales and exhales air (p. 601)
7. **(F)** Angina—Pain in the chest, occurring when blood supply to the heart is reduced and a portion of the heart muscle is not receiving enough oxygen (p. 604)
8. **(D)** Glucose—Form of sugar, the body's basic source of energy (p. 603)

MULTIPLE-CHOICE REVIEW

1. **(A)** EMTs do not normally administer fluids to patients unless they have received special training. (p. 602)
2. **(C)** When a patient presents with more than one condition or a familiar condition but under unusual circumstances, the EMT should assess the patient as usual and then seek advice if necessary. (p. 602)
3. **(A)** When a patient tells you that he has a disease with which you are unfamiliar, it is best to respond by saying "I'm not familiar with that disease. Could you tell me more about it?" (pp. 601–602)
4. **(C)** When a patient has two or more medical conditions that are presenting symptoms at the same time, it is good to consult with medical direction for advice. (p. 601)
5. **(D)** The patient with slurred speech may have had a cardiovascular accident, an overdose, or a seizure. (pp. 602–603)
6. **(C)** Patients who have had a seizure generally do not have chest pain. (p. 604)
7. **(A)** A patient who is vomiting coffee-ground-like colored material probably has internal bleeding (such as a gastrointestinal bleed). (pp. 604–605)
8. **(D)** A wheeze is a common breathing sound found in patients having an asthma attack, an allergic reaction, or bronchospasm. (pp. 605–606)
9. **(B)** There is no specific EMT intervention for the patient with abdominal pain (aside from oxygen administration). (pp. 605–606)
10. **(C)** The EMT has been trained to cool down and apply oxygen to the patient suspected of having hyperthermia. (p. 601)

COMPLETE THE FOLLOWING

1. Examples of EMT interventions for medical patients include the following: (p. 607)
   - Assisting a patient in using his own inhaler (respiratory difficulty)
   - Assisting a patient in taking his own nitroglycerin (cardiac compromise)
   - Application of an automated defibrillator (cardiac arrest)
   - Administration of oral glucose (diabetics with altered mental status)
   - Assisting a patient in using his own epinephrine auto-injector (allergic reaction)
   - Administration of activated charcoal (overdose or poisoning)
   - Talking down and restraining (behavioral emergencies)
   - Assisting in delivery of an infant (patient in labor)
   - Cooling or warming (environmental emergency)

STREET SCENES DISCUSSION

1. Standard Precautions should include gloves, mask, and eye-shield if you suspect an infectious disease.

2. Patients with dizziness should be encouraged to go to the hospital for evaluation, since there are many serious problems associated with the symptom.

3. If the patient is a diabetic, he might be having a "silent MI." Be very careful to encourage sick diabetics to seek medical attention.

Interim Exam 2

1. **(D)** The initial assessment includes assessing the airway, mental status, and circulation, as well as breathing. Blood pressure is a vital sign taken during the focused history and physical exam. (p. 210)

2. **(B)** Evaluating extremity mobility is not part of the initial assessment. Determining patient priority, forming a general impression, and assessing breathing are all part of the initial assessment. (p. 210)

3. **(B)** Environmental clues during the general impression of a child would include recognizing that the child is holding pieces of a toy (perhaps he or she swallowed one of the pieces). Vital signs and associated signs or symptoms like nausea are not part of the general impression. (p. 210)

4. **(C)** The patient's position, age, sex, sounds he or she is making, and smells from the environment are part of the general impression. Vital signs are not. (pp. 210, 212)

5. **(B)** Assessing mental status is the step of the initial assessment that comes after the general impression. (p. 210)

6. **(C)** AVPU stands for <u>A</u>lert, response to <u>V</u>erbal stimulus, response to <u>P</u>ainful stimulus, <u>U</u>nresponsive. (p. 213)

7. **(B)** See answer 6. (p. 213)

8. **(D)** The lowest and most serious mental status is U, or unresponsive. (p. 213)

9. **(B)** If a patient's level of responsiveness is lower than Alert, you should at least administer high-concentration oxygen by nonrebreather mask. Consider this patient a high-priority transport. (p. 214)

10. **(C)** If a patient is talking or crying, assume an open airway. However, this condition may change, so you need to monitor the patient. (p. 214)

11. **(C)** If the patient is not alert and breathing rate is slower than 8 breaths per minute, use a bag-valve mask to assist the ventilations. (p. 214)

12. **(B)** Pale and clammy skin indicates poor circulation, or hypoperfusion. (p. 214)

13. **(A)** A patient who gives a poor general impression is a *high* priority. (p. 215)

14. **(B)** The patient whose only complaint is nausea and vomiting is not generally considered a high priority. (p. 215)

15. **(A)** The initial assessment varies depending on the age of the patient and whether there is a medical or trauma problem. The medical history does not change the initial assessment. (pp. 215–216)

16. **(C)** The capillary refill test is used to evaluate the circulation of infants and children but is no longer advocated as an effective, reliable test for adults. (p. 221)

17. **(B)** Check the mental status of an unconscious infant by talking to the infant and flicking the infant's feet. The sternal rub would be too aggressive and could cause injury. (p. 221)

18. **(B)** A fever and a rash are not generally considered high priority. However, don't forget to take Standard Precautions and consider the need for a mask when treating such conditions. (p. 215)

19. **(A)** The difference between the general impression steps for a medical patient and that of a trauma patient is the need to provide manual stabilization of the head if you suspect spine injury in the trauma patient. (p. 216)

20. **(C)** Documenting examination findings that are negative (things that are not true) is called documenting a pertinent negative. (p. 340)

21. **(D)** When writing the PCR narrative section, do not state your personal opinion of the patient's condition. Only relevant facts, not subjective statements, should be documented. (pp. 339–341)

22. **(B)** An important concept of EMS documentation is "if it is not written down, you did not do it." (The presumption is that at the time of the incident you had the opportunity to document everything that you observed and treated.) (p. 341)

23. **(A)** If a patient does not wish to go to the hospital, document with a refusal-of-care form. Be sure to consult medical direction whenever there is a patient refusal. (pp. 342–345)

24. **(B)** Failure to perform an important part of patient assessment or care is an error of omission. Errors of commission are performing actions that are wrong or improper. (p. 345)

25. **(C)** Making up vitals is falsification and could endanger the patient's care. (p. 345)

26. **(C)** An objective statement describes something that is measurable, observable, or verifiable, such as vital signs. (p. 339)

27. **(A)** Stating that "the patient is alert and oriented" is an example of objective information that you observe but the patient does not tell you. (p. 339)

28. **(D)** Statements from patients, bystanders, or family should be put in quotes on the PCR. (p. 340)

29. **(A)** Statements about the rudeness of the family members are usually not relevant or needed on the PCR. (pp. 339–341)

30. (A) After establishing unresponsiveness in the initial assessment, proceed to open the airway. (p. 214)

31. (A) The EMT's "sixth sense" refers to clinical judgment, which is developed with experience. (p. 212)

32. (B) The vital signs are pulse, respirations, blood pressure, pupils, and skin condition, color, and temperature. (p. 226)

33. (B) The normal adult pulse rate at rest is between 60 and 100. (p. 228)

34. (D) The initial pulse rate for patients 1 year and older is normally taken at the radial pulse. (p. 228)

35. (D) When the pulse force is weak and thin, it is described as thready. (p. 228)

36. (B) Normal adult at-rest respiration rates vary from 12 to 20 breaths per minute. (p. 230)

37. (D) Crowing is a noisy, harsh sound heard during inhalation that indicates a partial airway obstruction. A gurgling sound is caused by fluid in the airway, which requires suctioning. (p. 231)

38. (C) The systolic blood pressure is the arterial pressure created when the left ventricle of the heart contracts. (p. 234)

39. (B) Diastolic blood pressure is the arterial pressure created by relaxation and refilling of the left ventricle of the heart. (p. 234)

40. (B) When a stethoscope is used along with a sphygmomanometer to take the blood pressure, this technique is called auscultation. (p. 236)

41. (A) Determining blood pressure by palpation is not as accurate as the auscultation method. This procedure is used when there is lots of noise around a patient. It is documented as the systolic reading. (p. 236)

42. (A) Information that you see, hear, feel, and smell are called signs and can be measured. Information the patient tells you are symptoms. (p. 242)

43. (B) When asking the patient "Have you recently had any surgery or injuries?", you are inquiring about the patient's pertinent past history. (p. 242)

44. (A) When you ask the patient "Are you on birth control pills?" you are inquiring about the patient's medications. This may give some clues about the patient's present problem. (p. 242)

45. (C) An acronym used to remember what questions to ask about the patient's present problem and past history is SAMPLE. AVPU is the level of responsiveness, PEARL is the status of the pupils, and DCAP-BTLS helps remind the EMT what to look for in a soft tissue exam. (p. 242)

46. (D) When conducting a patient interview on an adult patient, the EMT should position himself close to the patient, identify himself and reassure the patient, and gently touch the patient's shoulder or rest a hand over the patient's. It *is* necessary to ask the patient's age. (pp. 242–243)

47. (D) Normal diastolic pressures range from 60 to 90 mmHg. See Table 9-6. (p. 235)

48. (C) Using the formula presented in the text, a 36-year-old man would have an estimated systolic blood pressure of 136 mmHg (100 + age). See Table 9-6. (p. 235)

49. (B) Using the formula presented in the text, a 26-year-old woman would have an estimated systolic blood pressure of 116 mmHg (90 + age). See Table 9-6. (p. 235)

50. (A) The stethoscope should *not* be placed under the cuff and then inflated when evaluating the blood pressure because it may give a false reading. (pp. 237–238)

51. (C) When taking a patient's blood pressure, the stethoscope is placed over the brachial artery. The femoral artery is in the leg. (pp. 237–238)

52. (C) The mechanism of injury is the best indication of potential injury. (p. 197)

53. (B) When there are no apparent hazards at the scene of a collision, the danger zone should extend 50 feet in all directions from the wreckage. (p. 192)

54. (C) In the up-and-over head-on injury pattern, the patient is most likely to sustain head injuries. Chest and neck injuries are also common. Leg, knee, and hip injuries are usually the result of a down-and-under injury pattern. (pp. 198–199)

55. (C) A keen awareness that there may be injuries based on the mechanism of injury is called index of suspicion. (p. 204)

56. (C) The purpose of the initial assessment is to discover and treat life-threatening conditions. (p. 210)

57. (C) The first step in the focused history and physical exam of *any* trauma patient is to reconsider the mechanism of injury. (p. 250)

58. (C) The "A" in DCAP-BTLS stands for abrasions. (p. 251)

59. (D) Clues to determining the patient's need for a cervical collar include mechanism of injury, level of responsiveness, and location of injuries. The breathing rate will not assist in determining the need for a cervical collar. (pp. 253–254)

60. (B) The rapid assessment evaluates areas of the body where the greatest threats to the patient may be. (p. 265)

61. (A) The detailed physical exam is most often performed on the trauma patient with a significant mechanism of injury. (p. 273)

62. (A) To obtain a history of a patient's present illness, ask the OPQRST questions. These will focus on the chief complaint and potential causes. (p. 293)

63. (C) The "P" in OPQRST stands for *provokes*, which refers to questions such as "Can you think of anything that might have triggered this pain?" (p. 293)

64. (A) The correct order in the focused history and physical exam of the unresponsive medical patient is conduct a rapid physical exam, obtain baseline vital signs, gather the history of the present illness (OPQRST) from bystanders and family, and gather a SAMPLE history from bystanders and family. (pp. 296–298)

65. (C) For a stable patient, the EMT should perform the ongoing assessment every 15 minutes. For an unstable patient, perform the ongoing assessment every 5 minutes. (p. 312)

66. (A) During the ongoing assessment, whenever you believe there may have been a change in the patient's condition, you should repeat the initial assessment. (pp. 308–309)

67. (D) Cool, clammy skin most likely indicates hypoperfusion (shock). Exposure to cold causes dry, cold skin. Fever results in clammy and warm or hot skin. (p. 232)

68. (D) As an EMT, your overriding concern at all times is your own safety. Certainly your crew's safety is a priority, but your personal safety MUST come first. (p. 189)

69. (A) During the detailed physical exam of the head of a trauma patient, inspect the ears and nose for blood or clear fluids. (pp. 274–276)

70. (C) Infants and young children under the age of 8 are abdominal breathers. (p. 812, Chapter 31)

71. **(B)** Repeaters are devices used when radio transmissions must be carried over long distances. (p. 320)

72. **(C)** If possible, position yourself at or below the patient's eye level. This will be less threatening to the patient. (pp. 326–327)

73. **(B)** The first item given to the hospital in your medical radio report to the receiving facility is your unit identification/level of provider. (p. 323)

74. **(D)** The patient's attitude is not an essential component of the verbal report to the receiving hospital. (p. 326)

75. **(C)** Medical radio reports should paint a picture of the patient's problem in words. (pp. 324–325)

76. **(D)** Always question orders from medical direction that you do not understand. (p. 325)

77. **(A)** Medications that are carried on the ambulance and that EMTs can administer include activated charcoal, oxygen, and oral glucose. Nitroglycerin, epinephrine, and the prescribed inhaler are medications that the EMT may assist the patient with administration. (p. 355)

78. **(D)** Any action of a drug other than the desired action is called a side effect. (p. 360)

79. **(D)** When a drug is administered subcutaneously, this means the drug is injected under the skin. (p. 363)

80. **(D)** Infants and children depend more on the diaphragm for respiration than adults do. (p. 812, chapter 31)

81. **(A)** The order of preference for providing artificial ventilation are pocket face mask with supplemental oxygen; two-person bag-valve mask with supplemental oxygen; flow-restricted, oxygen-powered ventilator; and one-person bag-valve mask with supplemental oxygen. (p. 371)

82. **(B)** The adequate rate of artificial ventilation for a non-breathing adult patient is 10–12 breaths per minute. (p. 372)

83. **(C)** The adequate rate of artificial ventilation for a nonbreathing infant or child patient is 12–20 breaths per minute. (p. 372)

84. **(A)** If an unresponsive adult makes snoring or gurgling sounds, he most likely has a serious airway problem requiring immediate intervention. (pp. 370–371)

85. **(D)** The skin of a patient with inadequate breathing may be blue (or pale) in color and will feel cool and clammy. (pp. 370–371)

86. **(C)** If a patient is experiencing breathing difficulty, but is breathing adequately, it is usually best to place him in a position of comfort. This is generally a sitting-up position. (p. 376)

87. **(D)** The cause of adult chest pain due to a decreased blood supply to the heart is angina pectoris. Arrhythmia is an irregular heart rhythm. (pp. 401–402)

88. **(C)** Most heart attacks are caused by narrowing or occlusion of a coronary artery. The coronary arteries supply the heart muscle with blood. (pp. 400–401)

89. **(D)** Acute myocardial infarction is the condition in which a portion of the heart muscle dies because of oxygen starvation. (pp. 402–403)

90. **(B)** An irregular or absent heart rhythm is called arrhythmia. (p. 401)

91. **(A)** A pulse slower than 60 beats per minute is called bradycardia. (p. 393)

92. **(C)** An at-rest heart beat faster than 100 beats per minute is referred to as tachycardia. (p. 393)

93. **(A)** Congestive heart failure is the condition caused by excessive fluid buildup in the lungs and/or other organs and body parts because of the inadequate pumping of the heart. (p. 403)

94. **(D)** A conscious patient with a possible heart attack is best placed in the position of comfort. For ease of breathing, this is usually a sitting position. (p. 396)

95. **(A)** A diabetic found with a weak, rapid pulse and cold, clammy skin who complains of hunger pangs is probably suffering from hypoglycemia. Hyperglycemic patients often have warm, red, dry skin and an acetone breath. (pp. 449–450)

96. **(B)** In hyperglycemia, the patient will have acetone smelling breath. (pp. 449–450)

97. **(A)** A conscious hypoglycemic patient who is able to swallow is frequently administered oral glucose, with permission given by medical direction or standing orders. (p. 455)

98. **(C)** If you cannot administer glucose to the diabetic patient because she is not awake enough to swallow, you should treat her like any other patient with altered mental status. Secure the airway, provide artificial ventilations if necessary, and be prepared to perform CPR if needed. (p. 455)

99. **(C)** The first time a person is exposed to an allergen, the person's immune system forms antibodies. (p. 474)

100. **(C)** To be considered a severe allergic reaction, a patient must have signs and symptoms of shock or respiratory distress. (p. 474)

101. **(B)** If a patient has no history of allergies and is having his first allergic reaction, you should treat for shock and transport immediately. (pp. 478–479)

102. **(C)** Carbon monoxide, chlorine, and ammonia are examples of inhaled poisons. (p. 491)

103. **(A)** It is important for the EMT to determine when the ingestion of a poison occurred because different poisons act on the body at different rates. (p. 493)

104. **(B)** The principal prehospital treatment of a patient who has inhaled poison is administering high-concentration oxygen. (p. 499)

105. **(B)** If mixing alcohol and other drugs, the patient will exhibit with depressed vital signs. (p. 506)

106. **(D)** Activated charcoal is contraindicated for patients who have ingested alkalis, gasoline, or acids. (p. 496)

107. **(C)** Most cases of poisoning involve young children. (p. 490)

108. **(C)** Poisons that are swallowed are ingested poisons. (p. 493)

109. **(B)** A patient with hot and dry or hot and moist skin is experiencing a true emergency that requires rapid cooling and immediate transport. (p. 527)

110. **(A)** As frostbite progresses and exposure continues, the skin will turn from white and waxy to blotchy and grayish yellow and finally to grayish blue. (pp. 523–524)

111. **(C)** To treat a patient with deep frostbite, cover the frostbitten area, handle it as gently as possible, and transport patient. Do not rub the area or apply cold. Do not rewarm the area unless you can ensure it will not refreeze. (p. 524)

112. **(D)** With frostbite, the affected area feels frozen, but only on the surface. (p. 523)

113. (A) The initial sign of hypothermia is shivering. (p. 519)

114. (A) Extreme hypothermia is characterized by unconsciousness and absence of discernible vital signs. If there is shivering, numbness, and drowsiness, the patient is not yet in severe hypothermia. (pp. 518–520)

115. (D) The emergency care steps for a hypothermic patient include keeping the patient still and dry and applying heat to raise the patient's core body temperature. Do not encourage the patient to walk. (pp. 521–522)

116. (C) After calming a snakebite victim and treating for shock, you locate the fang marks. Next, you should cleanse the wound site with soap and water. (p. 542)

117. (A) When a patient who was working in a hot environment complains of severe muscle cramps in the legs and feels faint, you should move the patient to a cool place and begin care by administering oxygen by nonrebreather. (p. 527)

118. (C) The first step in caring for a rescued near-drowning victim is to establish an airway and evaluate the need for CPR. (p. 531)

119. (D) Your first step when called to care for any attempted suicide victim is to ensure your own safety. This may mean waiting for police assistance, depending on the circumstances of the suicide attempt. (p. 553)

120. (C) If you are unable to perform normal assessment and care procedures because the patient is aggressive and hostile, you should seek advice from medical direction. (p. 555)

121. (B) The EMT is allowed to use reasonable force to defend against attack by an emotionally disturbed patient. (p. 555)

122. (B) The developing unborn baby is called a fetus. (p. 564)

123. (C) The muscular organ in which the fetus develops is the uterus. (p. 564)

124. (A) The organ of pregnancy in which exchange of oxygen, nutrients, and wastes occurs between mother and fetus is the placenta. (p. 564)

125. (C) While developing, the fetus is protected by a thin, membranous "bag of waters" called the amniotic sac. (p. 565)

126. (A) When the presenting part of the baby first bulges from the vaginal opening, this is called crowning. (p. 565)

127. (C) The first stage of labor begins with uterine contractions. (p. 565)

128. (B) The second stage of labor ends with infant delivery. (p. 565)

129. (C) The third stage of labor ends with delivery of the placenta. (p. 565)

130. (D) If a woman is having her first baby, the first stage of labor will usually last 16 hours on the average. (p. 566)

131. (B) During the most active stage of labor, the uterus usually contracts every 2 to 3 minutes (with contractions commonly lasting 30 seconds to 1 minute). (p. 565)

132. (C) If the amniotic sac does not break during delivery, the EMT should puncture it with a finger; then remove the membranes from the baby's nose and mouth. (p. 572)

133. (B) To assist the mother in delivering the baby's upper shoulder, gently support the baby's head. Do not pull on the infant. (p. 574)

134. (B) After delivery, first position the newborn on his side, then suction the baby's nose and mouth before clamping the cord. We do not slap infants on their buttocks as this may injure them, or worse, you may drop the slippery child. (p. 576)

135. (C) If spontaneous respiration does not begin after suctioning the baby's mouth and nose, the EMT should vigorously rub the baby's back; then • consider mechanical ventilatory assistance. (p. 576)

136. (C) The first clamp placed on the umbilical cord should be about 10 inches from the baby. (p. 578)

137. (A) If bleeding continues from the umbilical cord after clamping and cutting, the EMT should clamp the cord again, close to the original clamp. (p. 578)

138. (A) The maximum amount of time to wait for the placenta to be delivered before transporting is 20 minutes. (p. 579)

139. (A) Delivery of the placenta is usually accompanied by the loss of no more than 500 cc of blood. (p. 580)

140. (B) The first step to control vaginal bleeding after birth is to place a sanitary napkin over the vaginal opening. Do not pack the vagina. Consider massaging the uterus if bleeding persists. Allow the mother to nurse the baby, which will control bleeding by stimulating contraction of the uterus. (p. 580)

141. (B) The presenting part of the baby in a breech birth is the buttocks or legs. (p. 582)

142. (B) If upon viewing the vaginal area, you see the umbilical cord presenting first (a prolapsed cord delivery), you should gently push up on the baby's head or buttocks to keep pressure off the cord. Do not cut the cord since it is the infant's blood supply. Never attempt to push the cord back into the vagina. (p. 583)

143. (C) If an arm presentation without a prolapsed cord is noted, the EMT should transport immediately, providing high-concentration oxygen. (p. 584)

144. (C) A baby is considered premature if the baby weighs less than 5 pounds or is born before the 37th week. (p. 586)

Chapter 26: Bleeding and Shock

MATCH TERMINOLOGY/ DEFINITIONS

▶ **PART A**

1. (J) Artery—blood vessel with thick, muscular walls that carries oxygen-rich blood away from the heart (p. 616)

2. (A) Brachial artery—major artery of the upper arm (p. 625)

3. (C) Capillary bleeding—bleeding that is characterized by a slow, oozing flow of blood (p. 619)

4. (H) Cardiogenic shock—lack of perfusion brought on by inadequate pumping action of the heart (p. 632)

5. (B) Compensated shock—when the patient is developing shock, but the body is still able to maintain perfusion (p. 631)

6. (E) Decompensated shock—condition that occurs when the body can no longer compensate for low blood volume or lack of perfusion; late signs, such as falling blood pressure, develop (p. 633)

7. (F) Femoral artery—major artery supplying the thigh (p. 625)

8. (I) Golden hour—optimum time limit between time of injury and surgery at the hospital; survival rates are best if surgery takes place within this time period (pp. 633–634)

9. **(G)** Hemorrhage—severe bleeding; a major cause of shock (p. 617)

10. **(D)** Hemorrhagic shock—shock resulting from blood loss (p. 632)

▶ **PART B**

1. **(J)** Hypoperfusion—inadequate circulation of the blood in which the body's cells and organs do not receive adequate supplies of oxygen and nutrients and dangerous waste products build up (p. 617)

2. **(H)** Hypovolemic shock—shock resulting from uncontrolled bleeding or plasma loss (p. 632)

3. **(E)** Irreversible shock—when the body has lost the battle to maintain perfusion to the organ systems; cell damage occurs, especially to the liver and kidneys (p. 633)

4. **(I)** Neurogenic shock—shock resulting from uncontrolled dilation of blood vessels due to nerve paralysis (sometimes caused by spinal cord injuries) (p. 632)

5. **(C)** Perfusion—adequate circulation of blood throughout the body, filling the capillaries and supplying cells and tissues with oxygen and nutrients (p. 617)

6. **(G)** Pressure dressing—bulky dressing held in position with a tightly wrapped bandage to help control bleeding (p. 621)

7. **(D)** Pressure point—site where a large artery lies near the surface of the body and directly over a bone; pressure on such a location can control profuse bleeding in the extremities (p. 623)

8. **(F)** Shock—another name for hypoperfusion (p. 617)

9. **(A)** Tourniquet—device that closes off all blood flow to and from an extremity (p. 626)

10. **(B)** Vein—blood vessel that has one-way valves and carries blood back to the heart (p. 617)

MULTIPLE-CHOICE REVIEW

1. **(B)** Blood that has been depleted of oxygen and loaded with carbon dioxide empties into the veins, which carry it back to the heart. (p. 617)

2. **(A)** Cells and tissues of the brain, spinal cord, and kidneys are the most sensitive to inadequate perfusion. (p. 617)

3. **(B)** The use of Standard Precautions is essential whenever bleeding is discovered or anticipated. (p. 621)

4. **(C)** Bleeding is classified as arterial, venous, and capillary. There is no category called cellular bleeding. (p. 618)

5. **(B)** Arterial bleeding is often rapid and profuse. Blood in arteries is maintained under high pressure by thick, muscular walls. For this reason, arterial hemorrhage is *more* difficult to control. Clot formation is also difficult because of this pressure. (p. 618)

6. **(B)** A steady flow of dark red or maroon blood is a result of venous bleeding. Deoxygenated blood travels back to the heart through veins. (p. 618)

7. **(C)** Bleeding described as oozing is usually a result of capillary bleeding. (p. 619)

8. **(B)** When a large bleeding vein in the neck sucks in debris or an air bubble (embolism), this can cause heart stoppage or damage the brain or lungs. An evisceration occurs when an organ or part of an organ protrudes through a wound opening. (p. 619)

9. **(D)** Sudden blood loss of 1,000 cc in an adult is considered serious. This is double the amount that a blood donor gives. (pp. 619–620)

10. **(D)** Sudden blood loss of 500 cc in a child is considered serious. (pp. 619–620)

11. **(D)** Sudden blood loss of 150 cc in a 1-year-old infant is considered serious. (pp. 619–620)

12. **(D)** The body's natural responses to bleeding are constriction of the injured blood vessel(s) and clotting. However, a serious injury may prevent effective clotting, allowing continued bleeding. (p. 619)

13. **(B)** Do not wait for signs and symptoms of shock to appear before beginning treatment. Any patient with a significant amount of blood loss should be treated to *prevent* the development of shock. Many signs and symptoms of shock appear late in the process. (p. 621)

14. **(D)** The major methods used to control external bleeding include direct pressure, elevation, and pressure points. Vessel clamps are used in surgery. (p. 621)

15. **(B)** Administering supplemental oxygen improves oxygenation of the tissues. Blood loss decreases perfusion, which means that less oxygen is delivered to the tissues. Supplemental oxygen increases the oxygen saturation of the blood still present in the circulatory system. (p. 621)

16. **(D)** The most common and effective way to control external bleeding is direct pressure. This can be done with your gloved hand, a dressing and your gloved hand, or by a pressure dressing and a bandage. (p. 621)

17. **(C)** The initial, or first, dressing should not be removed from a bleeding wound because it is a necessary part of clot formation. Removing it may destroy developing clots or cause further injury. (p. 621)

18. **(B)** After controlling bleeding from an extremity using a pressure bandage, be sure to check the distal pulse to make sure the bandage is not too tight. If administering oxygen, use a nonrebreather mask at 15 liters per minute. (p. 623)

19. **(D)** Elevation is used to assist in bleeding control for the following reasons: it slows bleeding, raises the limb above the heart, and helps to reduce blood pressure in the limb. Actually, shock speeds up the pulse. (p. 623)

20. **(C)** It is inappropriate to use elevation to assist in bleeding control if you suspect musculoskeletal injuries because you could further injure the patient. (p. 623)

21. **(A)** A pressure point is a site where a main artery lies near the surface of the body directly over the bone. Any site where a pulse can be felt is a pressure point. (p. 623)

22. **(C)** Use of a pressure point may not be effective if the wound is at the distal end of a limb. Blood is being sent to this area of the limb from many other smaller arteries. (p. 625)

23. **(A)** An air splint is most effective for controlling venous and capillary bleeding. It is not usually effective for arterial bleeding, at least not until the arterial pressure has decreased below that of the pressure in the splint. An air splint may be used to maintain pressure on a bleeding wound *after* other manual methods have already controlled the bleeding. (p. 625)

24. **(D)** Do not insert the ice directly into the wound. When applying cold to a bleeding area, wrap the ice pack/cold pack in a cloth or towel, do not apply directly onto the skin, and do not leave the ice pack/cold pack in place for more than 20 minutes. (p. 625)

25. (B) Many experts agree that the pneumatic anti-shock garment is useful for controlling bleeding from areas the garment covers. It is contraindicated for penetrating chest trauma and the patient in cardiogenic shock. (p. 626)

26. (A) Bleeding from a clean-edged amputation is usually initially cared for with a pressure dressing. This is because injured blood vessels seal themselves shut as a result of spasms produced by the muscular walls of the vessels. (p. 626)

27. (C) Rough-edged amputations, usually produced by crushing or tearing injuries, often bleed heavily because the nature of the injury does not allow for vasoconstriction. Bleeding from these wounds are difficult to control and in some isolated cases require a tourniquet as a last resort. (p. 626)

28. (A) Once a tourniquet is in place, it must not be removed or loosened unless ordered by medical direction. Do not loosen, as toxins will flow into the bloodstream. Never cover the extremity because you must visually monitor the wound site and the effectiveness of the tourniquet. (p. 626)

29. (C) A blood pressure cuff can be used as a tourniquet if inflated to 150 mmHg or more. (p. 628)

30. (D) Allow the drainage to flow freely. The head injury has resulted in increased pressure within the skull, which is forcing fluid out of the cranial cavity. Do not attempt to stop this bleeding or fluid loss; this may increase the pressure in the skull. (p. 628)

31. (B) The medical term for a nosebleed is epistaxis. (p. 628)

32. (D) A cold pack applied to the bridge of the nose, by itself, will not control bleeding. To stop a nosebleed, place the patient in a sitting position, leaning forward; apply direct pressure by pinching the nostrils; and keep the patient calm. (p. 628)

33. (A) The leading cause of internal injuries and bleeding is blunt trauma. (p. 629)

34. (A) A blast injury is *not* usually considered penetrating trauma, unless the blast propels sharp flying objects that penetrate the patient. (p. 629)

35. (B) Bradycardia and a flushed face are not commonly associated with internal bleeding. Signs of internal bleeding include vomiting a coffee-ground-like substance; dark, tarry stools; and a tender, rigid, or distended abdomen. (pp. 629–630)

36. (D) A laceration to the forearm would be considered external, not internal, bleeding. A patient who has internal bleeding may have painful, swollen, or deformed extremities (from bleeding within the limb); signs and symptoms of shock; or bright red blood in the stool. (pp. 629–630)

37. (C) Inadequate perfusion is referred to as shock or hypoperfusion. (p. 631)

38. (D) You will learn that an isolated injury to the head does not commonly produce shock because there is not enough room within the adult skull to permit enough bleeding to cause shock. Shock may develop from pump failure, lost blood volume, or dilated blood vessels. (p. 633)

39. (D) Hypovolemic (hemorrhagic) shock caused by uncontrolled bleeding is the type of shock most often seen by EMTs. (p. 632)

40. (C) The heart attack patient is in shock as a result of pump failure, not the other mechanisms described. (p. 632)

41. (C) Neurogenic shock may result from the uncontrolled dilation of blood vessels due to nerve paralysis caused by spinal cord injuries. Septic shock may also result in the massive dilation of blood vessels. (p. 632)

42. (A) When a patient is in shock but the body is still able to maintain perfusion to the vital organs, this is called compensated shock. (pp. 631–632)

43. (D) Early signs of shock that show the body is compensating are increased heart rate; increased respirations; pale, cool skin; and *increased* capillary refill time in infants and children. (p. 633)

44. (D) When the body has lost the battle to maintain perfusion to the organ systems, this is called irreversible shock. (p. 632)

45. (A) The patient in shock feels nauseated because blood flow is diverted from the digestive systems to the vital organs. Digestion of food is not a priority for the patient in shock. (p. 633)

46. (C) The pulse of a patient in shock will increase in an attempt to pump more blood. (p. 633)

47. (D) A drop in blood pressure is a late sign of shock. The falling blood pressure signifies that the patient has entered the decompensated stage of the shock process. (p. 633)

48. (D) Additional signs of shock may include thirst, dilated pupils, and cyanosis around the lips and nail beds. The shock patient will present with pale, cool, clammy skin, *not* flushed, warm skin, because blood is quickly directed away from the skin and sent to organs such as the heart and brain. (p. 633)

49. (B) The EMT should be especially careful when evaluating pediatric shock patients because they may have very few signs until a large percentage of their blood volume (approximately 50%) is lost. There is no problem giving them high-concentration oxygen. (p. 632)

50. (A) "Platinum 10 minutes" is the optimum on-scene time limit when treating a trauma patient. The golden hour is the time from injury to surgical treatment (pp. 633–634)

COMPLETE THE FOLLOWING

1. The major types of shock include: (p. 632)
- hypovolemic
- cardiogenic
- neurogenic

2. The signs and symptoms of shock include: (p. 633)
- altered mental status
- pale, cool, clammy skin
- nausea and vomiting
- vital sign changes such as increased pulse, decreased blood pressure, and increased respirations
- thirst
- dilated pupils
- cyanosis
- delayed capillary refill in children

STREET SCENES DISCUSSION

1. The rib cage protects the stomach, spleen, liver, gall bladder, pancreas, and parts of the intestine.

2. Yes. If it is available, ALS should be requested to intercept if it is not on scene when you are ready to transport.

3. Changes to mental status due to hypoperfusion or internal bleeding are indicators that the patient may be decompensating and needs surgery right away to stop the blood loss.

CASE STUDY—CONVENIENCE STORE SHOOTING

1. It ensures that the shooter is no longer on the scene.

2. Safety issues, number of patients, the need for additional resources

3. Internal and external bleeding are present. He is going into decompensated shock. This is recognized by the fast, weak radial pulse. Estimate his blood pressure at less than 90 systolic.

4. He is in decompensating hypovolemic, or hemorrhagic, shock from blood loss.

5. His brain interprets his blood loss (fluid) as "low fluid volume." Therefore, he asks for fluids. In this case, it is too late to restore his fluid volume by asking him to drink fluids. He needs IV fluids and whole blood in the trauma center.

6. Bullet fragments can easily ricochet into the chest. (Always listen to the lung sounds on a trauma patient to prevent missing potential injuries to the lungs.)

7. Use a nonrebreather mask at 15 liters per minute. Monitor his ventilations closely in case you need to switch to a BVM.

8. Call for ALS immediately. If ALS has not arrived when you are ready to transport, then arrange an intercept en route to the hospital.

9. A "platinum 10 minutes" on the scene

10. A "golden hour" from the time of the injury to the surgery

11. Insert an oral airway if he has no gag reflex. Switch to assisted ventilations if required. When the paramedics arrive, he should be tubed (unless your EMT training included endotracheal intubation).

12. That's controversial and dependent on your local protocols. However, since he has internal bleeding and no penetrating chest wound or pulmonary edema, some protocols would allow PASG use.

13. Because this patient is being ventilated (at this time), he is considered critical. And in fact, he is in decompensated shock and moving to irreversible shock.

14. Two large-bore IVs of normal saline or Ringer's lactate, endotracheal intubation, monitor ECG, consider PASG, and assisted ventilations.

15. Review your sample radio report with your instructor.

Chapter 27: Soft-Tissue Injuries

MATCH TERMINOLOGY/ DEFINITIONS

▶ PART A

1. **(N)** Abrasion—scrape or scratch in which the outer layer of the skin is damaged but all layers are not penetrated (p. 648)

2. **(K)** Air embolus—air bubble in the bloodstream (p. 658)

3. **(O)** Amputation—surgical removal or traumatic severing of a body part, usually an extremity (p. 651)

4. **(H)** Avulsion—flap of skin or other soft tissue torn loose or pulled off completely (p. 650)

5. **(C)** Bandage—any material used to hold a dressing in place (p. 683)

6. **(F)** Closed wound—internal injury in which there is no open pathway from the outside to the injured site (p. 645)

7. **(M)** Contusion—bruise (p. 646)

8. **(J)** Crush injury—injury caused when force is transmitted from the body's exterior to its internal structures (p. 647)

9. **(L)** Dermis—layer of the skin below the epidermis; it is rich in blood vessels, nerves, and specialized structures such as sweat glands, sebaceous (oil) glands, and hair follicles (p. 645)

10. **(I)** Dressing—any material used to cover a wound in an effort to control bleeding and help prevent further contamination (p. 683)

11. **(B)** Epidermis—outer layer of the skin (p. 645)

12. **(E)** Evisceration—intestine or other internal organ protruding through a wound in the abdomen (p. 668)

13. **(G)** Full thickness burn—burn in which all the layers of the skin are damaged; also called a third-degree burn (p. 673)

14. **(A)** Hematoma—swelling caused by the collection of blood under the skin or in damaged tissues as a result of an injured or broken blood vessel (p. 647)

15. **(D)** Laceration—cut that can be smooth or jagged (p. 648)

▶ PART B

1. **(H)** Occlusive dressing—any dressing that forms an airtight seal (p. 663)

2. **(F)** Open wound—injury in which the skin is interrupted, or broken, exposing the tissue underneath (p. 648)

3. **(D)** Partial thickness burn—burn in which the epidermis is burned through and the dermis is damaged; also called a second-degree burn (p. 672)

4. **(J)** Puncture wound—open wound caused by a sharp, pointed object that tears through the skin and destroys underlying tissues (p. 649)

5. **(B)** Rule of nines—method for estimating the extent of a burn area in which areas on the body are assigned certain percentages of the body's total surface area (p. 674)

6. **(I)** Rule of palm—method for estimating the extent of a burn area; the palm of the patient's hand, which equals about 1% of the body's surface area, is compared with the patient's burn to estimate its size (p. 674)

7. **(G)** Subcutaneous layers—layers of fat and soft tissues below the dermis (p. 645)

8. **(C)** Sucking chest wound—open chest wound in which air is sucked into the chest cavity (p. 663)

9. **(E)** Superficial burn—burn that involves only the epidermis, the outer layer of the skin; also called a first-degree burn (p. 671)

10. **(A)** Universal dressing—large bulky dressing (p. 685)

11. **(K)** Flail chest is a fracture of two or more adjacent ribs in two or more places that allows for free movement of the fractured segment (p. 660)

12. **(L)** Paradoxical motion is the movement of ribs in a flail segment that is opposite the rest of the chest wall (p. 661)

13. (M) Pneumothorax is air in the chest cavity (p. 633)

14. (N) Tension pneumothorax is a type of pneumothorax in which air that enters the chest cavity is prevented from escaping (p. 663)

MULTIPLE-CHOICE REVIEW

1. (C) The teeth, bones, and cartilage are *not* considered soft tissue. The soft tissues of the body include skin, blood vessels, fatty tissues, muscles, fibrous tissues, nerves, glands, and membranes. (p. 644)

2. (D) Blood insulation is a distracter. The functions of the skin include protecting the body by providing a barrier to germs, debris, and unwanted chemicals; shock (impact) absorption; and temperature regulation. (p. 644)

3. (D) Epithelial cells comprise the tissue that covers the respiratory tract. The layers of the skin are the epidermis, dermis, and subcutaneous layers. (p. 645)

4. (A) The layer of the skin called the epidermis is composed of dead cells, which are rubbed off or sloughed off and are replaced continuously. See answers 3, 5, 6. (p. 645)

5. (B) Specialized nerve endings in the skin layer called the dermis are involved with the senses of touch, cold, heat, and pain. (p. 645)

6. (C) Shock absorption and insulation are major functions of the subcutaneous layers of the skin. See answers 3, 4, 5. (p. 645)

7. (C) Wounds that usually result from the impact of a blunt object are called closed. Wounds resulting from stabbings, lacerations, and perforations are open wounds. (p. 645)

8. (B) A closed wound that involves a large amount of tissue damage and a collection of blood at the injury site is called a hematoma. A contusion is relatively minor. See answer 9 for crush injury. A penetration is a puncture wound. (p. 647)

9. (C) A soft-tissue injury caused by a force that can cause rupture or bleeding of internal organs is called a crush injury. (p. 647)

10. (C) An open wound is an injury in which the skin is interrupted, exposing the tissues underneath. See answer 9 for crush injury. See answer 8 for hematoma. (p. 647)

11. (B) A minor ooze of blood from capillary beds is from an injury called an abrasion. An amputation occurs when an extremity or digit is cut or torn completely off. A laceration is a cut, and a puncture is a penetration or hole made with a sharp object. (p. 648)

12. (C) A cut caused by a sharp-edged object such as a razor blade or broken glass is called a laceration. See answer 11 for abrasion. See answer 13 for puncture. See answer 14 for avulsion. (pp. 648–649)

13. (B) When a sharp, pointed object passes through the skin or other tissue, a puncture wound has occurred. (p. 649)

14. (A) When the tip of the nose is cut or torn off, this is an avulsion. Attempt to preserve any avulsed part, since it may be possible to surgically restore the part or to use it for skin grafts. (p. 650)

15. (A) The priority when treating severe open wounds is to control bleeding. While cleaning the wound, preventing contamination, and bandaging are important, it is necessary to first control bleeding by direct pressure (with elevation if necessary). (p. 653)

16. (D) Care for a laceration includes checking the pulse distal to the injury. Also check sensory and motor function. The patient may need stitches, plastic surgery, or a tetanus shot at the hospital, so do not put on butterfly bandages and release the patient. Never pull apart the edges of a laceration. (p. 653)

17. (C) Various types of guns fired at close range can cause burns around the entry wound, injection of air into the tissues (causing severe damage), and damage underlying tissue. Generally the patient would not present with a contusion unless he or she had on a bulletproof vest, which spreads the energy of the impact. (p. 654)

18. (D) Never remove an impaled object. Care in the field for a patient with an impaled object includes stabilizing the object, using direct pressure, and leaving the object in place (unless it is impaled in the cheek). See answer 16. (pp. 655–656)

19. (C) Never apply pressure to the object; rather, stabilize it with a bulky dressing. An impaled object may be plugging bleeding from a major artery while it is in place. To remove it may cause severe bleeding. Removal could also cause further injury to nerves, muscles, and other soft tissue. (pp. 655–656)

20. (A) To control profuse bleeding resulting from an impaled object, position your gloved hands on either side of the object and exert downward pressure. Be careful not to push the actual object in any further. (pp. 655–656)

21. (A) If you can see both ends of the object impaled in the cheek, pull it out in the direction it entered the cheek. However, never twist the object. If it is impaled into a deeper structure, stabilize it. The object may go into the oral cavity and create an airway obstruction or bleeding into the mouth may interfere with breathing or cause nausea or induce vomiting. (pp. 656–657)

22. (C) If a patient has an impaled object in the eye, your care should include use of 4 × 4s to stabilize the object and a paper cup to cover the impaled object. Make sure to cover the uninjured eye. Never use plastic foam cups as the particles may flake into the eye. (p. 657)

23. (D) In cases where an avulsed flap of tissue has been torn loose but not off, the EMT should fold the skin back to its normal position, clean the wound surface, control bleeding, and dress the wound. Do not tear off the remainder of the flap. (p. 658)

24. (C) Avulsed parts should be treated by placing in a plastic bag and then placing on top of a sealed bag of ice. Do not put the part directly on ice or in dry ice. Follow local protocols with regard to use of saline. (p. 658)

25. (C) When treating an amputation, be sure to place a snug pressure dressing over the stump. A tourniquet should only be used if other methods fail. The amputated part should not be placed directly on ice nor should ice be used on the stump. (p. 658)

26. (B) When treating an amputation, whenever possible transport the patient and the amputated body part in the same ambulance. This will avoid delays and possibly save the person's limb. (p. 658)

27. (A) An air bubble sucked into a large vein in the neck is called an air embolus. The "bends," or decompression sickness, involves nitrogen bubbles in the joints that do not enter the body through an external opening. (pp. 658–659)

28. (A) The treatment of neck vein injury is aimed at preventing an embolus, preventing shock, and stopping bleeding. Do not compress the neck as you can injure the trachea or compress the arteries. (p. 659)

29. **(D)** To treat a neck laceration, the EMT should use an occlusive dressing to ensure material is not sucked into the wound. Do not use an ACE bandage as it could restrict breathing and arterial flow in the neck. (p. 659)

30. **(B)** When applying pressure to a neck wound, be sure you do not compress both carotids at the same time. This could cut off the blood supply to the brain and cause a stroke or other brain injury. (p. 659)

31. **(D)** The chest can be injured in a number of ways, including blunt trauma, penetrating objects, and compression. (p. 659)

32. **(C)** When the driver of a motor vehicle pitches forward after a head-on collision and strikes the chest on the steering column, this is called a compression injury. The heart can be severely squeezed, the lungs can be ruptured, and the sternum and ribs fractured. (pp. 660–661)

33. **(B)** All open wounds to the chest should be considered life-threatening. Such open wounds impede the patient's breathing ability. (p. 662)

34. **(C)** An injury that has both an entrance and an exit is called a perforating puncture wound. (p. 650)

35. **(B)** When the delicate pressure balance within the chest cavity is compromised, initially the lung on the injured side will collapse. The patient will limit chest expansion due to the pain involved in breathing. (p. 665)

36. **(C)** When the chest cavity is open to the atmosphere, this is referred to as a sucking chest wound. A hemothorax is a condition in which the chest cavity fills with blood. (p. 663)

37. **(B)** Binding the chest will make it even harder for the patient to breathe. The treatment for an open chest wound includes maintaining an open airway, administering high-concentration oxygen, and sealing the open wound. (p. 663)

38. **(D)** When air becomes trapped in the chest cavity, it will *not* increase the ventilatory volume of the chest. Trapped air in the chest can put pressure on the unaffected lung and heart, reduce cardiac output, and affect oxygenation of the blood. (p. 665)

39. **(D)** The signs and symptoms of a pneumothorax or tension pneumothorax include tracheal deviation to the uninjured side, distended neck veins, and uneven chest wall movement. The depth of respiration is *not* increased. (p. 667)

40. **(B)** Coughed-up frothy blood is *not* a sign of traumatic asphyxia. The signs and symptoms include distended neck veins; head, neck, and shoulders that appear dark blue; and bloodshot and bulging eyes. (p. 667)

41. **(B)** When taping a four-sided occlusive dressing in place, have the patient forcefully exhale as you tape. (pp. 663–664)

42. **(B)** When an open wound to the abdomen is so large and deep that organs protrude, this is called an evisceration. (p. 668)

43. **(D)** Contusions over the upper ribs are signs of chest injury but not abdominal injuries. The signs of an abdominal injury include lacerations and puncture wounds to the lower back, large bruises on the abdomen, and indications of developing shock. (pp. 668–669)

44. **(B)** Partially digested blood that is vomited looks like coffee grounds. (p. 669)

45. **(C)** Headache is not normally a symptom of an abdominal injury. The symptoms of an abdominal injury include cramps, nausea, and thirst. Patients may also experience pain that is initially mild and then rapidly becomes intolerable. (pp. 668–669)

46. **(B)** Consider positioning the patient with an abdominal injury supine, with legs flexed at knees. This position relaxes the abdominal muscles and reduces pain. (p. 669)

47. **(C)** The treatment of an evisceration should *never* include replacing or touching the exposed organ. This could cause serious damage to the part and increase the chance of infection. (p. 669)

48. **(C)** When covering an exposed abdominal organ, apply a saline-moistened dressing directly over the wound site. Do not use aluminum foil since it can cut eviscerated organs. (pp. 669–670)

49. **(D)** Burn injuries often involve structures below the skin, such as muscles, nerves, bones, and blood vessels. (p. 671)

50. **(B)** In addition to physical damage caused by burns, patients often suffer emotional and psychological problems due to the lengthy recovery process and possibility of permanent disfigurement. (p. 671)

51. **(A)** When caring for a burn patient, think beyond the burn. Was there a possible medical emergency that caused the burn or did the burn aggravate an existing injury? (p. 671)

52. **(A)** When caring for burn patients, do not neglect assessment in order to begin burn care. A decision to transport immediately would be based on other injuries found. (p. 671)

53. **(D)** At normal temperature, distilled water is not a chemical that can burn a patient. Examples of agents causing burns are AC current, hydrochloric acid, and dry lime. (p. 671)

54. **(A)** A burn that involves only the epidermis is called a superficial burn. Epi-thickness is a distracter. (pp. 671–672)

55. **(B)** A burn that results in deep, intense pain, blisters, and mottled skin is called a partial thickness burn. (p. 672)

56. **(C)** To distinguish between a partial thickness burn and a full thickness burn, look for dry and white areas, which indicate a full thickness burn. Charred black or brown areas are also indicative of full thickness burns. (pp. 671–672)

57. **(B)** Electrical burns are of special concern since they pose a great risk of severe internal injuries. Chemical burns may remain on the skin and continue to burn for hours. Radiation burns may cause the patient to lose his hair over time. (p. 681)

58. **(C)** Chemical burns are of special concern since they may remain on the skin and continue to burn for hours. Superheated gases are usually present in a room with a fire in which the ceiling temperature is very hot. Electrical burns may travel from one extremity to the other and pose a great potential for internal injury. (p. 679)

59. **(D)** Burns to the face are of special concern because they may involve airway injury. They may also involve eye injury. (p. 674)

60. **(C)** Burns that can interrupt circulation to distal tissues are called circumferential burns. The resulting encircling scarring tends to limit normal functions. (p. 674)

61. **(B)** You are treating an adult patient who has partial-thickness burns to the entire left arm (9), chest (9), face, and neck (4½). The size of the burn area is 22.5%. (p. 675)

62. **(D)** You are treating an adult patient who has partial-thickness burns totally covering the legs (18 + 18), chest (9), and abdomen (9). The size of the burn area is 54%. (p. 675)

63. **(A)** A burn the size of five palms would cover approximately 5% of the body surface area. (p. 674)

64. **(B)** The age of the patient is an important factor in burns. Patients under 5 and over 55 years of age have the most

severe responses to burns. They also have a greater risk of death from burns. (p. 673)

65. **(A)** A partial thickness burn that involves less than 15% of the body surface is classified as a minor burn per Table 27-3 in the text. (p. 676)

66. **(B)** A partial thickness burn that involves between 15% and 30% of the body surface area is classified as a moderate burn per Table 27-3 in the text. (p. 676)

67. **(C)** A partial thickness burn that involves more than 30% of the body surface area is classified as a critical burn per Table 27-3 in the text. (p. 676)

68. **(D)** Partial thickness burns on the wrist would not be considered critical unless the hand was involved. Critical burns include circumferential burns, moderate burns in an infant or elderly patient, and burns complicated by musculoskeletal injuries. (p. 676)

69. **(B)** A partial thickness burn that involves between 10% and 20% of the body surface area of a child under 5 years of ages is classified as a moderate burn per Table 27-4 in the text. (p. 676)

70. **(C)** A full thickness burn to the front of the right forearm would not be considered a critical burn since it is only a small percentage of the body surface area. (p. 676)

71. **(A)** If a patient has a partial thickness burn to the entire back, the patient should be wrapped in a dry, sterile burn sheet. (p. 678)

72. **(B)** The primary care for a patient with a chemical burn is to wash away the chemical with flowing water. (p. 679)

73. **(C)** You are treating a patient who was burned. The patient is having visual difficulties, is restless and irritable, has an irregular pulse rate, and muscle tenderness. This patient probably has an electrical burn. (p. 682)

74. **(A)** If dry lime is the burn agent, brush it from the patient's skin and then flush with water. (p. 679)

75. **(A)** An occlusive dressing is used to form an airtight seal. (p. 685)

COMPLETE THE FOLLOWING

1. The signs of abdominal injury include: (any eight) (pp. 668–669)
   - pain, cramps, nausea, weakness, thirst
   - obvious lacerations and puncture wounds
   - lacerations and puncture wounds to the pelvis and middle or lower back or chest wounds near the diaphragm
   - indications of blunt trauma
   - indications of developing shock
   - coughing up or vomiting blood
   - rigid and/or tender abdomen
   - distended abdomen
   - the patient tries to lie very still with legs drawn up

2. The parts of the adult body that account for 9% each in the rule of nines are: (p. 675)
   - head and neck
   - each upper extremity
   - chest
   - abdomen
   - upper back
   - lower back and buttocks
   - front of each lower extremity
   - back of each lower extremity

3. The signs and symptoms of an electrical injury include: (any five) (p. 682)
   - burns where energy enters and exits
   - disrupted nerve pathways displayed as paralysis
   - respiratory difficulties or respiratory arrest
   - irregular heartbeat or cardiac arrest
   - muscle tenderness with or without muscular twitching
   - elevated blood pressure or low blood pressure with signs and symptoms of shock
   - restlessness or irritability if conscious, or loss of consciousness
   - visual difficulties
   - fractured bones and dislocations from severe muscle contractions or from falling
   - seizures

LABEL THE DIAGRAM (p. 672)

1. Superficial
2. Partial thickness
3. Full thickness
4. Skin reddened
5. Blisters
6. Charring

STREET SCENES DISCUSSION

1. Apply direct pressure as you elevate the arm. If that doesn't control the bleeding, hold a pressure point until the bleeding stops. Then firmly wrap the wound with a pressure bandage.

2. If the patient has an impaled object, do not attempt to remove it. Instead, stabilize the object in place with bulky dressings, applying pressure as each layer is positioned. Then secure the dressings in place with adhesive strips or tape. Be careful not to move the piece of glass.

3. If the patient already has low blood pressure, she is in very serious condition and needs rapid transport. Administer high-concentration oxygen, place her in a Trendelenburg position, keep her warm, and arrange for an ALS intercept en route to the hospital if possible.

Chapter 28: Musculoskeletal Injuries

MATCH TERMINOLOGY/ DEFINITIONS

1. **(A)** Bones—hard but flexible living structures that provide support for the body and protection for vital organs (p. 694)

2. **(I)** Cartilage—connective tissue that covers the outside of the bone ends and acts as a surface for articulation, allowing for smooth movements at joints (p. 699)

3. **(N)** Closed extremity injury—injury to an extremity in which the skin is not broken (p. 702)

4. **(E)** Crepitus—grating sensation or sound caused when broken bone ends rub together (p. 704)

5. **(B)** Dislocation—disruption or "coming apart" of a joint (p. 701)

6. **(H)** Extremities—portion of the skeleton that includes the clavicles, scapulae, arms, wrists, hands, pelvis, thighs, legs, ankles, and feet (p. 694)

7. **(G)** Fracture—any break in a bone (p. 701)

8. **(L)** Joints—places where bones articulate, or meet (p. 694)

9. **(O)** Ligaments—connective tissue that supports joints by attaching the bone ends and allowing for a stable range of motion (p. 699)

10. **(K)** Manual traction—process of applying tension to straighten and realign a fractured limb before splinting (p. 706)

11. **(C)** Open extremity injury—extremity injury in which the skin has been broken or torn through from the inside by an injured bone or from the outside by something that has caused a penetrating wound with associated injury to the bone (p. 702)

12. **(M)** Sprain—stretching and tearing of ligaments (p. 702)

13. **(J)** Strain—muscle injury caused by overstretching or over-exertion of the muscle (p. 702)

14. **(F)** Tendons—bands of connective tissue that bind muscles to bones (p. 699)

15. **(D)** Traction splint—special splint that applies constant pull along the length of the leg to help stabilize the fractured femur and reduce muscle spasms (p. 701)

MULTIPLE-CHOICE REVIEW

1. **(B)** As we age, our bones become deficient in calcium. (p. 695)

2. **(C)** The strong white fibrous material covering the bones is called the periosteum. (p. 696)

3. **(B)** In children, the majority of the long bone growth occurs in the growth plate (located at the ends of bones). Fractures in this area can be very serious and can lead to a shortening of a limb. (p. 699)

4. **(D)** Musculoskeletal injuries are caused by indirect, direct, and twisting forces. (p. 700)

5. **(B)** Fractures of the femur typically cause a 2-pint blood loss over the first 2 hours. If there are additional complications, such as an artery laceration, blood loss could be more severe. Blood loss from a fracture of tibia/fibula would be about 1 pint; and a pelvis fracture would cause a 3- to 4-pint loss. (p. 701)

6. **(C)** The death rate from closed fracture of the femur dropped from 80% to 20% in the post-WWI period due to the invention of the traction splint. The PASG was extensively used in the Vietnam conflict. (p. 701)

7. **(A)** The coming apart of a joint is referred to as a dislocation. A fracture is a break in a bone. See answer 8 for definitions of sprain and strain. (p. 701)

8. **(C)** The stretching or tearing of ligaments is called a sprain. A strain is caused by overstretching or overexertion of the muscle. (p. 702)

9. **(B)** A break in the continuity of the skin of a painful, swollen, deformed extremity is considered an open bone or joint injury. A simple fracture and a closed fracture have no break in the skin. Grating is not a type of fracture. (p. 702)

10. **(C)** Proper splinting of a possible closed fracture is designed to prevent closed injuries from becoming open ones. (p. 705)

11. **(C)** The signs and symptoms of a bone or joint injury include grating, swelling, and bruising. If shock develops, vomiting may occur. (pp. 703–704)

12. **(A)** When a joint is locked into position, the EMT should splint the joint in the position found. Do *not* disregard splinting and transport immediately unless the patient is a high priority for some other reason. If this is the case, then a long backboard would be used as a splint. (p. 705)

13. **(C)** The procedure, which is done at least twice whenever a splint is applied, is assessment for pulses, motor function, and sensation (PMS) distal to the injury. Once traction is applied, it is not reapplied. (pp. 706–707)

14. **(B)** The treatment of a painful, swollen extremity includes these steps: take Standard Precautions, splint the injury, elevate the extremity, and apply a cold pack. Do not elevate the extremity until it is splinted. (pp. 704–705)

15. **(C)** Multiple fractures, especially of the femur, can cause life-threatening external and internal bleeding. (pp. 704–705)

16. **(A)** Applying a cold pack to a possible fracture will help to reduce the swelling. It does not stop bleeding from the bone, nor does it stop all pain and discomfort. Do not use a pressure bandage at the site of a fracture since it may damage the bone ends. (pp. 704–705)

17. **(D)** If the initial assessment of a patient with a musculoskeletal injury reveals the patient is unstable, do *not* take time to splint each individual injury. It is not in the patient's best interest to waste the "Golden Hour" treating minor injuries. (pp. 703–705)

18. **(D)** A splint properly applied to a closed bone injury should help prevent damage to muscles, nerves, or blood vessels caused by broken bones, as well as prevent an open bone injury and motion of bone fragments. The splint should not prevent circulation to the extremity. (p. 705)

19. **(D)** Complications of bone injuries include excessive bleeding, increased pain from movement, and paralysis of the extremity. Distal circulation usually decreases. (p. 707)

20. **(C)** The objective of realignment is to assist in restoring circulation and to fit the extremity into a splint. (p. 705)

21. **(A)** If there is a severe deformity of the distal extremity or it is cyanotic or pulseless, the EMT should align with gentle traction before splinting. The PASG should not be used for alignment. If you delay splinting until en route to the hospital, the circulation to the extremity could be hindered. (p. 705)

22. **(A)** The types of splints generally carried by EMTs include rigid, formable, and traction. Other listings are examples of the three types of splints. (p. 706)

23. **(D)** Rigid splints are seldom used to immobilize joint injuries in the position found, except for triangulation. Formable splints are used for this purpose. (p. 706)

24. **(C)** Traction splints are used specifically for fractures of the femur. (p. 709)

25. **(D)** When splinting, the EMT should immobilize the injury site and joints above and below. Do not leave open wounds exposed as they may get infected. Sometimes protruding bone ends fall back into place when the limb is placed in a splintable position. However, it is not the EMT's responsibility to reduce a fracture in the field. (pp. 707, 709)

26. **(C)** To ensure proper immobilization and increase patient comfort when using a rigid splint, pad the spaces between the body part and the splint. (pp. 704–705)

27. **(B)** The method of splinting is always dictated by the severity of the patient's condition and the priority decision. If the

patient is a high priority for "load and go" transport, choose a fast method of splinting. If the patient is a low priority for transport, choose a slower-but-better splinting method. (pp. 706–707)

28. **(D)** If the patient with a musculoskeletal injury is unstable, the EMT should care for life-threatening problems first, consider aligning the injuries to an anatomical position, and secure the entire body to a long spine board. In the case of a critical patient, consider using a long backboard as a total body splint and lifting/spinal immobilization device. (pp. 704–705)

29. **(D)** Hazards of improper splinting include aggravation of a bone or joint injury, reduced distal circulation, and delay in transport of patient with life-threatening injury. (p. 707)

30. **(C)** If the lower leg is cyanotic or lacks a pulse when a knee joint injury is assessed, the EMT should realign with gentle traction if no resistance is met. Call medical direction if you need some encouragement. An attempt at restoring a pulse must be made, otherwise the patient could lose the lower leg. (p. 707)

31. **(B)** Examples of a bipolar traction splint include Hare, Fernotrac, and half-ring. (p. 709)

32. **(B)** The amount of traction the EMT should pull when applying a Sager traction splint is about 10% of the body weight up to 15 pounds. (pp. 709–710)

33. **(B)** The indications for a traction splint are a painful, swollen, deformed mid-thigh with no joint or lower leg injury. (p. 710)

34. **(B)** Whenever possible, three rescuers should be used to apply a traction splint. This allows one rescuer to support the injury site when the limb is lifted to position the traction splint. (p. 711)

35. **(C)** If the patient has multiple leg fractures and exhibits signs of shock (hypoperfusion), the EMT should apply the PASG as a splint. The patient will most likely be in shock so the PASG will serve a dual purpose. Be sure to follow your local protocols (p. 717)

36. **(D)** Signs and symptoms of a knee injury include pain and tenderness, swelling, and deformity. (p. 721)

37. **(A)** Elderly patients are more susceptible to hip fractures because of brittle bones or bone weakened by disease. (p. 718)

38. **(B)** When a patient has a fractured hip, the injured limb may appear shorter. (p. 718)

39. **(C)** When a patient who was involved in a serious fall has an unexplained sensation of having to empty his or her bladder, the patient may have a pelvic fracture. (p. 715)

40. **(D)** When securing a patient who has a pelvic injury, you should not raise the lower legs. (pp. 715–716)

COMPLETE THE FOLLOWING

1. Signs and symptoms of a musculoskeletal injury include: (pp. 703–704)
   - pain and tenderness
   - deformity or angulation
   - grating, or crepitus
   - swelling
   - bruising
   - exposed bone ends
   - joints locked into position
   - nerve and blood vessel compromise

2. Signs and symptoms of a hip fracture include: (pp. 718–719)
   - localized pain
   - sensitive to pressure on the lateral prominence of the hip
   - surrounding tissues discolored (delayed sign)
   - swelling
   - unable to move the limb while on the back
   - unable to stand
   - foot on the injured side is turned outward
   - injured limb may appear shorter

LABEL THE DIAGRAM (p. 695)

1. Skull	16. Clavicle
2. Cervical spine	17. Scapula
3. Manubrium	18. Ribs
4. Sternum	19. Humerus
5. Xiphoid process	20. Elbow
6. Thoracic spine	21. Ulna
7. Costal cartilage	22. Radius
8. Lumbar spine	23. Sacral spine
9. Iliac crest	24. Femur
10. Pelvis	25. Patella
11. Femur head	26. Tibia
12. Acetabulum	27. Fibula
13. Pubis	28. Tarsals
14. Medial malleolus	29. Metatarsals
15. Lateral malleolus	30. Phalanges

STREET SCENES DISCUSSION

1. You would have observed an open cut or laceration with bleeding where the bone exited the skin.

2. Yes. In order to apply a splint to a grossly deformed long bone, it will be necessary to move the bone into a splintable (straight) position with gentle traction on the extremity.

3. If the patient does not have a distal pulse, contact medical direction, who may allow you to gently manipulate the extremity once try to restore the pulse.

4. If the patient's vital signs are stable and there is no evidence of multiple fractures, as ALS unit is probably not needed.

Chapter 29: Injuries to the Head and Spine

MATCH TERMINOLOGY/ DEFINITIONS

1. **(O)** Autonomic nervous system—nervous system that consists of nerves that control involuntary functions such as the heartbeat and breathing (p. 751)

2. **(K)** Central nervous system—brain and spinal cord (p. 749)

3. **(I)** Cerebrospinal fluid (CSF)—fluid that surrounds the brain and spinal cord (p. 752)

4. **(B)** Concussion—mild closed head injury without detectable damage to the brain (p. 753)

5. **(J)** Contusion—bruised brain caused when the force of a blow is great enough to rupture blood vessels (p. 753)

6. **(H)** Cranium—bony structure making up the forehead, top, back, and upper sides of the skull (p. 751)

7. **(D)** Malar—cheekbone; also called the zygomatic bone (p. 751)

8. **(M)** Nasal bones—bones that form the upper third, or bridge, of the nose (p. 751)

9. **(C)** Nervous system—body system that is divided into two subsystems and that provides overall control of thought, sensation, and the voluntary and involuntary motor functions of the body. (The major components of the nervous system are the brain and the spinal cord.) (p. 749)

10. **(N)** Orbits—bony structures, or sockets, around the eyes (p. 751)

11. **(A)** Peripheral nervous system—pairs of nerves that enter and exit the spinal cord between the vertebrae, twelve pairs of cranial nerves that travel between the brain and organs without passing through the spinal cord, and all of the body's other motor and sensory nerves (p. 749)

12. **(E)** Spinous process—bony bump on the vertebra that you can feel on a person's back (p. 752)

13. **(L)** Temporal bones—bones that form part of the side of the skull and floor of the cranial cavity (p. 751)

14. **(G)** Temporomandibular joint—movable joint formed between the mandible and the temporal bones; also called the TM joint (p. 751)

15. **(F)** Vertebrae—bones of the spinal column (p. 752)

MULTIPLE-CHOICE REVIEW

1. **(B)** The function of the spinal column is to protect the spinal cord. (pp. 751–752)

2. **(C)** The spine is made up of 33 vertebrae. (p. 752)

3. **(C)** When a patient has a scalp injury, expect profuse bleeding since the scalp is very vascular. Do not try to determine the wound depth or palpate the site with fingertips. (p. 752)

4. **(C)** A bruise behind the ear is called Battle's sign. (p. 755)

5. **(B)** Discoloration of the soft tissues under both eyes is called raccoon's eyes. (p. 755)

6. **(A)** The signs and symptoms of a skull or brain injury include blood or fluid leakage from the ears and/or nose. (p. 755)

7. **(B)** Skull or brain injury may result in altered mental status and unequal pupils. Difficulty moving below the waist is a sign of a spine injury. (p. 755)

8. **(A)** Temperature increase is a late sign of brain or skull injury. It is due to inflammation, infection, or damage to temperature-regulating centers. (p. 755)

9. **(C)** Shock (hypoperfusion) from blood loss is generally *not* a sign of head injury, except in infants. There simply is not enough room within the adult skull to permit enough bleeding to cause shock. If there is a head injury with shock, evaluate for blood loss occurring elsewhere. Neurogenic shock is possible with spinal injury accompanying head injury, though rarely seen in the field. (p. 755)

10. **(B)** The significance of an increase in carbon dioxide in the injured brain is that it causes brain tissue swelling. Hyperventilating the patient with supplemental oxygen at a rate of at least 25 ventilations per minute may reduce brain tissue swelling, although it is controversial (pp. 753–754)

11. **(A)** A patient with a GCS of less than 8 should be taken to a trauma center. (pp. 758–759)

12. **(D)** If an object has penetrated a patient's skull, stabilize the object with bulky dressings. This will minimize accidental movement of the object. (p. 757)

13. **(B)** The primary concern for emergency care of facial fractures or jaw injuries is the patient's airway. Such fractures create the potential for bleeding into the airway and difficulty maintaining a patent airway. (pp. 757–758)

14. **(D)** The cervical and lumbar vertebrae are most frequently injured because they are not supported by other bony structures. (p. 760)

15. **(C)** When the spine is excessively pulled, which commonly occurs during a hanging, this is called a distraction injury. (p. 760)

16. **(C)** On your size-up of an automobile collision, you notice that both sides of the windshield have a spider-web crack. It is wise to call for a backup ambulance because both the driver and the passenger will need to be treated for spinal injury. (p. 776)

17. **(D)** A fall from *three* times the patient's height is considered a high index of suspicion for a spinal injury. The EMT should also maintain a high degree of suspicion for a spinal injury when the patient has been involved in a motor vehicle collision, motorcycle crash, or has open fractures to the ankles that resulted from a fall. (p. 761)

18. **(D)** Lateral bending injuries are caused by using improper lifting techniques. Diving accidents commonly cause flexion, extension, or compression injuries of the cervical spine. (p. 761)

19. **(A)** The unconscious trauma patient should be treated as if he has a spine injury. (pp. 762–763)

20. **(D)** The most reliable sign of spinal cord injury in the conscious patient is paralysis of the extremities. (p. 762)

21. **(B)** A lack of spinal pain does not rule out the possibility of spinal cord injury because other painful injuries may mask it. (pp. 762–763)

22. **(A)** When assessing a suspected spine-injured patient and you note a reversal of the normal breathing pattern, this is likely a result of damage to the nerves that control the rib cage. (p. 762)

23. **(D)** If a patient is found on her back with arms extended above the head, this may indicate a cervical-spine injury. (pp. 762–763)

24. **(A)** If a patient is up and walking around at the scene of a high-speed collision, the EMT should assess for a potential spinal injury. (pp. 776–777)

25. **(A)** If a patient has the mechanism of injury for a spinal injury, do not assess for spinal pain by asking the patient to move. Keep the patient as still as possible, and assess for equality of strength and tingling in the extremities. (p. 762)

26. **(A)** After performing the initial assessment and rapid trauma exam on a spine-injured patient, your next step is to determine the patient's priority, since this will be important in deciding how to immobilize him. (pp. 762–763)

27. **(B)** If a patient complains of pain when you are attempting to place the head in a neutral in-line position, steady the head in the position found. (p. 764)

28. **(B)** When treating a patient with a spine injury, one EMT should maintain constant manual in-line stabilization until the patient is secured to a backboard. (p. 764)

29. **(C)** The cervical collar does not completely eliminate neck movement. All other answer choices are true. (p. 766)

30. **(C)** If a stable patient is found in a sitting position on the ground and is complaining about back pain, the EMT should immobilize with a short spine board or an extrication vest. This will immobilize the head, neck, and torso until he can be transferred to a long spine board. (pp. 772–776)

31. (B) The rapid extrication procedure is *not* used for stable, low-priority patients. All other answer choices are true. (p. 769)

32. (A) When immobilizing a 6-year-old or younger child on a long backboard, provide padding beneath the shoulder blades. This eliminates the void behind the shoulders caused by the child's large head. (p. 786)

33. (B) If a helmet has a snug fit that allows little or no movement of the patient's head within the helmet, the helmet may be left in place. (pp. 777, 781)

34. (B) The correct order of steps for applying a short spine immobilization device: position device behind the patient; secure the device to patient's torso; evaluate torso fixation and pad behind the neck as necessary; secure the patient's head to the device. (pp. 771–772)

35. (D) Prior to and after immobilization, the EMT should assess distal pulses, motor function, and sensation (PMS) in all extremities. (p. 764)

COMPLETE THE FOLLOWING

1. Signs of skull fracture or brain injury include: (any six) (p. 755)
   - visible bone fragments
   - altered mental status
   - deep laceration or severe bruise or hematoma
   - depressions or deformity of the skull
   - any severe head pain
   - Battle's sign
   - raccoon's eyes
   - unequal pupils
   - one "sunken" eye
   - clear fluid from ears and/or nose
   - increase in blood pressure
   - equilibrium problems
   - paralysis or disability on one side of body
   - bleeding from the ears or nose
   - personality changes
   - temperature increase
   - blurred or multiple image vision
   - impaired hearing
   - projectile vomiting
   - seizures
   - deteriorating vital signs
   - posturing
   - irregular breathing patterns

2. Types of brain injuries include: (pp. 753–754)
   - concussion
   - contusion
   - hematoma (subdural, epidural)

LABEL THE DIAGRAM (p. 752)

1. Cervical
2. Thoracic
3. Lumbar
4. Sacral
5. Coccyx

STREET SCENES DISCUSSION

1. The airway is always the highest priority for assessment and treatment.

2. The decision to immobilize him is based on the mechanism of injury, not on whether or not he has neck pain.

3. Serious head injuries are associated with irregular breathing patterns, high blood pressure, and a pulse rate under 60.

CASE STUDY—DEEP DIVE IN A SHALLOW POOL

1. You would want to know if the patient struck his head, where he entered the pool, if there was any loss of consciousness, exactly how he flipped over, and whether the patient at any point had any movement or sensation in his arms or legs.

2. As long as the patient is floating with assistance and manual stabilization of his head and neck is being maintained, you can float him to the shallow end of the pool where it will be easier to apply a long backboard.

3. Equipment needed includes a long backboard that floats, a rigid cervical collar, a head immobilizer, some padding, and straps or cravats.

4. Ask him if he remembers what happened, if he is having trouble breathing, and if he has feeling or sensation in his arms and legs. You should ask the OPQRST questions about his chief complaint.

5. Tell the patient that you are going to do everything you can to properly immobilize his spine and get him to the most appropriate hospital as quickly as possible.

6. Your partner should complete the initial assessment, take baseline vital signs, make sure the patient is securely immobilized, and reassess distal pulses, motor function, and sensation.

7. Many spine injury calls go to court, so make sure the prehospital care report is very accurate. Be sure to document the actions of the bystander who was in the pool when you arrived and how the injury was reported to have occurred (MOI). Be very specific that the patient stated that he had no sensation or movement in his arms and legs prior to your arrival and that distal pulses, motor function, and sensation were checked and rechecked before and after immobilization.

Chapter 30: Putting It All Together for the Trauma Patient

MATCH TERMINOLOGY/ DEFINITIONS

1. **(D)** Multiple-trauma patient—a patient with more than one serious injury (p. 793)

2. **(C)** Teamwork—cooperation of crew members, each knowing their role and working together to manage the serious patient (pp. 794–795)

3. **(B)** Rapid trauma assessment—quick assessment of the head, neck, chest, abdomen, pelvis, extremities, and posterior of the body to detect signs and symptoms of injury (p. 795)

4. **(G)** Hypoperfusion—inability of the body to adequately circulate blood to the body's cells to supply them with oxygen and nutrients (p. 796)

5. **(A)** Golden Hour—the optimum limit of time between the moment of injury and surgery at the hospital (p. 797)

6. **(H)** Emergency move—procedure designed to move a patient quickly when the situation of safety warrants it (p. 798)

7. **(F)** Hematoma—swelling caused by a collection of blood under the skin or in damaged tissues as a result of an injured or a broken blood vessel (p. 795)

8. **(E)** Mechanism of injury—action or forces that may have caused or contributed to the injury (p. 793)

MULTIPLE-CHOICE REVIEW

1. (B) The patient with a fractured right leg and a crushed pelvis is called a multiple-trauma patient. (p. 793)

2. (C) When a patient has an obvious angulated forearm and is unresponsive, your assessment and treatment priority is the airway. (p. 793)

3. (C) The multiple-trauma patient most likely will be stabilized in the surgical suite. (p. 793)

4. (A) The three "Ts" involved in the management of a multiple-trauma patient are timing, transport, and teamwork. (p. 793)

5. (C) A reasonable goal for scene time when dealing with a critical trauma patient is 10 minutes. (p. 797)

6. (B) When a trauma patient is making gurgling sounds as he breathes, you should suction his airway. (p. 794)

7. (D) Sometimes a long backboard can act as a full body splint when the critical patient must be immobilized quickly. (p. 797)

8. (D) When a patient has two fractured femurs, a crushed pelvis, and a possible abdominal injury, you should not apply a traction splint. Do consider applying a PASG (if local protocol allows), and request an ALS intercept en route to the hospital. (pp. 797–798)

9. (C) When trying to minimize the on-scene care of a multiple-trauma patient, do not take the time to bandage all lacerations. (pp. 797–798)

10. (C) Even when you are trying to cut scene time for a multiple-trauma patient, the one thing you do not cut out is scene safety—no matter how serious the patient is. (pp. 797–798)

COMPLETE THE FOLLOWING

1. Treatments that would be appropriate on the scene of a critical trauma patient include: (p. 797–798)
   - Suctioning the airway
   - Inserting an oral or nasal airway
   - Restoring a patent airway by sealing a sucking chest wound
   - Ventilating with a bag-valve mask
   - Administering high-concentration oxygen
   - Controlling bleeding
   - Immobilizing the patient with a cervical collar and a long backboard
   - Inflating a pneumatic antishock garment

STREET SCENES DISCUSSION

1. Yes, if you suspect supine hypotensive syndrome due to compression of the vena cava by the uterus.

2. You should consider turning the patient and backboard on the side to help clear the airway.

3. No, not with her other problems. Application of a traction splint would take too long.

4. Make sure additional units are responding and that all other patients are assessed and treated.

MATCH TERMINOLOGY/ DEFINITIONS

1. (A) Adolescent—child from 12 to 18 years of age (p. 808)

2. (C) Blow-by oxygen—flowing oxygen over the face of a small child so it will be inhaled (p. 833)

3. (N) Central line—intravenous line that is placed close to the heart (p. 859)

4. (L) Croup—group of viral illnesses that cause inflammation of the larynx, trachea, and bronchi (p. 840)

5. (I) Epiglottitis—bacterial infection that produces swelling of the epiglottis and partial airway obstruction (p. 840)

6. (K) Febrile seizure—complication of a rapidly rising temperature (p. 844)

7. (B) Fontanelle—"soft spot" at the front of an infant's skull where bones have not yet fused together (p. 821)

8. (F) Gastrostomy tube—feeding tube placed through the abdominal wall directly into the stomach (p. 860)

9. (G) Newborn or infant—child between birth and 1 year of age (p. 808)

10. (H) Preschooler—child from 3 to 6 years of age (p. 808)

11. (D) School-aged child—child from 6 to 12 years of age (p. 808)

12. (O) Shunt—drainage device that runs from the brain to the abdomen to relieve excess cerebrospinal fluid (p. 860)

13. (J) SIDS—sudden unexplained death during sleep of an apparently healthy baby in the first year of life (p. 848)

14. (E) Toddler—child from 1 to 3 years of age (p. 808)

15. (M) Tracheostomy tube—tube placed through the neck into the trachea to create an open airway (p. 858)

MULTIPLE-CHOICE REVIEW

1. (B) A toddler is between 1 and 3 years old. (p. 808)

2. (C) A school-aged child is between 6 and 12 years old. (p. 808)

3. (D) When assessing the toddler, examine the head *last*, not first. Toddlers fear having their head or face touched by strangers; to build confidence, examine heart and lungs first, then the head. (p. 809)

4. (C) Until about age 6, a child's head is proportionately larger and heavier than the adult's. This is why padding needs to be placed behind the shoulders when the child is immobilized. It is also the reason why children fly head first when involved in auto collisions or fall out of a window. (p. 810)

5. (B) The soft spot on an infant's skull is called a fontanelle. (p. 810)

6. (A) A sunken fontanelle may indicate dehydration. See answer 7. (p. 810)

7. (B) A bulging fontanelle may indicate elevated intracranial pressure. It is also a sign of meningitis. It may also bulge when the infant cries. (p. 810)

8. (D) Newborns usually breathe through their noses. This is why secretions in and obstruction of the nasal passageways can cause breathing problems. (p. 810)

9. (B) In an infant, hyperextension of the neck may result in airway obstruction because hyperextension can close off the flexible trachea. (p. 812)

10. (D) If the EMT suctions a child's airway for longer than a few seconds at a time, this could lead to cardiac arrest. Suctioning temporarily cuts off the body's oxygen supply; if it is prolonged, it is especially dangerous to infants and children. (p. 812)

11. (A) The tongues of infants and children are more likely than an adult's to fall back into and block the airway because their tongues are proportionately larger than the adult's. (p. 812)

12. (B) The insertion procedure for an oropharyngeal airway in an infant or child is done with the tip pointing toward the tongue and throat, which is the same position it will be in after insertion. Flipping it over the tongue may cause a tear in the soft palate. (pp. 828–829)

13. (A) When assessing the capillary refill of a child 5 years old or younger, peripheral perfusion is considered satisfactory if the color returns in less than 2 seconds. (p. 831)

14. (D) Loss of consciousness is not a sign of a mild airway obstruction in an infant or child. (p. 831)

15. (C) A child with a severe airway obstruction, or severe partial one, *cannot* cry and the cough becomes ineffective. (p. 831)

16. (C) The effects of hypoxia on an infant or a child is slowed heart rate and altered mental status. Hypoxia is the underlying reason for many of the most serious medical problems with children. (p. 833)

17. (D) Always use infection control barriers even when ventilating infants and children. Guidelines to use when ventilating the infant or child include: avoid breathing too hard through the pocket face mask or using excessive bag pressure and volume; use properly sized face masks to assure a good mask seal. Also remember if ventilation is not successful in raising the patient's chest, perform procedures for clearing an obstructed airway, then try to ventilate again. (p. 818)

18. (B) The flow-restricted, oxygen-powered ventilation device is contraindicated in infants and children. There are special units that are designed for pediatric patients, which require additional training, but they are not used in the field by EMTs. (p. 833)

19. (C) Common causes of shock in a child include infection, trauma, blood loss, and dehydration. (pp. 835–836)

20. (D) Croup is not a cause of shock. Less common causes of shock in a child include allergic reactions, poisoning, and cardiac events (rare). (pp. 835–836)

21. (B) The blood volume of infants and children is approximately 8% of the total body weight. (p. 836)

22. (D) Children decompensate very rapidly, not very slowly! When children are in shock, they compensate very well, appear better than they actually are, and "go sour quickly" once they decompensate. (p. 836)

23. (C) When a child is bleeding internally, the EMT should avoid waiting for signs of decompensated shock before treating for shock. At this point, the child has approximately 30% blood loss. (p. 836)

24. (B) Decreased urine output and absence of tears are signs of shock in infants and children. (p. 836)

25. (B) When treating a child in shock, unless there are injuries that would contraindicate it, the EMT should elevate the patient's legs. (p. 837)

26. (A) Because children have a large skin surface area in proportion to their body mass, they can easily become victims of hypothermia. (p. 837)

27. (B) If a child has an airway respiratory disease, it is very important that the EMT *avoid* inserting a tongue blade into the mouth, which could stimulate laryngospasms. Administering blow-by oxygen is an appropriate action. (pp. 838–839)

28. (A) Stridor on inspiration is an upper airway problem. The signs of an airway disease in a child include breathing effort on exhalation, rapid breathing, and wheezing. (pp. 838–839)

29. (C) A viral illness that causes inflammation of the upper airway and bronchi, which is often accompanied by a "seal bark" cough, is called croup. Epiglottitis is a bacterial infection that produces swelling of the epiglottis that usually develops in an older child; the patient exhibits with drooling due to the inability to swallow. (p. 840)

30. (C) About one-third of all pediatric trauma deaths are related to airway mismanagement. (p. 841)

31. (B) Hypothermia does *not* cause fever. Causes of fever in children include upper respiratory infection, pneumonia, and infection. (p. 841)

32. (A) Rectal or oral thermometers generally are *not* used in the prehospital setting unless permitted by local medical direction. (p. 842)

33. (C) When treating an infant or child with a high fever, monitor for shivering while cooling with tepid water. Do not use alcohol as it is a fire hazard and can be absorbed by the skin. Do not cover with a towel soaked in ice water, which can rapidly cause hypothermia. (p. 842)

34. (B) Infants are more susceptible to dehydration because, compared to adults, a greater percentage of their body is water. (p. 844)

35. (C) Fevers are the *most common* cause of seizures in infants and children. While they are rarely life-threatening in children who have them, they should be considered life-threatening by the EMT. (p. 844)

36. (B) Severe aspirin poisoning does not cause dehydration. It can cause seizures, shock, and coma. (p. 846)

37. (A) A common cause of lead poisoning in children is ingesting chips of lead-based paint. Eating fish from freshwater lakes is generally not a problem unless the lake is polluted. (p. 846)

38. (C) If you are treating a child who accidentally ingested a handful of her mother's vitamin tablets, you should be concerned because many vitamin pills contain iron, which can be fatal to a child. (p. 847)

39. (D) The majority of meningitis cases occur between the ages of 1 month and 5 years. (p. 843)

40. (D) In cases of sudden infant death syndrome, the EMT should provide resuscitation and transport to the hospital. You should avoid accusatory actions such as looking for evidence of neglect. Instead, be supportive, since parents who lose a child to SIDS often suffer intense guilt feelings. (p. 848)

41. (B) The number one cause of death in infants and children is trauma. Much trauma to infants and children occurs because they are curious and learning about their environment. (p. 848)

42. (C) The child who has been struck by a vehicle may present with a triad of injuries that include head injury, lower extremity injury (possibly a fractured femur), and abdominal injury (with possible internal bleeding). (p. 849)

43. (D) The most frequent sign of head injury is altered mental status. Respiratory arrest is a common secondary effect. Head injury itself is seldom a cause of shock except in infants. Suspect internal injuries whenever a head-injured child presents with shock. (p. 850)

44. (D) Because the musculoskeletal structures of the chest are less developed in infants and children, they are more likely to incur injury to structures beneath the ribs. (p. 850)

45. (C) Because the abdominal muscles of infants and small children are immature, there is less protection for underlying organs. (pp. 850–851)

46. (B) When using PASG on a pediatric patient, the EMT should remember the abdominal section is not generally used on children. (p. 851)

47. (D) You must keep the infant or child covered to prevent a drop in body temperature. Burned patients who become hypothermic have a higher death rate. (p. 851)

48. (D) A parent's concern about the child's injuries is normal and to be expected. Indications that child abuse may be occurring include repeated responses to provide care for the same child or family, poorly healing wounds or improperly healed fractures, and indications of past injuries. (pp. 854–855)

49. (C) Torn clothing on the child is not necessarily an indication of child abuse. When you respond to the home of a person that you think may be a child abuser, observe for a family member who has trouble controlling anger, indications of alcohol and drug abuse, and any adult who appears in a state of depression. (pp. 854–855)

50. (C) While you should talk with the child separately about how an injury occurred, it is not your role to ask the child if he or she has been abused. Always report your suspicions to the emergency department staff and in accordance with local policies. (pp. 856–857)

51. (D) When treating a child who you suspect is suffering from epiglottitis, it is important to: immediately transport the child, not place anything in the child's mouth, and constantly monitor the respiratory status. (p. 841)

52. (C) The primary cause of cardiac arrest in children is a respiratory disorder. (p. 841)

53. (A) Do not use rubbing alcohol to bring down a fever as it is flammable and can get absorbed through the child's skin. (p. 842)

54. (B) Children can easily be poisoned by taking too much acetaminophen. (p. 846)

55. (D) When a young child is struck by a car, he or she often will receive leg injuries at the bumper level, abdomen and chest injuries as he or she strikes the car hood, and then get thrown from the car and land on the head. (p. 849)

COMPLETE THE FOLLOWING

1. Signs of respiratory distress in a child include: (any ten) (pp. 838–839)
   - nasal flaring
   - retraction of the muscles above, below, and between the sternum and ribs
   - use of abdominal muscles
   - stridor
   - audible wheezing
   - grunting
   - breathing rate greater than 60

- cyanosis
- decreased muscle tone
- poor peripheral perfusion
- delayed capillary refill
- altered mental status
- decreased heart rate

COMPLETE THE CHART (p. 832)

1. 1 second
2. 1 second
3. 1 second
4. 10 to 12
5. 12 to 20
6. 12 to 20

STREET SCENES DISCUSSION

1. The child may have had a seizure.

2. If the mental status did not improve and you suspected the child had a temperature as well as a rash, there may be an infectious disease involved. Be sure to use a face mask, eye shield, and disposable gloves.

3. Follow up in case there is an infectious disease to which you may have been exposed.

CASE STUDY—THE CASE OF THE POISONED JUICE

1. Use gloves, eye shield, and mask.

2. Find out exactly who drank the juice. Separate the healthy children from the juice drinkers to limit the "sympathy" sickness.

3. Dehydration

4. A shunt is a tube to drain excess cerebrospinal fluid in the head into the abdomen. Shunts are used for children who are hydrocephalic.

5. Pulse of 90 to 140, respirations of 25 to 40; BP is usually not taken on a child under 3.

6. Pulse of 80 to 130, respirations of 20 to 30; BP is usually not taken on a child under 3.

7. Pulse of 80 to 120, respirations of 20 to 30, and BP of 99 systolic

8. Have the caretaker hold the child. Be sure to keep the infant warm; warm your stethoscope and hands prior to touching the child. Observe the breathing from a distance.

9. Have the caretaker hold the child. Assure the child that he was not bad. Remove an article of clothing, examine, and then replace the clothing. Examine in a trunk-to-head approach to build confidence.

10. Use a toy, let them help you, and approach from toes to head.

11. In a child safety car seat

12. Ask the parent if this is how the infant normally reacts to this stimuli.

13. The juice can be analyzed to determine what organism caused the problem.

CASE STUDY—ABUSER OR LOVING PARENT?

1. At a motor vehicle collision scene, traffic is usually your greatest hazard.

2. Yes, since the limping driver could change his mind. You would not want to delay transporting the child in order to call for another ambulance later in the call.

3. Your initial concerns for the child are mental status and the status of his ABCs.

4. Yes, it is a significant finding. His mental status is probably deteriorating.

5. One way to determine a child's mental status is to ask the parent what is "normal" for the child.

6. The cracks are evidence that the both of patients' heads impacted the windshield. This is a very significant mechanism of injury.

7. In addition to helping you determine what happened to the child, the mother's statement also tells you that the patient is normally very active and expressive. He is not now.

8. Yes. Also evaluate the need for assisting ventilation.

9. Yes, request an ALS intercept. The patient may need to be intubated and the extra hands would be helpful.

10. Just provide the facts. The mother may have broken at least two laws: She may have been driving while legally intoxicated and she did not use the proper restraints on the child. If she had followed the laws that are designed to protect children, the injuries probably would not have been so severe.

Chapter 32: Special Needs Patients

MATCH TERMINOLOGY/ DEFINITIONS

1. **(J)** Central IV catheter—a catheter surgically inserted for long-term delivery of medications or fluids into the central circulation (p. 875)

2. **(B)** Ventilator—a device that breathes for a patient (p. 870)

3. **(A)** Congenital disease/condition—a disease or condition that is present at birth (p. 867)

4. **(N)** Pacemaker—a device that uses electrical impulses to regulate rhythms of the heart, usually implanted under the skin (p. 870)

5. **(G)** Stoma—a surgically created opening into the body, as with a tracheostomy, colonostomy, or ileostomy (p. 869)

6. **(M)** Acquired disease/condition—a disease or condition that occurs after birth (p. 867)

7. **(D)** Automatic implanted cardiac defibrillator (AICD)—a device implanted under the skin that can detect life-threatening cardiac dysrhythmias and respond by delivering one or more high-energy shocks to correct the rhythm (p. 871)

8. **(C)** Left ventricular assist device (LVAD)—a battery-powered mechanical pump implanted in the body to assist a failing left ventricle in pumping blood to the body (p. 872)

9. **(L)** Continuous positive airway pressure (CPAP)—a device that exerts constant pressure through a tube and mask worn by a patient to keep airway passages from collapsing at the end of a breath (p. 868)

10. **(K)** Ostomy bag—an external pouch that collects fecal matter diverted from the colon or ileum through a surgical opening (colostomy or ileostomy) in the abdominal wall (p. 874)

11. **(I)** Dialysis—the process of filtering the blood to remove toxic or unwanted wastes and fluids (p. 874)

12. **(H)** Urinary catheter—a tube inserted into the bladder through the urethra to drain urine from the bladder (p. 873)

13. **(F)** Tracheostomy—a surgical opening in the neck into the trachea (p. 869)

14. **(E)** Feeding tube—a tube used to provide delivery of nutrients of the stomach. A nasogastric feeding tube is inserted through the nose and into the stomach; a gastric feeding tube is surgically implanted through the abdominal wall into the stomach (p. 873)

MULTIPLE-CHOICE REVIEW

1. **(D)** To ensure proper care for the patient with special needs, the EMT must be able to recognize, understand, and evaluate the patient's specific special health-care needs in addition to the chief complaint. (p. 865)

2. **(A)** The EMT may find patients with special care needs when responding to calls in any of the following locations, except the emergency department. (pp. 865–866)

3. **(C)** One of the best resources to help you when confronted with a special needs patient who is on a specific device would be to use the family member with the patient. (pp. 865–867)

4. **(C)** A condition that is present at birth of the special needs patient is considered congenital. (p. 867)

5. **(B)** A device designed to keep the air passages from collapsing at the end of a breath is called a CPAP. (p. 868)

6. **(D)** A patient who has a tracheostomy tube may need to be suctioned occasionally. This is especially common during times of distress, the first few weeks after the tube insertion, and if the patient has an infection. (p. 869)

7. **(C)** A device that is programmed to take over the functions of timing and rate of the patient's breathing is called a ventilator. (p. 870)

8. **(C)** If the patient on the device in question 7 has an electrical or battery failure, the EMT will need to begin bag-mask ventilation. (p. 870)

9. **(D)** A cardiac device that is occasionally implanted in the patient's left upper abdominal quadrant is called a pacemaker. (p. 870)

10. **(C)** A cardiac chamber that pumps blood through the aorta to the body is called a left ventricular assist device. (p. 872)

11. **(B)** A tube that is inserted into a patient who has lost the ability to regulate his urine is called a urinary catheter. (p. 873)

12. **(A)** When a patient tells you he needs to go for dialysis every other day, this is done to detoxify the blood. (p. 874)

13. **(C)** Examples of devices commercially available as a Groshong®, Hickman®, or a Broviac® would be called a central venous line. (p. 876)

14. **(D)** A special needle is required to access a device called an implanted port, Port-a-Cath®, and Mediport®. (p. 876)

STREET SCENES DISCUSSION

1. The ambulance was called because Amber was experiencing a fever and beginning to look gray. What is most likely wrong with the patient?

   She has a respiratory infection that is getting worse and affecting her ability to breathe.

2. Why is it necessary to suction Amber's trach tube?

When a patient has a trach tube, she cannot clear her throat by simply coughing or spitting. If it becomes partially obstructed with secretions, it is necessary to suction the tube to keep it clear.

3. What do you suppose was causing the gurgling sounds when Amber was breathing?

Initially when Amber was breathing, gurgling sounds could be heard. This sound was due to the partial obstruction of the tube from secretions.

Chapter 33: Geriatric Patients

MATCH TERMINOLOGY/ DEFINITIONS

1. **(B)** Alzheimer's disease—chronic disorder resulting in dementia (p. 884)

2. **(C)** Confabulation—when an elderly person replaces lost circumstances with imaginary ones (p. 886)

3. **(E)** Hypothermia—abnormally low body temperature (p. 890)

4. **(F)** Pneumonia—an inflammation in the tissue of the lung (p. 890)

5. **(G)** Aortic dissection—a separation of the layers of the artery described as a tearing sensation (p. 890)

6. **(A)** Geriatric—elderly person, generally considered 65 years of age or older (p. 882)

7. **(D)** Dysrhythmia—an abnormal heart rhythm (p. 885)

8. **(H)** Diverticulosis—an outpouching of the intestine provides a sac where food can lodge and cause inflammation (p. 891)

MULTIPLE-CHOICE REVIEW

1. **(C)** Starting at age 30, our organ systems lose about 1% function each year. (p. 882)

2. **(C)** Common causes of traumatic injuries in the older patient are car crashes or falls. (p. 882)

3. **(D)** Assessing the airway of an older patient is often difficult because of dentures and because of arthritic changes in the bones of the neck. (p. 885)

4. **(B)** Since older patients are less likely to show severe symptoms in certain conditions, it can be difficult to determine the patient's priority. (p. 885)

5. **(C)** When interviewing, if the patient tells you he was wrong in some responses this is sometimes the result of neurological condition as well as taking multiple medications. (pp. 885–887)

6. **(B)** When a patient replaces lost circumstances with imaginary ones, this is known as confabulation. (p. 887)

7. **(D)** All of the above as patients have high, low, and decreased sensitivity to pain. (p. 887)

8. **(B)** As a person ages, the systolic blood pressure has a tendency to increase. (p. 887)

9. **(D)** Hip fractures are common in elderly patients, especially women, due to loss of calcium. (p. 887)

10. **(C)** An EMT should consider that any injury of an elderly person could be a sign of abuse or neglect. (pp. 892–893)

COMPLETE THE FOLLOWING

The Physiological Effects of Aging and Implications for Assessment (p. 883)

1. Increased risk of heart attack and stroke, hypertension

2. Diminished activity and tolerance of physical stress

3. Decreased ability to clear foreign substances from lungs

4. Difficulty chewing and swallowing; less enjoyment of eating; difficulty digesting and absorbing food; constipation; early feeling of fullness when eating

5. Increased toxicity from alcohol and medications; diminished ability of blood to clot

6. Decreased energy and tolerance of heat and cold

7. Decreased strength

8. Many different medications, sometimes prescribed by different physicians

9. Depression; loss of social support

10. Thin, dry, wrinkled skin

STREET SCENES DISCUSSION

1. If you decide that the patient's condition is serious enough to use the ambulance lights and siren, you probably should call for ALS.

2. Many elderly people are on fixed incomes. Some feel they cannot pay big heating bills, so they keep the temperature down and wear lots of clothing instead. Since older people cannot regulate body temperature very well, this could cause medical problems.

3. The elderly patient may be afraid of losing his independence, of being left in the care of strangers, or just going to the hospital where he has lost friends and loved ones. You can help ease this transition by treating the patient in a respectful, dignified manner, acknowledging his fears and concerns, and attempting to put them in perspective.

Chapter 34: Ambulance Operations

MATCH TERMINOLOGY/ DEFINITIONS

1. **(G)** AED—automated external defibrillator (p. 903)

2. **(I)** ATV—automatic transport ventilator (p. 904)

3. **(H)** CID—cervical immobilization device (p. 905)

4. **(A)** Due regard—legal term, which appears in most states' driving laws, referring to the responsibility of the emergency vehicle operator to drive safely and keep the safety of all others in mind at all times (p. 912)

5. **(B)** EMD—Emergency Medical Dispatcher (p. 910)

6. **(E)** Hypothermia thermometer—special thermometer that is designed to go down to 82°F. (p. 903)

7. **(D)** Landing zone (LZ)—large, flat area without aerial obstruction in which a helicopter can land to pick up a patient (pp. 932–933)

8. **(F)** Sager®—traction splint for the immobilization of a painful, swollen, deformed thigh (p. 905)

9. **(J)** Thumper—mechanical compressor for performing CPR that is especially helpful to services with transport time to the hospital over 15 minutes (p. 904)

10. **(C)** True emergency—call in which the driver of the emergency vehicle responds with lights and siren because he is of the understanding that loss of life or limb may be possible (p. 913)

MULTIPLE-CHOICE REVIEW

1. **(C)** The federal agency that develops specifications for ambulance vehicle designs is the U.S. Department of Transportation. (p. 901)

2. **(B)** The purpose for carrying an EPA-registered, intermediate-level disinfectant on the ambulance is to destroy mycobacterium tuberculosis. (p. 902)

3. **(D)** The telemetry repeater is used in the ambulance to boost the radio signal. Equipment that should be in the portable first-in kit to be taken directly to a patient's side would include the suction unit, rigid cervical collar, and a blood pressure cuff. (p. 903)

4. **(D)** The suction unit is used in the "A" (airway) step of the initial assessment of a trauma patient. Supplies used for the "C" (circulation) step would include disposable gloves, occlusive dressings, and the AED. (p. 903)

5. **(A)** The rubber bulb syringe is a supply used for childbirth. Equipment used to obtain vital signs includes an adult and a pediatric stethoscope, sphygmomanometer kit, and a penlight. (p. 903)

6. **(A)** A device used to carry patients over a long distance is called a Stokes basket. The scoop stretcher is used to lift and move patients without a spine injury through tight places. See answer 7. (p. 903)

7. **(C)** A Reeves® stretcher is used for carrying a patient who must lie supine down stairs when a cot is too heavy or wide, *not* for spine injury. The Stokes, or basket stretcher, is used to carry patients in high-angle rescue. (p. 903)

8. **(D)** A typical fixed oxygen delivery system consists of a 3,000-liter reservoir, a two-stage regulator, and the necessary reducing valve and yokes. (p. 904)

9. **(C)** The automatic transport ventilator is *not* an essential item to carry on the ambulance for prehospital respiratory care. (p. 904)

10. **(D)** The fixed suction unit in the ambulance should reach a vacuum of at least 300 mmHg within 4 seconds. It should provide an air flow of *30* liters per minute and should be usable by a person at the *head* of the patient. Oxygen tanks require periodic hydrostatic testing. (p. 904)

11. **(B)** The mechanical CPR compressor is a helpful device but is not essential for assisting with cardiopulmonary resuscitation. (p. 904)

12. **(D)** Burn sheets are not used for immobilization. Equipment carried on an ambulance that is used for immobilization includes a Hare® traction splint, triangular bandages, and padded aluminum splints. (p. 905)

13. **(A)** Chemical cold packs are carried on an ambulance for use with musculoskeletal injuries. (p. 905)

14. **(D)** The Hare® traction device is for splinting. Supplies used for wound care should include sterile burn sheets, 5 × 9-inch combine dressings, and self-adhering roller bandages. (p. 905)

15. **(B)** Sterilized aluminum foil is used to maintain body heat or as an occlusive dressing. Body parts should be wrapped in a plastic bag and kept cool. Use a paper cup over an avulsed eye. Never use aluminum foil to directly cover an injury since it can cut the patient. (p. 905)

16. **(C)** Large safety pins are used with a sling. Supplies for childbirth include a rubber bulb syringe, sanitary napkins, and sterile surgical gloves. (p. 905)

17. **(C)** Every shift, both you and your partner should complete the equipment checklist. Preventative maintenance, oil changes, and waxing the ambulance are done routinely but not on each shift. (p. 907)

18. **(B)** The battery is checked with the engine off. (p. 909)

19. **(D)** It is not the EMD's job to advise the caller that an ambulance is not needed. The responsibilities of the Emergency Medical Dispatcher (EMD) include dispatching and coordinating EMS resources, interrogating the caller, prioritizing the call, and coordinating with other public safety agencies. (pp. 910–911)

20. **(C)** When an EMD questions a patient or caller, he or she does not routinely ask if the patient has been in the hospital recently. This is part of the EMT's SAMPLE history taken at the scene. (pp. 910–911)

21. **(B)** The brand of vehicle is not important to EMS, but would be for the police report. When speaking with a caller who is at the scene of a traffic collision, the EMD should ask if traffic is moving, how many lanes of traffic are open, and if any of the vehicles are on fire. (p. 911)

22. **(D)** To be a safe ambulance operator, the EMT should be tolerant of other drivers, always wear glasses or contact lenses if required, and have a positive attitude about his or her ability as a driver. (p. 912)

23. **(D)** Most state statutes prohibit passing of a school bus that has its red lights blinking. Stop and wait for the bus driver to shut off the red lights, which signals that all the children are in a safe position. Then proceed with caution. State statutes *do* allow emergency vehicle operators to do all of the following under certain conditions: park the vehicle anywhere so long as it does not damage personal property; proceed past red stop signals, flashing red stop signals, and stop signs; and exceed the posted speed limit as long as life and property are not endangered. (p. 916)

24. **(A)** At the scene of a collision, you examine a patient and find that he is stable. This situation is no longer considered a true emergency; further use of lights and siren would be inappropriate. (p. 913)

25. **(D)** Do not use the siren throughout the call. Use the siren sparingly. Never assume that all motorists will hear your signal, and be prepared for erratic movements of motorists. (pp. 913–914)

26. **(B)** The decision about the use of lights and sirens should always be made with the medical condition of the patient in mind. The continuous sound of a siren may cause a sick or an injured person to suffer increased fear and anxiety, and his condition may deteriorate as stress increases. (pp. 913–914)

27. **(B)** Escorts or multi-vehicle responses are a very dangerous means of response. Motorists often do not expect to see the second emergency vehicle and may collide with it. (pp. 914–915)

28. **(D)** The type of emergency (except MCIs) does not affect ambulance response; factors that do include time of the day, weather, and road maintenance and construction. See also Complete the Following answer 2. (pp. 915–916)

29. **(B)** Park in front of the wreckage if you are the first emergency vehicle on the scene so your flashing lights can warn

approaching motorists until flares and other signals can be placed. Park 100 feet and uphill from a wreckage that involves fire. (p. 917)

30. (B) Packaging is the sequence of operations required to ready the patient to be moved and to combine the patient and the patient-carrying device into a unit ready for transfer. (p. 918)

31. (A) An unconscious patient who has no potential spine injury should be positioned in the ambulance in the recovery position, which promotes maintenance of an open airway and the drainage of fluids. (p. 920)

32. (B) Forming a general impression of the patient is done when you first see the patient, *not* en route to the hospital. En route, the EMT rechecks bandages and splints, performs ongoing assessment, continues to monitor vital signs, and notifies the receiving facility of estimated time of arrival. (pp. 920–921)

33. (D) If a patient develops cardiac arrest en route to the hospital, the EMT's first action should be to tell the operator to stop the vehicle. (p. 922)

34. (B) When delivering the patient to the hospital, the EMT should *never* move a patient onto the hospital stretcher and leave. This is considered abandonment. (p. 923)

35. (C) When approaching a helicopter, first wait for the pilot or medic to wave you in. Then approach from the front or side of the craft. All other approach directions could cause injury or death. Remember to always follow the directions of the flight crew. (p. 933)

36. (C) Patients who are cardiac arrest victims are rarely candidates for helicopter transport. (pp. 931–932)

COMPLETE THE FOLLOWING

1. List the seven questions an EMD should ask a caller reporting a medical emergency. (p. 910)
   - What is the exact location of the patient?
   - What is your call-back number?
   - What's the problem?
   - How old is the patient?
   - What's the patient's sex?
   - Is the patient conscious?
   - Is the patient breathing?

2. List seven factors that can affect ambulance response. (p. 915)
   - day of the week
   - time of the day
   - weather
   - road maintenance and construction
   - railroads
   - bridges and tunnels
   - schools and school buses

3. List the four major ways the EMT on the scene of a collision should describe the landing zone to the air rescue service. (p. 933)
   - terrain
   - major landmarks
   - estimated distance to nearest town
   - other pertinent information

LABEL THE PHOTOGRAPHS (p. 930)

1. Low-level	3. High-level
2. Intermediate	4. Sterilization

STREET SCENES DISCUSSION

1. Notify the dispatcher, call the police, and assure that there are no injuries caused by the collision. While waiting for the police to respond, ask the dispatcher to reassign the initial call to another unit.

2. The driver of the emergency vehicle would be at fault.

3. Because you cannot stop the ambulance fast enough if an unsuspecting motorist drives in front of you. Even with emergency lights and sirens on, you cannot assume that other drivers will see you or hear you approach.

CASE STUDY—THE AMBULANCE COLLISION

1. Yes, by stopping before proceeding through the intersection.

2. Yes, by wearing a shoulder harness.

3. It was necessary to assign yet another ambulance to handle that call.

4. Do no harm.

5. The service may lose business. The EMS personnel may be ridiculed, and some patients may actually be afraid to get into your ambulance!

6. Because he is allowed to look into incidents of this nature with close scrutiny. This is especially true in the public sector, when injury has occurred.

7. Absolutely. Civilian motorists are not required to drive with "due regard for the safety of all others."

8. He does, unless his service is willing to assist him or unless he has some insurance or legal aid.

9. Yes, he could.

10. Proper driver screening and qualification, driver training, driving SOPs (which include always wearing shoulder harness in the front of the vehicle, how to negotiate an intersection, and proper use of emergency lights and siren), retraining, keeping the vehicles in good shape, and a good quality-improvement program.

Chapter 35: Gaining Access and Rescue Operations

MATCH TERMINOLOGY/ DEFINITIONS

1. **(H)** A Post—post in front of the driver's compartment that supports the roof and windshield (p. 949)

2. **(A)** B Post—when moving toward the rear of the vehicle, the second post you see, which supports the roof (pp. 949, 954)

3. **(L)** Complex—access that requires tools or special equipment to reach the patient (pp. 955–956)

4. **(J)** Cribbing—blocks of hardwood, usually 4 × 4 × 18-inch or 2 × 4 × 18-inch, used to stabilize a vehicle (p. 952)

5. **(M)** Disentanglement—three-part procedure used by rescue personnel to free a patient trapped in a vehicle (p. 956)

6. **(E)** Entrapment—when a patient is pinned and requires assistance, sometimes mechanical, to free him (p. 940)

7. **(N)** Extrication—process by which entrapped patients are rescued from vehicles, buildings, tunnels, or other places (p. 939)

8. **(O)** Glas-Master®—saw that is designed to cut laminated windshield glass (p. 956)

9. **(D)** Ground gradient—decreasing circles of voltage on the ground surrounding a point where a charged wire is down (p. 948)

10. **(K)** Inner circle—area immediately around and including the wrecked vehicle (p. 942)

11. **(I)** Laminated glass—safety glass used in automobile windshields; made of two sheets of plate glass bonded to a sheet of tough plastic (p. 956)

12. **(C)** Nader pin—named after a well-known consumer advocate, this case-hardened pin is held by the cams of an automobile's door locking system (p. 955)

13. **(G)** Personal protective equipment—gear designed to prevent the rescuer from being injured while working in the inner circle (p. 942)

14. **(F)** Stabilization—to crib or block a vehicle or structure to prevent further unintended, uncontrolled movement (p. 952)

15. **(B)** Tempered glass—glass used in an automobile's side and rear windows designed to break into small rounded pieces rather than sharp fragments (p. 956)

MULTIPLE-CHOICE REVIEW

1. **(B)** The correct term is specialty rescue teams. Such teams may be provided by a variety of agencies such as EMS, fire, police, industrial, or commercial services. (p. 939)

2. **(B)** Defining patient care is not a phase of extrication. The phases of extrication encompass ten steps that include gaining access to the patient, disentangling the patient, and sizing up the situation. See also Complete the Following answer 1. (p. 939)

3. **(A)** An important part of a rescue scene size-up is determining the extent of entrapment. Starting IVs on the patient is not a part of the size-up and is a paramedic skill. Removing shattered glass, if needed, should be done from as far away from the patient as is possible. Informing the patient about the extent of vehicle damage will make him more anxious. Don't lie if asked, but focus on treating the patient. (p. 941)

4. **(C)** During size-up of a collision, you must be able to read a collision and develop an action plan based on your knowledge of rescue operations and estimate of the patient's condition and priority. Knowledge includes previous experience; remember you were called to rescue the patient, not the vehicle! (p. 940)

5. **(B)** When developing an action plan for patient extrication, always keep in mind the "golden hour." The cost of vehicle damage or the type of vehicle is less relevant to the extrication as is the presence of bystanders, although they should not interfere with your operations. (p. 940)

6. **(C)** If a vehicle has an airbag that deployed, the manufacturer recommends lifting the bag and examining at the steering wheel and dash. If either is damaged, it is likely that patient's chest is damaged, which would mean great potential for internal injury. The use of a HEPA mask is not required; gloves and eye protection are recommended. (p. 941)

7. **(B)** The unsafe act that contributes most to collision scene injuries is failure to wear protective gear during rescue operations. (p. 942)

8. **(D)** By limiting the inner circle to rescuers who are in protective gear, you help to *decrease* potential injuries. Factors that may contribute to injuries of rescuers at a collision include a careless attitude toward personal safety, a lack of skill in tool use, and physical problems that impede strenuous effort. (p. 942)

9. **(D)** Plastic "bump hats" do not provide adequate protection; use quality headgear. Good protective gear at the scene of a collision includes fire-resistant trousers or turnout pants; steel toe, high-top work shoes; and firefighter or leather gloves. (pp. 944–945)

10. **(A)** To ensure eye protection at the collision scene, the EMT should wear safety goggles with a soft vinyl frame. Safety glasses can be worn, but they must have *large* lenses and side shields. Thermal masks are cold-weather gear. A hinged plastic helmet shield will allow particles to enter from under the shield. (p. 945)

11. **(C)** An aluminized rescue blanket may be used to protect your patient from poor weather and flying particles. The rescuer should be properly attired for cold weather conditions. (p. 945)

12. **(A)** When using flares, the EMT should watch for spilled fuel or other combustibles prior to igniting. Do not throw flares out of the moving vehicle or use as a traffic wand. Never turn your back on traffic; walk toward the traffic so you can observe oncoming vehicles. (p. 946)

13. **(C)** When there is an electrical hazard, the safe zone should be far enough away to assure an arcing wire does not cause injury. If you feel a ground gradient, you are already too close to the electricity. (p. 946)

14. **(D)** A material or an object that will carry electricity is called a conductor. (p. 946)

15. **(B)** If a vehicle collides with a broken utility pole with utility wires down, you should tell the vehicle's occupants to stay in the vehicle until the power company arrives. (p. 948)

16. **(B)** In wet weather, a phenomenon known as a ground gradient may provide your first clue that a wire is down. (p. 948)

17. **(A)** If you feel a tingling sensation in your legs and lower torso, you should turn 180 degrees and shuffle with both feet together (or hop on one foot) to safety. Either technique helps prevent your body from completing a circuit with the energized ground, which can cause electrocution. Hopping is much more dangerous, due to likelihood of falling, which may complete the circuit. (p. 948)

18. **(D)** Do *not* apply a short spine board to the driver as this is the time for a quick removal. If there is a fire in the car's engine compartment and people are trapped within the vehicle, you should quickly and carefully remove the patient, assure that the fire department has been called, and don protective gear and use your fire extinguisher. (pp. 949–951)

19. **(C)** When a vehicle's hood is closed and there is an engine fire, you should *not* attempt to open the hood as this will fuel the fire with oxygen and the fire will flare up. (p. 949–951)

20. **(A)** When a vehicle rolls off the roadway into dried grass in a field, it is possible that a fire may occur from the catalytic converter, which is under the car, and its temperature can reach over 1,200°F. (p. 951)

21. **(C)** "Try Before You Pry" is the foundation for the simple access procedure. Disentanglement is removing the vehicle from around the patient who is entrapped. Stabilization is ensuring the vehicle is less likely to roll or move during extrication efforts. (p. 955)

22. (D) Once a vehicle is stabilized and an entry point is gained, do *not* pull a patient out of an access hole prior to spinal immobilization. (p. 956)

23. (C) If an unconscious patient is in a sitting position behind the wheel with legs pinned by the vehicle, the best approach to disentanglement would be to cut the roof, displace the doors, then displace the dash. This allows for plenty of room to work and for vertical rapid extrication if the patient's condition deteriorates. (pp. 956–957)

24. (D) Removing the roof of a vehicle does *not* stabilize a vehicle. (pp. 956–957)

25. (C) When an extrication involves displacing the dash or steering wheel but the airbag has not yet deployed, disconnect the battery cable. Be aware that it can still deploy. (pp. 957, 959)

COMPLETE THE FOLLOWING

1. The ten phases of the rescue process are: (p. 939)
   - preparing for the rescue
   - sizing up the situation
   - recognizing and managing hazards
   - stabilizing the vehicle prior to entering
   - gaining access to the patient
   - providing initial patient assessment and rapid trauma exam
   - disentangling the patient
   - immobilizing and extricating the patient from the vehicle
   - providing a detailed physical exam, ongoing assessment, treatment, and transporting to the most appropriate hospital
   - terminating the rescue

2. The factors that can increase the potential for an injury at a collision site are: (any six) (p. 942)
   - a careless attitude toward personal safety
   - lack of skill in tool use
   - physical problems that impede strenuous effort
   - failure to eliminate or control hazards
   - using unsafe tools
   - failure to select the proper tool for the task
   - failure to recognize mechanisms of injury and unsafe surroundings
   - lifting heavy objects improperly
   - deactivating safety devices designed to prevent injury
   - failure to wear highly visible outer clothing, especially when exposed to highway traffic

LABEL THE PHOTOGRAPHS (pp. 950, 953, 958)

1. Extinguishing fire under vehicle
2. Extinguishing fire under the dash
3. Stabilizing car on wheels
4. Stabilizing car on its side
5. Stabilizing car on its roof
6. Car roof folded back

STREET SCENES DISCUSSION

1. The strategy depends on the abilities, training, and equipment available to the rescuers. However, taking the roof off first has an advantage; if the patient takes a turn for the worse, the patient could be removed through the roof on a long backboard.

2. This is a serious mechanism of injury. The patient should be transported to a trauma center.

3. ALS should be requested right away, due to the mechanism of injury and the patient's unresponsiveness.

Chapter 36: Special Operations

MATCH TERMINOLOGY/ DEFINITIONS

1. **(O)** Cold zone—area in which the command post and support functions that are necessary to control the incident are located (p. 967)

2. **(L)** EMS Command—senior EMS person on the scene who establishes an EMS command post and oversees the medical aspects of a multiple-casualty incident (p. 981)

3. **(M)** Hazardous material—any substance or material in a form that poses an unreasonable risk to health, safety, and property when transported in commerce (p. 964)

4. **(N)** Hot zone—area immediately surrounding a dangerous goods incident that extends far enough to prevent adverse effects from released dangerous goods to personnel outside the zone (p. 967)

5. **(K)** National Incident Management System (NIMS)—system used for the management of a large-scale multiple-casualty incident, involving assumption of responsibility for command and designation and coordination of such elements as triage, treatment, transport, and staging (p. 977)

6. **(J)** Multiple-casualty incident (MCI)—any medical or trauma incident involving three or more patients that places a great demand on EMS equipment and personnel (p. 976)

7. **(I)** Staging supervisor—person responsible for overseeing and keeping track of ambulances and ambulance personnel at a multiple-casualty incident and who directs ambulances to treatment areas at the request of the transportation officer (p. 989)

8. **(H)** Staging area—area in which ambulances are parked and other resources are held until needed (p. 989)

9. **(G)** Transportation supervisor—person responsible for communicating with area officers and hospitals to manage transportation of patients to hospitals from the scene of a multiple-casualty incident (p. 990)

10. **(F)** Treatment supervisor—person responsible for overseeing treatment of patients who have been triaged at a multiple-casualty incident (p. 987)

11. **(E)** Treatment area—area in which patient care is delivered at a multiple-casualty incident (p. 987)

12. **(C)** Triage—process of quickly assessing patients in a multiple-casualty incident and assigning each a priority for receiving emergency care or transportation to definitive care (p. 981)

13. **(D)** Triage supervisor—person responsible for overseeing triage at a multiple-casualty incident (p. 981)

14. **(B)** Triage area—area in which secondary triage takes place at a multiple-casualty incident (p. 987)

15. (A) Triage tag—color-coded tag indicating the priority group to which a patient has been assigned (p. 987)

MULTIPLE-CHOICE REVIEW

1. (A) Using the *North American Emergency Response Guidebook,* the EMT would find that ethyl acetate is a chemical that irritates the eyes and respiratory tract. See Table 36-1. (p. 965)

2. (B) Using the *North American Emergency Response Guidebook,* the EMT would find that Benzene (benzol) is a chemical that has toxic vapors that can be absorbed through the skin. See Table 36-1. (p. 965)

3. (D) The regulations that require training in hazardous materials for responders to hazmat incidents are OSHA 1910.120. (pp. 965–966)

4. (B) The level of training for those who initially respond to releases or potential releases of hazardous materials in order to protect people, property, and the environment is called First Responder Operations. (p. 966)

5. (A) The level of training for those who are likely to witness or discover a hazardous substance release is called First Responder Awareness. (p. 966)

6. (C) The standard that deals with competencies for EMS personnel at a hazardous materials incident is called NFPA 473. (p. 966)

7. (D) Pet stores generally are not hazmat locations. Examples of potential hazardous materials locations would include garden centers, chemical plants, and trucking terminals. (p. 966)

8. (C) Unless EMS personnel are trained to the level of Hazardous Materials Technician, they must remain in the cold zone. (p. 967)

9. (C) All victims leaving the hot zone should be considered contaminated until proven otherwise. (p. 967)

10. (A) The primary concern at the scene of a hazardous materials incident is the safety of the EMT and crew, patients, and the public. Stabilizing the incident often takes a long time. Exposed patients need to be removed but this, too, does not happen quickly, due to the need to identify the hazmat material and decontaminate the patients. (p. 967)

11. (B) Upon arrival at a tanker truck crash where the vehicle has overturned and is rapidly leaking its contents onto the street, the EMT should isolate the area and call for the appropriate backup assistance. Do not try to stop or seal the leak since this would expose many rescuers to the chemical. Sending in the least senior EMT to assess the patient is not an appropriate move as it could sacrifice a rescuer. (p. 967)

12. (B) The "safe zone" of a hazardous materials incident should be established in an upwind/same level location. If it was established downwind, you would increase the chance of being exposed to the chemicals. Zones established downhill may be contaminated by hazardous runoff. (p. 967)

13. (C) Initiating rescue attempts inside the hot zone are delayed until the product and proper protection needs are determined. The role of the incident commander at a hazardous materials incident is to delegate responsibility for directing bystanders to a safe area, establishing a perimeter, and evacuating people if necessary. (p. 967)

14. (A) When a contaminated victim of a hazardous-material incident comes in contact with other people who are not contaminated, this is referred to as secondary contamination. (p. 973)

15. (C) The designations on the sides of tanker trucks are called hazardous material placards. (pp. 967–969)

16. (B) The commonly used placard system for fixed facilities is called the NFPA 704 system. (p. 967)

17. (B) All employers are required to post in an obvious spot the information about all the chemicals in the workplace on a form called an MSDS (Material Safety Data Sheet). (p. 969)

18. (A) The NFPA rules are really only guidelines and do not detail how to manage an incident. Resources that the EMT should use at a hazardous-material incident include the local hazmat team, the *Emergency Response Guidebook,* and CHEM-TEL. (pp. 970–971)

19. (A) CHEMTREC is a 24-hour service for identifying hazardous materials that also provides instructions for handling spills. (p. 971)

20. (B) The responsibilities of EMS personnel at a hazardous materials incident are taking care of the injured and monitoring and rehabilitating hazmat team members. (p. 971)

21. (A) The rehab sector at a hazardous-material incident should be located in the cold zone, *not* the warm zone. It should also be protected from the weather, easily accessible to EMS, and free from exhaust fumes. (pp. 971–972)

22. (D) As soon as possible after a hazmat team member exits the hot zone, the EMT should reassess his vital signs. Remember that hazmat team members should have their baseline vitals taken while suiting up and both preentry and exit vitals should be tracked on a flow sheet. (pp. 971–972)

23. (C) Always try to contain the runoff water when it is necessary to decontaminate a patient before hazmat specialists arrive. Flushing water down the nearest drain could contaminate the area's entire water supply. (p. 974)

24. (D) A good local disaster plan is not generic, but rather should be written to address the events that are conceivable for a particular location (e.g., Florida needs to plan for hurricanes, Kansas for tornadoes). (p. 977)

25. (D) Upon arrival of the first EMS unit at the scene of an MCI, the crew leader should assume EMS command, conduct a scene walk-through, and call for backup. Do *not* begin patient treatment since even though this might save one or two lives, it would be at the expense of the majority of the patients because response would be delayed and disorganized. (p. 978)

26. (C) Once units arrive at an MCI, as much face-to-face communication as possible should be used, especially between Command and area supervisors and between area supervisors and subordinates. This will help to reduce radio channel crowding. (p. 980)

27. (C) If an MCI involves hazardous materials, a rehabilitation sector would be needed. (p. 981)

28. (A) The individual at an MCI who is responsible for the sorting and prioritizing of the patients is the triage supervisor. (p. 981)

29. (A) Patients who are assessed to have decreased mental status at an MCI are considered Priority-1. Other examples of Priority-1 patients are those with airway and breathing difficulties, uncontrolled or severe bleeding, severe medical problems, shock, and severe burns. (p. 984)

30. (A) Patients who are assessed to have shock (hypoperfusion) at an MCI are considered Priority-1. See answer 29. (p. 984)

31. (B) Patients who are assessed to have multiple bone or joint injuries at an MCI are considered Priority-2 unless they show signs of impending shock. Other examples of Priority-2 patients are those with burns without airway problems and back injuries with or without spinal cord damage. (p. 984)

32. (D) Patients who are assessed to have died at the MCI scene are considered Priority-4 (or zero). (p. 984)

33. (C) The individual at an MCI who is responsible for maintaining a supply of vehicles and personnel at a location away from the incident site is the staging supervisor. (p. 989)

34. (C) The individual at an MCI who is responsible for determining patient destinations and notifying the hospitals of the incoming patients is the transportation supervisor. (p. 990)

35. (D) Patient transport decisions at an MCI are based upon priority, destination facilities, and transportation resources. The patient's family preferences are not a consideration in a disaster situation. (p. 990)

COMPLETE THE FOLLOWING

1. The information you should be prepared to give when you call for assistance from CHEMTREC includes: (p. 971)
   - Give your name, your call-back number, and your FAX number.
   - Explain the nature and location of the problem.
   - Report the identification number(s) of the material(s) involved if there is a safe way for you to obtain this information.
   - Give the name of the carrier, shipper, manufacturer, consignee, and point of origin.
   - Describe the container type and size.
   - Report if the container is on rail car, truck, open storage, or housed storage.
   - Estimate the quantity of material transported and released.
   - Report local conditions (e.g., the weather, terrain, proximity to schools and/or hospitals).
   - Report injuries and exposures.
   - Report local emergency services that have been notified.
   - Keep the line of communication open at all times.

2. The characteristics of the rehab area must include the following: (any four) (p. 972)
   - located in the cold zone
   - protected from weather
   - large enough to accommodate multiple rescue crews
   - easily accessible to EMS units
   - free from exhaust fumes
   - allows for rapid re-entry into the emergency operation

COMPLETE THE CHART (p. 983)

1. EMS Staging Officer (Supervisor)
2. EMS Safety Officer (Supervisor)
3. Transportation Officer (Supervisor)
4. Triage Officer (Supervisor)
5. Rehab Officer (Supervisor)
6. P-2 Tx Leader

STREET SCENES DISCUSSION

1. Yes, a helicopter would be appropriate provided there is a nearby landing zone that will not keep ambulances from transporting patients.

2. With a short transport time, you could have the ambulances turn around and return to the scene to pick up additional patients.

3. Some EMS providers have used a school bus to transport low-priority patients to a hospital. If you ever do so, medically clear each patient on the bus to assure they are low priority and arrange for medical personnel to travel with them on the bus to the hospital.

CASE STUDY—THE SCHOOL BUS MCI

1. Size up the situation, establish EMS command, make contact with the fire and police command officers.

2. You should don the EMS Command or Medical Command vest. Your responsibilities are the overall management of the medical aspects of the incident, working directly with the chief officers of the police and fire departments, assuring the safety of all your personnel, and designating triage, treatment, transport, and staging area supervisors.

3. Triage supervisor

4. Set up the triage area and begin tagging patients and classifying into priority for removal from the scene to the treatment area.

5. Respond three to the scene and seven to a staging area about a mile away with easy access to the scene. The ambulances responding to the scene will help fill out the complement of command officers and provide personnel to triage patients.

6. The first crew leader at the staging area should be designated as the staging officer and be responsible for the release of ambulances and personnel to the scene as directed by command. If this is a lengthy operation, he should also attend to the human needs of the staging personnel by locating restrooms and food. He will need to be able to communicate with arriving mutual aid units, providing them with maps and directions to the scene and hospital as it becomes necessary.

7. Yes, but only upon direction of Command and/or the staging supervisor.

8. Transportation and treatment area supervisors would be helpful in managing the flow of patients.

9. On long backboards with rigid extrication collars applied

10. Take the patients to the respective section of the treatment area depending on their triage tag priority.

11. P-2

12. P-1

13. P-4 (or zero)

14. P-1

15. Allow one parent per child to assist and stay with the child in the treatment area if space permits.

16. Transportation area supervisor

17. Do a roll call of the hospitals for bed availability and the number of patients of each priority they can handle.

18. Consider the use of a medivac helicopter.

19. P-3 patients with minor injuries who are medically cleared. There will still need to be medical personnel on the bus just in case a patient's status changes.

20. Appoint a Public Information Officer, plan for rehab and a light meal after the incident, and consider setting up a critical incident stress debriefing for all personnel who were at the scene who are interested in talking about what they saw and did.

Chapter 37: EMS Response to Terrorism

MATCH TERMINOLOGY/ DEFINITIONS

1. **(E)** Permeation—the movement of a substance through a surface or, on a molecular level, through intact materials (p. 1004)

2. **(C)** Dissemination—spreading (p. 1006)

3. **(H)** Tactics—specific operational actions to accomplish assigned tasks (p. 1020)

4. **(A)** Contamination—contact with or presence of a material where it does not belong and that is somehow harmful to persons, animals, or the environment (p. 1004)

5. **(G)** Secondary devices—destructive devises, such as bombs, placed to be activated after an initial attack and timed to injure emergency responders who rush in to help care for those targeted by an initial attack (p. 998)

6. **(B)** Decontamination—a chemical and/or physical process used to remove and prevent the spread of a contaminant (p. 1006)

7. **(D)** Exposure—the dose of concentration of an agent multiplied by the time, or duration (p. 1003)

8. **(F)** Routes of entry—pathways into the body, generally by absorption, ingestion, injection, or inhalation (p. 1003)

MULTIPLE-CHOICE REVIEW

1. **(B)** CBRNE (p. 997)

2. **(C)** Domestic terrorist (pp. 996–997)

3. **(D)** OTTO (p. 998)

4. **(D)** Any of the above (pp. 998–1000)

5. **(B)** It is the anniversary of the Murrah building bombing in Oklahoma City. (p. 1000)

6. **(A)** Car crashes involving more than two patients with serious traumatic injuries. (p. 1000)

7. **(C)** Biological/Etiological (pp. 1000–1001)

8. **(B)** Radiological (p. 1001)

9. **(C)** Osmosis (p. 1003)

10. **(D)** All of the above (p. 1005)

11. **(B)** Mechanical (p. 1005)

12. **(B)** Standard Precautions (pp. 1005–1006)

13. **(C)** Inhalation (pp. 1007, 1010)

14. **(A)** Dermal (p. 1008)

15. **(D)** Any of the above (p. 1011)

16. **(C)** Virulence (p. 1012)

17. **(C)** Lethality of the agent (p. 1013)

18. **(D)** Smallpox (p. 1017)

19. **(A)** Demulsification (p. 975, Chapter 36)

20. **(C)** Dilution (p. 975, Chapter 36)

COMPLETE THE FOLLOWING

Decontamination for Responders Wearing PPE (pp. 975–976)

1. This is a limited list that may not require personal showers since the responders were wearing PPE. List six terms that would be found on the equipment list for decontamination.
   - Buckets
   - Brushes
   - Decontamination solution
   - Decontamination tubs
   - Dedicated water supply
   - Tarps or plastic sheeting
   - Containment vessel for water runoff
   - Pump to transfer wastewater from decontamination tubs to containment vessel
   - A-frame ladder
   - Appropriate-level PPE for responders performing decontamination

2. List six of the objectives of the responders assigned to decontamination. (p. 975)
   - Determine appropriate level of protective equipment based on materials and associated hazards.
   - Properly wear and operate in PPE.
   - Establish operating time log.
   - Set up and operate the decontamination line.
   - Prioritize the decontamination of victims according to a triage system.
   - Perform triage in PPE.
   - Be able to communicate while in PPE.

STREET SCENES DISCUSSION

1. This organization could be a potential threat to emergency service personnel because of the trouble in the world and America's position in the Middle East. Regardless of your personal opinion on this issue, it is clear that there are people who have strong feelings that would go to great lengths to hurt those who they feel have opposing views. Always be very careful when responding to any incident of this nature.

2. It is extremely unusual to find a motor vehicle collision in an isolated location such as an alleyway, with no one around, completely on fire. This "smells" of an arson job or a potential setup.

3. It is always the acceptable practice to stop and not proceed if the emergency services personnel feel they are in imminent danger. The first priority is always your safety and that of your crew!

4. Examples of groups or types of domestic terrorists that have been identified include: environmental terrorists, survivalists, militias, racial-hate groups, and groups with extreme political, religious, or other philosophies or beliefs.

MATCH TERMINOLOGY/ DEFINITIONS

▶ PART A

1. **(M)** Alveoli—microscopic sacs of the lungs where exchange of carbon dioxide and oxygen takes place (p. 1035)

2. **(K)** Bronchi—two large sets of branches that come off the trachea and enter the lungs (There are right and left mainstem bronchi.) (p. 1034)

3. **(A)** Carina—fork at the lower end of the trachea where the two mainstem bronchi branch (p. 1034)

4. **(J)** Cricoid cartilage—ring-shaped structure that circles the trachea at the lower portion of the larynx (p. 1034)

5. **(O)** EIDD—esophageal intubation detector device that may be used to detect incorrect placement (or to verify correct placement) of the endotracheal tube (p. 1049)

6. **(C)** Endotracheal tube—tube designed to be inserted into the trachea; oxygen, medication, or a suction catheter can be directed into the trachea through an endotracheal tube. (p. 1038)

7. **(I)** Epiglottis—leaf-shaped structure that acts as a covering to the opening of the trachea and that prevents food and foreign matter from entering it (p. 1034)

8. **(G)** Esophagus—tube that leads from the pharynx to the stomach (p. 1034)

9. **(F)** Glottic opening—opening to the trachea (p. 1039)

10. **(H)** Ventilate—to provide ventilations at a higher rate to compensate for oxygen not delivered during intubation or suctioning (p. 1038)

11. **(D)** Hypopharynx—area directly above the openings of both the trachea and the esophagus (p. 1034)

12. **(E)** Hypoxia—inadequate oxygenation, or oxygen starvation (p. 1038)

13. **(B)** Intubation—insertion of a tube (p. 1038)

14. **(N)** Laryngoscope—illuminating instrument that is inserted into the pharynx to permit visualization of the pharynx and larynx (p. 1038)

15. **(L)** Larynx—voicebox (p. 1034)

▶ PART B

1. **(E)** Mainstem bronchi—either of the two (right or left) large sets of branches that come off the trachea and enter the lungs (p. 1034)

2. **(G)** Nasogastric tube (NG tube)—tube designed to be passed through the nose, nasopharynx, and esophagus. It is used to relieve distention of the stomach in an infant or child patient. (p. 1055)

3. **(H)** Nasopharynx—area directly posterior to the nose (p. 1034)

4. **(I)** Oropharynx—area directly posterior to the mouth (p. 1034)

5. **(A)** Orotracheal intubation—placement of an endotracheal tube through the mouth and into the trachea (p. 1038)

6. **(J)** Cricoid pressure—pressure applied to the cricoid cartilage to suppress vomiting and bring the vocal cords into view; also called cricoid pressure (p. 1034)

7. **(D)** Stylet—long, thin, flexible metal probe (p. 1042)

8. **(B)** Trachea—"windpipe"; the structure that connects the pharynx to the lungs (p. 1034)

9. **(F)** Vallecula—groove-like structure anterior to the epiglottis (p. 1034)

10. **(C)** Vocal cords—two thin folds of tissue within the larynx that vibrate as air passes between them, producing sounds (p. 1034)

MULTIPLE-CHOICE REVIEW

1. **(C)** The area directly above the openings of both the trachea and the esophagus is called the hypopharynx. (p. 1034)

2. **(B)** The groove-like structure anterior to the epiglottis is called the vallecula. The carina is the location where the trachea bifurcates into the right and left mainstem bronchi. (p. 1034)

3. **(B)** Food is more apt to be aspirated into the right mainstem bronchus rather than the left mainstem bronchus because the right splits off the carina at less of an angle than the left. (p. 1034)

4. **(A)** The brain's center for respiratory control is located in the brainstem. The cerebellum controls fine-motor coordination, and the cerebrum contains the centers of higher cognitive abilities. The pons functions as a bridge between the cerebrum and cerebellum. (p. 1034)

5. **(C)** The endotracheal tube is primarily intended to be inserted into the trachea and functions to provide direct access to the trachea. This allows positive pressure ventilation without the hazards of aspiration. Medication administration and suctioning are also possible via the tube, although these are not the primary functions of the tube. (p. 1038)

6. **(A)** Orotracheal intubation allows direct ventilation of the lungs, bypassing the entire upper airway. (p. 1038)

7. **(C)** When placing the endotracheal tube, the EMT uses direct visualization. Rapid-sequence, blind, and surgical techniques are performed by paramedics. (p. 1038)

8. **(D)** Orotracheal intubation provides complete control of the airway and minimizes the risk of aspiration. It also provides for better oxygen delivery and allows for deeper suctioning of the airway. (p. 1038)

9. **(C)** During orotracheal intubation attempts, the heart rate may decrease, *not* increase, due to vagal nerve stimulation. Monitor the patient's heart rate closely. Complications of orotracheal intubation include hypoxia from prolonged attempts, soft-tissue trauma to the lips, gums, or airway structures, and gagging and vomiting. (pp. 1038–1039)

10. **(B)** When the endotracheal tube is advanced too deeply, right-mainstem intubation commonly occurs. (p. 1039)

11. **(C)** The *most* serious complication of endotracheal intubation is unrecognized esophageal intubation, which will rapidly result in death. Mainstem bronchus intubation, bradycardia, and airway trauma are also potential complications. (p. 1039)

12. **(A)** The EMT should reassess the location of the endotracheal tube each time the patient is moved to prevent complications from accidental extubation. The tube can easily be displaced just enough to remove it from the trachea. Be sure to reassess the tube position after each move. (p. 1039)

13. **(C)** Most adult patients can be intubated using a size 2 or 3 straight blade or size 3 curved blade. (p. 1039)

14. **(C)** The straight blade is designed so that the tip of the blade is placed under the epiglottis. (p. 1039)

15. **(D)** The curved blade is designed so the tip of the blade is placed into the vallecula. (p. 1039)

16. **(A)** The cuff at the distal end of the endotracheal tube usually seals with 8 to 10 cc of air. Infant tubes are cuffless. (p. 1040)

17. **(C)** When using an endotracheal tube on an infant or child less than eight years of age, do not expect to see a cuff on the tube in the out-of-hospital setting. In these pediatric patients, the cricoid cartilage serves as a "cuff." The AHA 2005 Guidelines do allow the use of cuffed tubes on children in the hospital. (p. 1040)

18. **(B)** No matter what the internal diameter of the endotracheal tube, it has a standard 15-millimeter adapter so the bag-valve mask can easily be attached. Infant and child tubes are cuffless, therefore, they do not have an inflation valve or pilot balloon. (p. 1040)

19. **(C)** It is generally accepted that the average-size adult male should receive either an 8.0 or 8.5 mm tube. (p. 1042)

20. **(C)** In an adult, the properly placed tube will have the 22 cm mark at the teeth. (p. 1042)

21. **(D)** Once the lubricated stylet is inserted, the endotracheal tube should be shaped like a hockey stick. This facilitates tube placement. (p. 1043)

22. **(D)** Prior to securing an endotracheal tube, insert an oral airway as a bite block, listen to both lungs, and listen over the epigastrium. Do not suction down the tube until it is properly taped into place or you may accidentally extubate the patient. (p. 1043)

23. **(C)** Endotracheal tube length is dependent upon the tube diameter; the tube length during placement is unimportant. Items that should be checked prior to an intubation attempt include the laryngoscope light bulb, cuff on the tube, and the shape formed by the stylet in the tube. (p. 1042)

24. **(C)** The laryngoscope is designed to be held in the left hand. Do not use it as a fulcrum as you may break the patient's teeth. (p. 1039)

25. **(A)** Cricoid pressure is designed to help reduce vomiting by indirectly compressing the esophagus. In addition, it often brings the vocal cords into view. (p. 1047)

26. **(B)** The correct order for verifying tube placement by auscultation for the presence of breath sounds is first the epigastrium, then left, then right chest apex. (p. 1049)

27. **(C)** If the breath sounds are diminished or absent on the left but present on the right, it is likely the tube has advanced into the right mainstem bronchus. (p. 1049)

28. **(B)** The EMT should make no more than *two* attempts at orotracheal intubation. If both attempts fail, insert an oral airway, continue to ventilate the patient with high-concentration oxygen via bag-valve mask, and aggressively suction the airway. (p. 1051)

29. **(D)** The narrowest portion of the infant's or small child's airway is the cricoid ring. The proper sizing of the uncuffed tube is critical to ensure an appropriate seal of the ET tube. (p. 1036)

30. **(B)** A #1 straight blade is preferred for use in infants and small children. (p. 1052)

31. **(C)** A nasogastric tube (NG) is commonly used in an infant or child patient to decompress the stomach and proximal bowel. (p. 1055)

32. **(B)** When you are unable to adequately ventilate the child or infant patient due to distention of the stomach, you should consider the use of a nasogastric tube. (p. 1055)

33. **(D)** The major contraindication for an NG tube placement would be head or major facial trauma due to the potential of placing the tube directly into the brain. (p. 1055)

34. **(A)** The NG tube should be measured from the tip of the nose around the ear to below the xiphoid process. (p. 1057)

35. **(D)** Do not hook the NG tube up to the suction unit. Once the NG tube is passed gently downward along the nasal floor, the EMT should confirm tube placement by aspirating stomach contents, secure the tube in place with tape, and confirm placement by auscultating the epigastrium while injecting 10–20 cc of air. (p. 1057)

COMPLETE THE FOLLOWING

1. The four indications for when to perform orotracheal intubation include: (p. 1043)
   - inability to ventilate the apneic patient
   - to protect the airway of a patient without a gag reflex or cough
   - to protect the airway of a patient unresponsive to any painful stimuli
   - cardiac arrest

2. The six complications of deep suctioning that can be avoided by preoxygenation include: (p. 1059)
   - cardiac dysrhythmias
   - hypoxia
   - coughing
   - damage to the lining (mucosa) of the airway
   - spasm of the bronchioles if catheter extends past the carina
   - spasm of the vocal cords during orotracheal suctioning

STREET SCENES DISCUSSION

1. Be prepared to extubate the patient, assuring that you have suction available at the patient's side.

2. Yes. The patient is critical, and ALS would be helpful.

3. Remove the tube, and reintubate the patient.

4. Yes. The tube needs to be placed with the patient's head and neck manually stabilized in an in-line position. You also should consider a straight blade.

Interim Exam 3

1. **(B)** The circulation of blood throughout the body, filling the capillaries and supplying the cells and tissues with oxygen and nutrients, is called perfusion. Physiology is the study of how the body functions. Metabolism is the process of all the physical and chemical changes within the body that are necessary for life. (p. 615)

2. **(D)** With one exception (the pulmonary artery), arteries carry oxygenated blood away from the heart. (pp. 616–617)

3. **(A)** With one exception (the pulmonary vein), veins carry deoxygenated blood back to the heart. (pp. 616–617)

4. **(D)** Once an adult loses approximately a liter of blood, his or her condition is considered serious. This is one-sixth of the total blood volume in a 150-pound patient. (p. 619)

5. **(C)** Once a child loses approximately 500 mL of blood, his or her condition is considered serious. (p. 619)

6. **(B)** Once an infant loses approximately 150 cc of blood volume, his other condition is considered serious. Note that a cc and an mL are equal measurements. (p. 619)

7. **(A)** Since internal bleeding is not visible, the EMT must base severity of blood loss on signs and symptoms exhibited. Mechanism of injury may also be a good clue to internal injury. What the patient tells you will not reveal how much blood has been lost. (p. 629)

8. **(D)** The patient's history of diabetes is *not* significant in determining bleeding severity. The factors on which severity of bleeding depends are the rate of bleeding and the amount of blood loss, the patient's age and weight, and the ability of the patient's body to respond and defend against blood loss. (p. 619)

9. **(B)** Blood that oozes and is dark red is most likely from a capillary. Venous bleeding will be a steady flow of dark red or maroon blood. Arteries spurt and blood is usually bright red. (p. 618)

10. **(C)** You are treating a patient who has a slashed wrist, which is spurting bright red blood. After trying direct pressure and elevation to control the bleeding, the next step would be to press on the brachial artery. See answer 11. (pp. 623–625)

11. **(D)** When all other methods have failed to control bleeding, the EMT should apply a tourniquet as the last resort. (p. 626)

12. **(C)** Vomiting bile is usually not a sign of internal bleeding. Signs of internal bleeding include painful, swollen, or deformed extremities; a tender, rigid abdomen; and bruising. (pp. 629–630)

13. **(C)** A fall from a height will usually produce a blunt injury, unless the patient falls onto something that penetrates, such as a fence. Examples of penetrating trauma include handgun bullet wounds, carving-knife wounds, and screwdriver stab wounds. (p. 629)

14. **(C)** Gunshot wounds are considered penetrating trauma. Examples of blunt trauma include blast injuries, auto-pedestrian collisions, and falls. (p. 629)

15. **(A)** The signs and symptoms of internal bleeding are the same as those of shock (hypoperfusion). Patients with these signs are difficult to stabilize in the field. (pp. 629–630)

16. **(B)** Hypovolemic, cardiogenic, and neurogenic are all types of shock. Hydrophobia is another name for rabies. (p. 632)

17. **(C)** At a point when the body can no longer compensate for the low blood volume, decompensated shock begins. Anaphylactic shock is a severe allergic reaction with respiratory distress and hypotension. (p. 632)

18. **(C)** The brain and spinal cord are the major components of the central nervous system. The peripheral nerves branch out from the spinal cord. (p. 749)

19. **(D)** The nervous system is divided into the central, peripheral, and autonomic nervous systems. Voluntary is a type of skeletal muscle that allows movement. (p. 749)

20. **(D)** The cranium consists of the forehead, top, back, and upper sides of the skull. The maxilla is the upper jaw, and the mandible is the lower jaw. (p. 751)

21. **(A)** The bones forming the face include the zygomatic, mandible, and maxillae. Vertebrae are bones of the spine. (p. 751)

22. **(A)** The brain and spinal cord are bathed in cerebrospinal fluid. Lymphatic fluid is responsible for maintaining our immune system. Synovial fluid lubricates the joints. (pp. 751–752)

23. **(B)** The spine is divided into sections called vertebrae. Coccygeal is the name of one section of the vertebrae. (p. 752)

24. **(B)** The lumbar area of the spine includes five vertebrae. (p. 752)

25. **(C)** The cervical area of the spine includes seven vertebrae. (p. 752)

26. **(B)** When a patient strikes her head and states she feels groggy and has a headache, she most likely has a concussion. (p. 753)

27. **(D)** While the patient most likely has a concussion, any altered mental status after striking the head, such as "just sitting there staring off into space for a few minutes," can be an early indication of a contusion, a concussion, or a coup injury. An attention deficit is not usually injury induced. (p. 753)

28. **(B)** When a patient has some memory loss after a head injury, this is referred to as amnesia. (p. 753)

29. **(C)** When a bruising of the brain occurs on the side of the injury, this is referred to as a coup injury. When bruising occurs on the opposite side, this is called contrecoup. A hematoma is a collection of blood within tissue. A hematoma in the cranium is usually named by its location such as epidural (outside the dura), subdural (below the dura), or intracerebral (within the brain). (p. 753)

30. **(D)** A collection of blood within the skull or the brain is called a subdural, epidural, and intracerebral hematoma depending on the specific location. See answer 29. (pp. 753–754)

31. **(D)** Decreased respiration does *not* lead to increased cellular perfusion; rather, it decreases perfusion. Head injury is made worse by limited room for expansion inside the skull. As pressure in the skull increases, it becomes more difficult for blood to flow into the head. This leads to carbon dioxide level increases in the brain. (p. 755)

32. **(B)** An assessment strategy used to check an extremity for injury or paralysis in the conscious patient is assessing equality of strength by checking hand grip or pushing against the patient's hands and feet. (pp. 762–763)

33. **(B)** Incubation period is the time between exposure and appearance of symptoms. (p. 1013)

34. **(D)** If a patient has a brain injury with skull fracture, the patient's pupils will tend to be unequal. (p. 755)

35. **(D)** The vitals of a patient with a brain injury are increased blood pressure, decreased pulse. (p. 755)

36. **(A)** Consider the possibility of a cranial fracture whenever you note deep lacerations or severe bruises to the scalp or forehead. (p. 755)

37. **(B)** The spinal column is made up of 33 irregularly shaped bones. (p. 752)

38. **(B)** Any blunt trauma above the clavicles may damage the *cervical* vertebrae. (p. 752)

39. **(A)** Priapism is a persistent erection of the penis. (p. 763)

40. (B) Often with a cervical spine injury, the patient in a supine position may have his arms stretched out above his head. (p. 763)

41. (C) Injuries to an elderly person should be considered as possibly due to abuse or neglect. (p. 892–893)

42. (C) Geriatric patients have decreased elasticity of the lungs and decreased activity of cilia that results in decreased ability to clear foreign substances from the lungs. (p. 883)

43. (D) As a normal process of aging, geriatric patients lose skin elasticity and sweat glands shrink. This results in thin, dry, wrinkled skin. (p. 883)

44. (B) Geriatric patients usually have diminished function of the thyroid gland that results in decreased energy and tolerance of heat and cold. (p. 883)

45. (C) When an elderly patient falls, this may indicate a more serious problem such as abnormal heart rhythm, which may cause a diminished cardiac output. (p. 892)

46. (C) An unstable object impaled in the cheek wall should be pulled out if easily done. This minimizes the potential for bleeding into the airway. (p. 656)

47. (A) If possible, a patient with facial fractures should be transported on a long spine board in the supine position. Then the patient and board can be rotated to the side to ensure drainage from the patient's mouth. (p. 757)

48. (D) The pressure point for controlling bleeding from the leg is the femoral artery. (p. 624)

49. (A) Do *not* pick embedded particles out of the cut. Care for an open wound includes controlling bleeding, bandaging the dressing in place, and cleaning the wound surface. (p. 653)

50. (B) The best method for control of nasal bleeding is pinching the nostrils together. (p. 628)

51. (C) The first step in caring for possible internal bleeding after ensuring respiration and circulation and controlling life-threatening external bleeding is treating for shock. Do not place the patient in a sitting position if you suspect shock. (p. 630)

52. (D) A razor blade cut is an example of a laceration. The term "incision" was used in the old curriculum. (pp. 648–649)

53. (D) The condition in which flaps of skin are torn loose or pulled off completely is called avulsion. (pp. 650–651)

54. (C) If a patient has an object impaled in the forearm, after the control of profuse bleeding, you should stabilize the object. Do not remove the object. (pp. 655–656)

55. (D) Pale, cool, clammy skin is a sign of shock. (p. 633)

56. (A) An object impaled in the eye should be stabilized with gauze and protected with a disposable cup. It is also important to cover the other eye to limit movement of the eyes. (p. 657)

57. (C) A lacerated eyelid or injury to the eyeball should be covered with folded 4 × 4s to carefully hold it in place. (p. 657)

58. (A) All open wounds to the chest should be considered life-threatening. (p. 662)

59. (C) Before moving a supine patient with possible spinal injuries onto a long spine board, you should always apply a rigid collar. A KED is not needed for a supine patient. (p. 764)

60. (A) The initial effort to control bleeding from a severed neck artery should be direct pressure or pinching. Then apply the occlusive dressing. Remember Standard Precautions. (p. 659)

61. (B) The most reliable sign of spinal cord injury in conscious patients is paralysis of extremities. Tenderness along the spine may indicate injury to the bones or muscles. (pp. 762–763)

62. (D) When caring for an open abdominal wound with evisceration, do not replace the organ but cover with a moistened dressing. (p. 669)

63. (C) A patient in acute abdominal distress without vomiting should be transported face up with the knees bent to relieve the pressure on the abdominal muscles. (p. 669)

64. (C) When a joint is locked into position, the EMT should splint it in the position found. Do not apply force to move a joint. (p. 705)

65. (A) A splint properly applied to an extremity should prevent an open bone injury, motion of bone fragments, and damage to muscles and blood vessels. It should *not* impede circulation. (p. 705)

66. (B) A fracture to the humerus shaft is best cared for by immobilizing with a rigid splint or sling and swathe, which limits movement in all directions. (pp. 707–709)

67. (D) A fracture to the proximal end of the humerus is best cared for by immobilizing with a sling and swathe. (p. 729)

68. (B) The best way to immobilize a fractured elbow when the arm is found in the bent position and there is a distal pulse is to keep the arm in its found position and apply a short paddled splint. Do not straighten fractured joints that have pulses. (p. 729)

69. (B) When splinting, if a severe deformity exists or distal circulation is compromised, you should align to the anatomical position with gentle traction. (pp. 705–706)

70. (C) The first step in immobilizing a fractured wrist with distal pulse is to place the broken hand in its position of function. (p. 731)

71. (A) A patient with a fractured pelvis should be immobilized on an orthopedic stretcher or long spine board with legs bound together with wide cravats. An antishock garment could be applied if local protocols permit. In many localities, application requires an order from a physician. (pp. 715–717)

72. (D) A fractured femur is best immobilized with a traction splint. (p. 721)

73. (A) Before immobilizing a fractured knee, assess for distal PMS function. If there is no pulse, you may need to manipulate the extremity. (pp. 721–722)

74. (B) The best method for immobilizing a suspected ankle fracture is a pillow splint. (pp. 724–725)

75. (B) A sprain is an injury in which ligaments are torn. (p. 702)

76. (C) Definitive care for open extremity injuries is *not* provided in the prehospital setting. All other choices are true. (p. 702)

77. (D) Muscle is attached to bone by tendons. (p. 699)

78. (B) A partial thickness burn involves the epidermis and dermis. (p. 672)

79. (A) The entire back of an adult patient's right upper extremity is 4.5% (the entire arm is 9, so half is 4.5%) and her entire chest (which is 9%) is therefore 9 + 4.5 = 13.5%. (p. 675)

80. (C) A moderate burn involves superficial burns covering more than 50% of the body surface. (p. 676)

81. (A) Partial thickness burns cause swelling and blistering. (p. 672)

82. (D) A patient suffering chemical burns to the skin caused by dry lime should be treated by first brushing away the lime. Also, if you look up the chemical, you would note it should not be mixed with water or phenol. (p. 679)

83. **(D)** Acid burns to the eyes should be flooded with water for at least 20 minutes. (p. 680)

84. **(A)** A method for estimating the extent of a burn is the rule of nines. (p. 674)

85. **(A)** The number one priority for all EMS personnel at a collision scene is safety of the crew, which includes wearing the appropriate protective clothing. The unsafe act that contributes most to collision scene injuries is failure to wear protective gear during rescue operations. (p. 942)

86. **(A)** When arriving at the scene of a collision, the *first* thing an EMT should do is evaluate hazards and calculate the need for additional support. (p. 940)

87. **(D)** The EMT cannot be responsible for protecting the patient from injuries sustained by not wearing a seatbelt. The EMT is responsible for protecting the patient from broken glass from the wrecked car, sharp metal in the wrecked car, and the environment. (p. 945)

88. **(D)** It is not your responsibility to describe extrication procedures to the bystanders; doing so could take too much valuable time. At the scene of an auto collision, the EMT should try to keep the patient's safety in mind, inform the patient of the unique aspects of the extrication, and keep his or her own personal safety in mind. (p. 945)

89. **(C)** A vehicle involved in a collision that is determined to be a simple access will not require equipment to get to the patient. (p. 955)

90. **(C)** When applying a short spine board, the EMT should *never* apply a chin strap to the patient. (p. 771)

91. **(D)** Do not pull the patient out the side windows. To assist with patient access, the EMT should initially try opening each car door, roll down windows, and ask the patient to unlock the doors. (pp. 956–957)

92. **(A)** Requirements for speed of removal dictate the specific technique used for spinal immobilization of a patient at a collision scene. (pp. 940–941)

93. **(D)** The steps should be (1) sizing up the situation, (2) stabilizing the vehicle, (3) gaining the access, (4) disentangling the patient. (p. 939)

94. **(D)** The number of ambulances in the region is *not* a consideration unless this is an MCI. Considerations for size-up of a collision include potential hazards, need for additional EMS units, and the number of patients involved. (pp. 940–941)

95. **(C)** To minimize injuries at a collision, EMTs should wear highly visible clothing so they do not get hit by a car while attending to their patient. Use the proper tools for the task and do not deactivate the safety guards on tools or you will be injured. It is not always feasible to wait until the police arrive on the scene. (pp. 942–943)

96. **(B)** The vehicle's catalytic converter can be a source of ignition at a collision because it is often over 1,200°F. (p. 951)

97. **(A)** The three-step process of disentanglement described in the text includes creating exitways by displacing doors and roof posts, disentangling occupants by displacing front end, and gaining access by disposing of the roof. Opening the trunk and disconnecting the battery cable are not priority tasks. (pp. 956–959)

98. **(B)** If a vehicle's electrical system must be disrupted, disconnect the ground cable from the battery. (p. 957)

99. **(D)** When positioning flares, use a formula that includes the stopping distance for the posted speed plus the margin of safety. (p. 946)

100. **(C)** Once the vehicle has been stabilized, the *second* part of an extrication procedure for patient rescue is to displace doors and roof posts. The first part is to dispose of the roof. (pp. 956–959)

101. **(A)** The Emergency Medical Dispatcher (EMD) has told you the exact location of a collision, how many and what kinds of vehicles are involved, and any known hazards. Other information that would be helpful from the EMD concerning this collision would be how many persons are injured. (p. 910)

102. **(C)** The EMD does not need to ask the person's name. All other questions are pertinent. (p. 910)

103. **(A)** When operating a siren, be aware that the continuous sound of a siren could worsen a patient's condition. All motorists will *not* hear and honor your signal. If you use the siren continuously, there should be a valid reason for doing so. The noise from the siren can damage your ears over a period of time. (pp. 913–914)

104. **(D)** Factors that affect an ambulance's response to a scene include day of the week, time of the day, and detours. Danger zones usually cannot be planned for. (pp. 915–916)

105. **(B)** If a patient develops cardiac arrest during transport, have the operator of the ambulance stop the ambulance so you can begin defibrillation. Also alert the hospital about the arrest. (p. 922)

106. **(C)** When transferring a nonemergency patient to the emergency department personnel, you should check to see what is to be done with the patient. (p. 923)

107. **(C)** The last step when transferring a patient is to obtain your release, which often takes the form of a thank-you for the information provided. (p. 923)

108. **(C)** At the hospital, as soon as you are free from patient-care activities, you should prepare the prehospital care report. (pp. 923–927)

109. **(D)** Suction catheters, contaminated dressings, and blood-soaked linens are considered biohazards; unopened gauze bandages are not. (p. 925)

110. **(D)** Completeness and operability of equipment is *not* always ensured in the EMS/hospital equipment exchange program. Always inspect it; if you find parts are broken or incomplete, notify someone in authority so the device can be repaired or replaced. (p. 925)

111. **(D)** Vigorous cleaning of the ambulance while parked at the hospital is prevented or restricted by time, equipment, and space. There is, however, no law against it. (pp. 930–931)

112. **(D)** You should air the ambulance en route to quarters. When you return to quarters, replenish oxygen cylinders, clean the interior of the ambulance, and prepare yourself for service. (pp. 927–931)

113. **(D)** Antivenin solution is not routinely carried in an ambulance as it needs to be refrigerated, is expensive, and is rarely used. A poison-control kit should include paper cups, activated charcoal, and drinking water. (p. 906)

114. **(C)** The fixed suction system is *not* part of the first-in kit. All other answer choices are correct. (p. 904)

115. **(A)** The first thing to inspect on the ambulance when the engine is off is the body of the vehicle. (p. 907)

116. **(B)** Rescue tools should always be examined for rust and dirt. (pp. 909–910)

117. **(B)** Along with physical and mental fitness, ambulance operators should be able to perform under stress. (p. 912)

118. **(D)** When driving an ambulance, you should realize that there are no state laws that grant the absolute right of way. (pp. 912–913)

119. **(B)** The headlights of an ambulance should be turned on whenever the vehicle is on the road so it can easily be seen. (p. 914)

120. **(D)** To assume that there is no electrical hazard would be very dangerous. When a car collides with a utility pole, the EMT should assume obviously dead wires could be energized at any moment, that severed conductors may be energizing every wire, and wires may be charged at the highest voltage present. (p. 949)

121. **(B)** The easiest way to break tempered window glass is with a spring-loaded center punch. (p. 956)

122. **(D)** Airway passages *do* swell when a child has airway disease. All other signs listed are indications of a respiratory disease. (p. 838)

123. **(C)** The soft spot on top of an infant's head is called the fontanelle. (p. 811)

124. **(B)** Small children are referred to as abdominal breathers because they use their diaphragm for breathing. (p. 812)

125. **(C)** A child's compensating mechanism for shock fails at approximately 30% blood loss. (pp. 813–814)

126. **(D)** In cases of sudden infant death syndrome, the EMT should provide resuscitation and transport to the hospital. (p. 848)

127. **(C)** Injuries to the center of the back and upper arms might lead you to consider child abuse. Multiple skinned knees and sprained ankles are common in children. (pp. 854–855)

128. **(A)** A child who is hypoxic will have a slowed heart rate. (p. 828)

129. **(D)** Artificial ventilations for an infant or child under 8 years of age should be provided at a rate of 20 per minute. (p. 833)

130. **(B)** If you suspect respiratory distress in a conscious toddler, you should not insert anything in the patient's mouth. This could set off spasms along the upper airway that will totally obstruct the airway. (p. 839)

131. **(C)** Common causes of shock in children include infection, trauma, blood loss, and dehydration. (pp. 835–836)

132. **(C)** A sunken fontanelle may indicate dehydration. (p. 810)

133. **(A)** Flowing oxygen over the face of a small child so it will be inhaled is referred to as the blow-by technique. (p. 833)

134. **(B)** A complication of a rapidly rising temperature in a child is often a seizure. (p. 842)

135. **(D)** A group of viral illnesses that cause inflammation of the larynx, trachea, and bronchi is called croup. (p. 840)

136. **(D)** The strong, white, fibrous material covering the bones is called the periosteum. (p. 696)

137. **(C)** The coming apart of a joint is referred to as a dislocation. (p. 701)

138. **(A)** Overstretching or overexertion of a muscle is called a strain. (p. 702)

139. **(B)** Proper splinting of a closed fracture is designed to prevent closed injuries from becoming open ones. (p. 705)

140. **(B)** Any force strong enough to fracture the pelvis also can cause injury to the spine. (p. 715)

141. **(D)** The Sager® is a unipolar splint. Examples of bipolar traction splints include Hare®, Fernotrac®, and half-ring. (p. 709)

142. **(C)** The indications for a traction splint are painful, swollen, deformed mid-thigh with no joint or lower leg injury. (p. 709)

143. **(C)** The Hazardous Materials Technician actually plugs, patches, or stops the release of a hazardous material. First Responder Awareness rescuers are trained only to recognize the problem and initiate a response from the proper organizations. First Responder Operations rescuers are trained to initially respond to releases or potential releases of hazardous materials in order to protect people, property, and the environment. The most advanced level of training is for the Hazardous Materials Specialist; this level rescuer is expected to have advanced knowledge and skills and to command and support activities at the incident site. (p. 966)

144. **(C)** The "safe zone" should be established on the same level as and upwind from the hazardous materials accident site. This positioning prevents flowing liquids or burning gases from spreading into the "safe zone." (p. 967)

145. **(B)** A resource that must be maintained at the work site by the employer and that must be available to all employees working with hazardous materials is called the Material Safety Data Sheet. This sheet generally names the substance, its physical properties, fire and explosion hazard information, health hazard information, and emergency first-aid treatment. (p. 969)

146. **(B)** EMS personal at a hazmat incident are responsible for caring for the injured and monitoring and rehabilitating the hazmat team members. (p. 972)

147. **(D)** When a patient is categorized as Priority-1 at an MCI, this means the patient has treatable life-threatening illness or injuries. (p. 986)

148. **(A)** The MCI officer responsible for communicating with each treatment area to determine the number and priority of the patients in that sector is called the staging supervisor. (pp. 989–990)

149. **(C)** A Priority-2 patient at an MCI would be color-coded yellow. Priority-1 patients would be red, Priority-3 would be green, and Priority-4, black or gray. (p. 986)

150. **(C)** Patients at an MCI who are assessed to have minor injuries are categorized as Priority-3. See answer 149. (p. 986)

Appendix A ALS-Assist Skills

MATCH TERMINOLOGY/ DEFINITIONS

1. **(G)** Cricoid pressure—gently pressing the thumb and index finger just to either side of the medial throat and over the cricoid cartilage to bring the patient's vocal cords into view (p. 1070)

2. **(C)** Drip chamber—chamber from which the drops of IV fluid flow (p. 1075)

3. **(E)** ECG—measurement of the electrical activity of the heart on a graph (p. 1073)

4. **(B)** Flow regulator—stopcock located below the drip chamber that can be pushed up or down to start, stop, or control the flow rate (p. 1075)

5. **(F)** Infiltration—when an IV needle has either punctured a vein and exited the other side or has pulled out of the vein and the fluid is flowing into the surrounding tissues instead of into the vein (p. 1077)

6. (H) IV—intravenous line inserted into a vein so that blood, fluids, or medications can be administered directly into a patient's circulation (p. 1075)

7. (D) Macro drip—drip chamber used when a higher flow of fluid is needed (for a multi-trauma victim in shock, for example) (p. 1075)

8. (A) Mini drip—drip chamber used when minimal flow of fluid is needed (with children, for example) (p. 1075)

9. (I) Needle port—opening below the flow regulator on an IV set into which medication is injected (p. 1075)

MULTIPLE-CHOICE REVIEW

1. (C) Traditionally, the "gold standard" of airway care has been the endotracheal tube because it can be inserted directly into the trachea, forming an open pathway for air, oxygen, or medications to be blown into the lungs. The AHA 2005 Guidelines do state that LMA and Combitube are equivalents to ET. (p. 1069)

2. (D) Typical patients who need an advanced airway inserted include patients in pulmonary or cardiopulmonary arrest, patients in need of airway control, and those in respiratory failure due to overdose (or fluid in the lungs, asthma, asphyxia, or allergic reaction). A patient with full thickness burns to the extremities would not need such assistance unless his level of responsiveness diminished. (p. 1069)

3. (A) Prior to an intubation attempt, you may be asked to ventilate the patient. During the attempt, you may be asked to press on the neck to help bring the vocal cords into view. (p. 1070)

4. (A) You do not shock a patient during an intubation attempt. During the intubation attempt, you may be asked to stand by and be prepared to begin ventilations, to gently press on the sides of the cricoid cartilage, and maintain neck stabilization. (pp. 1069–1070)

5. (B) Once the endotracheal tube is inserted in the trachea and the cuff is inflated, the paramedic should confirm placement by first using an esophageal intubation detector and then auscultating. See answer 6. (p. 1070)

6. (D) We do not listen over the lower abdomen. After inserting the tube, the intubator should listen with his stethoscope over the left lung, the right lung, and the epigastrium to confirm placement. Once the intubator assures the proper placement, then the ET tube is taped into place using an oral airway as a bite block. (p. 1070)

7. (A) If during the movement of the patient the advanced airway is moved, you should notify the paramedic, who will immediately recheck placement. If an ET tube is pushed in, it will most likely enter the right mainstem bronchus, preventing oxygen from entering the patient's left lung. If the tube is pulled out, it can easily slip into the esophagus and send all the ventilations directly to the stomach, denying the patient oxygen. This is a fatal complication if it goes unnoticed before an ET tube is anchored in place. (pp. 1071–1072)

8. (B) If you are ventilating a breathing patient with a BVM, you should time your ventilations with the patient's respiratory efforts. Do not decrease the oxygen concentration. (pp. 1071–1072)

9. (C) If, when ventilating, you feel a sudden change in the resistance, this could be caused by air escaping through a hole in the lungs and filling the space around the lungs, which is called a tension pneumothorax. (p. 1072)

10. (B) When ventilating a patient in cardiac arrest with a BVM, with each defibrillation attempt you should remove the bag from the tube. If you do not do this, the weight of the unsupported bag may accidentally displace the tube. (p. 1072)

11. (B) It is important to note the mental-status changes of patients who are intubated because they may wake up and bite on the tube, or they may attempt to pull out the tube. (p. 1072)

12. (A) After the paramedic injects some medication down the tube, if you are assigned to ventilations, you may be asked to ventilate the patient to increase the rate at which medication enters the bloodstream through the respiratory system. ET meds are still allowed but being replaced by the IO route. (p. 1072)

13. (C) If the patient has a suspected cervical spine injury, your role will be to maintain in-line spinal stabilization throughout the procedure. (p. 1072)

14. (C) A standard procedure used to alert EMS personnel to life-threatening heart rhythm disturbances is the ECG. (p. 1073)

15. (D) Interpreting the ECG is the responsibility of personnel with additional training in its interpretation. The EMT should know how to turn on the ECG monitor and change the battery, change the roll of paper, and record an ECG strip. (p. 1073)

16. (B) When assisting with an ECG, you should try to get in the habit of applying the leads to the electrode and then to the patient. If you apply the electrodes to the leads while they are on the patient, this creates some discomfort. (p. 1073)

17. (D) When preparing the patient's skin for ECG electrodes, dry the area, remove oil, and shave the patient's skin. You may also apply an antiperspirant to the patient who is sweating. Do not apply alcohol to the skin as it could burn the patient if defibrillation is necessary. (p. 1073)

18. (D) In the most common electrode configuration, the red electrode is placed on the left lower chest. White is right, and red is ribs. (p. 1073)

19. (B) In the most common electrode configuration, the green or black electrode is placed under the center of the left clavicle. (p. 1073)

20. (D) A mini-drip IV administration set produces 60 drops for every cc. (p. 1075)

21. (A) A macro-drip IV administration set produces 10 to 15 drops for every cc. (p. 1075)

22. (D) When inspecting an IV fluid bag, always check for expiration date, clarity of the fluid, and leaks in the bag. (p. 1076)

23. (A) When removing the protective covering from the port of the fluid bag and the protective covering from the spiked end of the tubing, be very careful to maintain sterility. If these parts touch the ground, they must *not* be used. (p. 1076)

24. (B) The IV line is flushed prior to using it on a patient because it prevents introducing an air embolism into the patient's vein. (p. 1076)

25. (C) The patient's blood pressure has nothing to do with the IV flow rate. Interruptions in the flow of an IV can be caused by a closed flow regulator, a constricting band left on the patient's arm, and kinked tubing. (p. 1077)

26. (C) CPAP or continuous positive airway pressure is a method of treating patients with certain respiratory diseases that is now found in the field. The other choices are all equipment that has been around for some time (intermittent positive pressure ventilation device and bag mask). (pp. 1077–1078)

27. (B) CPAP produces PEEP, or positive end expiratory pressure, which in turn helps to expand collapsed alveoli, thus preventing atelectasis, which is collapse of the small air sacs in the lungs. (p. 1078)

28. (A) Masks for CPAP must fit to the face with a tight and complete seal to be effective. (p. 1078)

COMPLETE THE FOLLOWING

1. You may be asked to carry out four steps in the process of applying electrodes: (p. 1073)
   - Turn on the ECG monitor.
   - Plug in the monitoring cables or "leads."
   - Attach the monitoring cables to the electrodes.
   - Apply the electrodes to the patient's body.

Appendix B Basic Cardiac Life Support Review

MATCH TERMINOLOGY/ DEFINITIONS

1. **(G)** Biological death—when brain cells die (p. 1080)

2. **(K)** Brachial pulse—pulse measured by feeling the major artery of the arm; the absence of this pulse is used as a sign, in infants, that heartbeat has stopped and CPR should begin. (p. 1087)

3. **(L)** Cardiopulmonary resuscitation—actions you take to revive a person—or at least temporarily prevent biological death—by keeping the person's heart and lungs working (p. 1080)

4. **(D)** Carotid pulse—pulse felt between the groove of the Adam's apple and the muscles located along the side of the neck (p. 1086)

5. **(C)** Clinical death—when breathing and heartbeat stop (p. 1080)

6. **(E)** 50:50 rule—requirement that the amount of time you spend compressing the patient's chest should be the same as the time spent for release (p. 1088)

7. **(F)** Gastric distention—bulging of the stomach that may be caused by forcing air into the patient's stomach during rescue breathing (p. 1084)

8. **(J)** Head-tilt, chin-lift maneuver—maneuver that provides for maximum opening of the airway (p. 1082)

9. **(B)** Abdominal thrusts—manual thrusts to the abdomen used to dislodge an airway obstruction (p. 1093)

10. **(M)** Jaw-thrust maneuver—maneuver used to open the airway of a patient with a suspected spine injury (p. 1084)

11. **(N)** Line of lividity—red or purple skin discoloration that occurs when gravity causes the blood to sink to the lowest parts of the body and collect there (p. 1092)

12. **(O)** Recovery position—lying the patient on the side to allow for drainage from the mouth and to prevent the tongue from falling backward (p. 1086)

13. **(A)** Rescue breathing—providing artificial ventilations to a person who has stopped breathing or whose breathing is inadequate (p. 1081)

14. **(I)** Substernal notch—general term for area of the lower border of the sternum (p. 1088)

15. **(H)** Xiphoid process—short triangular piece of cartilage (tough, elastic gristle) that extends from the bottom of the sternum (p. 1088)

MULTIPLE-CHOICE REVIEW

1. **(B)** When a patient's breathing and heartbeat stop, the *brain* cells will begin to die after 4 to 6 minutes. Heart, liver, and kidney cells begin to die after about 1 hour. (p. 1080)

2. **(D)** Once clinical death occurs, brain cells begin to die within 4 to 6 minutes. However, it usually takes 10 minutes for biological death to occur. (p. 1080)

3. **(C)** In the ABC method of cardiopulmonary resuscitation, the "A" stands for airway. (p. 1080)

4. **(C)** In the ABC method of cardiopulmonary resuscitation, the "C" stands for circulation. (p. 1080)

5. **(D)** To determine if an adult or child is pulseless, the EMT should check for a pulse at the carotid artery. (p. 1081)

6. **(A)** To determine pulselessness in an infant, the EMT should use the brachial artery. This is because the carotid pulse is difficult to determine in an infant. (p. 1081)

7. **(B)** If you are alone, after determining unresponsiveness in the adult, the next thing you should do before starting CPR is to activate EMS. (p. 1081)

8. **(C)** When an unconscious patient's head flexes forward, the *tongue* could cause an airway obstruction. (p. 1082)

9. **(C)** One of the best ways way to relieve an airway obstruction due to the positioning of the patient's tongue is the head-tilt, chin-lift maneuver. The jaw-thrust maneuver is used on a trauma patient. (pp. 1082–1084)

10. **(C)** The head-tilt, chin-lift maneuver should not be used on a diving accident victim due to the potential for cervical-spine injury. The jaw-thrust is taught only to health-care providers. (pp. 1082–1084)

11. **(A)** The recommended maneuver for opening the airway of a patient with possible cervical spine injury is the jaw-thrust maneuver. (p. 1084)

12. **(B)** After opening the airway in a patient who requires rescue breathing, the EMT should inflate the patient's lung with two breaths 1 second each. (p. 1084)

13. **(C)** Initial ventilations did not result in chest rise. Your next step is to perform the steps of CPR. (p. 1084)

14. **(B)** A common problem in the resuscitation of infants and children caused by improper head position or too quick ventilations is gastric distention. (p. 1084)

15. **(B)** In adult rescue breathing, the EMT provides 10–12 breaths every minute. (p. 1084)

16. **(A)** Infants should be ventilated at the rate of one breath every 3 seconds (60 seconds/20 breaths per minute = 3 seconds). (p. 1084)

17. **(C)** When a patient has a distended abdomen due to air being forced into the stomach, the EMT should be prepared to suction should the patient vomit. Do not decrease the oxygen concentration; pressing on the abdomen would produce vomiting. (p. 1086)

18. **(A)** The recovery position is used because it protects the airway and allows for drainage from the mouth. It also prevents the tongue from blocking the airway. (p. 1086)

19. **(C)** When delivering chest compressions during CPR, avoid using a stabbing motion to deliver compressions. Use a rhythmic 50% compression–50% relaxation motion. (p. 1088)

20. **(D)** The adult CPR compression point is located on the middle of the sternum, centered from side to side. (p. 1088)

21. (A) Before beginning artificial ventilation, assess the patient's breathing for 5 seconds. (p. 1089)

22. (D) For an adult, the one-rescuer compression-to-ventilations ratio is 30:2. (p. 1091)

23. (C) The adult CPR compression rate in one-rescuer CPR is 100 times a minute. (p. 1091)

24. (B) The adult CPR compression rate in two-rescuer CPR is 100 times a minute when an advanced airway is in place. (p. 1091)

25. (B) The compression depth for an adult or older child (beyond puberty) should be 1.5 to 2 inches in the middle of the chest between the nipples at 100 times a minute. (p. 1091)

26. (C) The compression depth for a young child (who has not yet reached puberty) or infant should be ⅓ to ½ the depth of the chest at a rate of 100 times a minute. (p. 1091)

27. (B) The compression to ventilation ratio for a young child or infant when there are two rescuers should be 15:2. This provides additional ventilation with the presumption that the arrest may have been a primary respiratory event, as compared to adults, in which the arrest is usually due to an electrical event (VF/pulseless VT). Note that the two-person CPR procedure is not taught to the citizens, only to health care providers. (p. 1091)

28. (C) The compression to ventilation ratio for a young child or infant when there is only one rescuer doing the CPR is 30:2. This is the ratio taught in all the citizen courses and as such it is the universal compression-to-ventilation ratio, since only the health care courses address two-rescuer CPR. (p. 1091)

29. (D) The compression rate when performing CPR on an infant is at least 100 times a minute. (p. 1091)

30. (C) When opening the airway of an infant, use a slight head-tilt. Full hyperextension of the neck can cause the airway to close. (p. 1090)

31. (B) With effective CPR, the patient's pupils may constrict. Dilation occurs when the patient is hypoxic. (pp. 1091–1092)

32. (D) CPR compressions are delivered to children with the heel of one hand. The fingertips are used to deliver compressions for infants. (pp. 1090–1091)

33. (A) With the exceptions of advanced airway placement and defibrillation, CPR should not be interrupted for more than 10 seconds. (p. 1092)

34. (B) If you are treating a patient with a partial airway obstruction, poor air exchange, and gray skin, you should treat the patient for a complete airway obstruction. (p. 1093)

35. (B) Complete airway obstruction in a conscious patient is indicated by an inability to speak. Crowing, gurgling, and snoring are all sounds of partial airway obstruction. (p. 1093)

36. (C) When you have recognized complete airway obstruction in a conscious adult patient, you should deliver a series of manual abdominal thrusts. Only unconscious patients are placed in a supine position when ventilations are attempted. (p. 1093)

37. (D) To deliver chest thrusts to an unconscious patient, place the patient in the supine position. (p. 1094)

38. (D) You are treating an unresponsive adult patient with a complete airway obstruction. You have been unsuccessful in your initial two attempts to ventilate the patient. You should continue with chest compressions, look in mouth, ventilations. (p. 1094)

39. (C) When treating an 8-month-pregnant female who has a complete airway obstruction, the EMT should use chest thrusts. (pp. 1094–1095)

40. (B) If a patient has a partial airway obstruction and is able to speak and cough forcefully, you should carefully watch the patient. Do not interfere with the patient's attempts to expel the foreign body. However, be prepared to provide help if the partial airway obstruction becomes a complete obstruction. (p. 1093)

41. (B) The major difference between the adult and infant procedure for foreign body airway obstruction when you suspect a severe or complete obstruction is that infants receive a combination of back slaps and chest compressions. Adults do not receive the back slaps, only the chest compressions. For all ages the rescuer should look in the mouth but not automatically sweep it out unless an obstruction is actually seen. (pp. 1094–1095)

42. (A) While you are trying to clear an obstructed airway in an adult, the patient loses consciousness. You open the airway, look in the mouth, and attempt to ventilate. If this fails, begin CPR compressions. (pp. 1093–1094)

43. (B) You have been unsuccessful in initially ventilating an unconscious infant. You reposition the head and attempt to ventilate again but are unsuccessful. Your next step is to perform back blows and chest thrusts. (pp. 1094–1095)

44. (D) Signs of choking in an infant are *lack* of a strong cry, ineffective cough, agitation, wheezing, blue color, and breathing difficulty. (p. 1096)

45. (B) In health care provider CPR training, infants are up to 1 year of age, children are from 1 year to puberty, and adults are from puberty till death. Remember that citizen CPR courses do not teach this distinction and will still define a child as age 1 to 8. (p. 1090)

COMPLETE THE FOLLOWING

1. The special circumstances in which the EMT should not initiate CPR even though the patient is pulseless include: (p. 1092)
 • A line of lividity
 • Decomposition
 • Mortal injury
 • Rigor mortis
 • Stillbirth

2. Situations in which the EMT may stop CPR include: (p. 1092)
 • Spontaneous circulation occurs (then provide rescue breathing as needed)
 • Spontaneous circulation and breathing occur
 • Another trained rescuer can take over for you
 • You turn care of the patient over to a person with a higher level of training
 • Upon order of Medical Director or patient's physician
 • If you become physically exhausted (e.g., backcountry rescue)

3. List the information missing from following the chart. (p. 1091)
 (A) 1.5 to 2 inches
 (B) 100/minute
 (C) 1-second duration
 (D) Carotid artery
 (E) 30:2
 (F) 30:2
 (G) 15:2